Stroke

Epidemiology, evidence, and clinical practice

Stroke

Epidemiology, evidence, and clinical practice

Second Edition

Shah Ebrahim

Professor of Epidemiology and Ageing
Department of Social Medicine
University of Bristol
and

Rowan Harwood

Consultant in Geriatric Medicine
Department of Health Care of the Elderly
University Hospital, Nottingham

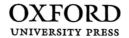

OXFORD
UNIVERSITY PRESS

This book has been printed digitally and produced in a standard specification
in order to ensure its continuing availability

OXFORD
UNIVERSITY PRESS

Great Clarendon Street, Oxford OX2 6DP

Oxford University Press is a department of the University of Oxford.
It furthers the University's objective of excellence in research, scholarship,
and education by publishing worldwide in

Oxford New York

Auckland Bangkok Buenos Aires Cape Town Chennai
Dar es Salaam Delhi Hong Kong Istanbul Karachi Kolkata
Kuala Lumpur Madrid Melbourne Mexico City Mumbai Nairobi
São Paulo Shanghai Taipei Tokyo Toronto

Oxford is a registered trade mark of Oxford University Press
in the UK and in certain other countries

Published in the United States
by Oxford University Press Inc., New York

ISBN 0-19-263075-X

Preface to second edition

Almost a decade has passed since the first edition of *Clinical epidemiology of stroke* came out and the explosion of new research in stroke is very apparent. Several important themes have coloured medicine during this time: the development of evidence-based health care, optimism for acute drug treatments for stroke, the growth of new information about the human genome, a dramatic increase in the number of stroke clinicians and researchers, both in Great Britain and also internationally, and the establishment of the Cochrane Collaboration.

All of these trends are relevant in revising a book of this nature. Clinical epidemiology remains an essential foundation for the practice of evidence-based health care. The enthusiasms of the pharmaceutical industry have resulted in a large number of new trials, often too small to detect clinically important differences, and have increased the number of clinicians actively engaged in stroke research. However, it seems even more important that these clinicians should have a good understanding of the design of trials, the rationale for randomization and blinding, and the importance of selecting the most appropriate outcomes. Surprisingly little of practical importance has resulted from a decade of exploration of the human genome—the best indication of a person's risk remains their phenotype and not their genotype. The impetus to organize stroke medicine into a defined speciality, with an emphasis on acute stroke, is ever stronger—but it is essential to bear in mind the importance of interdisciplinary working, the value of primary care, geriatric medicine, psychiatry, and rehabilitation in the prevention, treatment, rehabilitation, and long-term care of stroke patients. The Cochrane Collaboration is currently grappling with a task of enormous size—the compression of the tens of thousands of randomized controlled trials and other scientific evidence—into systematic reviews of the effects of interventions.

In producing this new edition, the volume of work was too great for a single author so Rowan Harwood and I joined forces. Scanning the reference list at the end of the book demonstrates the explosion in 'essential' published work. Not surprisingly, the book is bigger than before, and has an extra opening section titled 'Epidemiology' which comprises the nuts and bolts of the subject and reviews the purposes of health care for stroke patients. The remaining sections follow the format of the first edition: Diagnosis, Management, and Prognosis. All the chapters have been substantially updated—and it is gratifying to see how many of the areas in desperate need of research have now been covered by a new cohort of bright and capable stroke researchers.

The book aims to retain its focus on epidemiology that is relevant to the clinician and attempts to use examples from stroke to illustrate many aspects of epidemiological thinking. The book is not intended to be an authoritative encyclopaedia of stroke—others have done an excellent job here—but aims to stimulate readers to think about their own practice, the nature of scientific evidence, and the vast areas of clinical uncertainty that remain the target for research over the coming decades.

Shah Ebrahim
Rowan Harwood
1999

Foreword

Being asked by the authors to write a Foreword to their book on stroke gives me the feeling not so much of having arrived, but of being on the way out. Nonetheless it is both an honour and a pleasure to welcome the second edition of *Clinical Epidemiology of Stroke*, now retitled *Stroke: epidemiology, evidence, and clinical practice*. And this new edition is not before time. Although I have used, and quoted from, and made slides from the first edition a great deal, and still do, stroke is moving so fast now that an update was clearly needed. This is not so much because the epidemiological principles have greatly changed, but because we know so much more of stroke prevention and treatment. Also, in these days of ever increasing specialization, and sub-specialization, Shah Ebrahim has teamed up with Rowan Harwood, a geriatrician, to make the second edition wisely not just a one but a two man band effort.

Epidemiology has something of a glum reputation with medical students, probably because it is usually taught in the classroom. It gets in the way of getting on with seeing the next patient. Also, to the average student it doesn't seem terribly relevant to day-to-day doctoring, but one keeps being told it is important, so it must be. And it doesn't seem to quite fit comfortably anywhere in the course. Too soon and it doesn't make sense and is quickly forgotten through lack of use (like the arcane corners of biochemistry). Too late, and it is literally too late.

What I didn't realize as a student, and I don't think times have changed much for the present generation, was that the methodologies and ways of thinking wrapped up in the discipline of 'epidemiology' actually underpin so much of clinical practice. Epidemiology is not just about epidemics, drains, and atmospheric pollution. It is the science of clinical common sense. Whilst the basic scientists produce hypotheses (this is how we think the world works, so this ought to be so), the epidemiologists test them in real life (is it actually so? are we sure? how should our clinical practice be changed?).

Epidemiological principles permeate this book on stroke, and they are made transparent. It is not just a 'how to do it' book but also a 'why to do it this way' book. And the 'how to do it' is as much about how to do, or at least understand, the epidemiological techniques themselves, as to provide evidence-based health care. Rather than having to go to some heavy epidemiological tome, the stroke care provider can find clear explanations of how a diagnostic test should be evaluated, what exactly regression-dilution bias is, what makes a good trial, how to sort out clinical disagreement, a bit of health economics, how to construct a decision analysis tree, and more. Don't understand the difference between an odds ratio and a risk ratio? Then go to Table 2.1. And, reassuringly for someone like myself who gave up science to do medicine because I wasn't good enough at maths, the explanations are easy to understand. No natural logarithms and not too many uncomfortable numbers under one. It is all this 'epidemiology' which actually underpins what we clinicians, doctors or nurses or the professions allied to medicine, do every day in our care of stroke patients. We may not recognize the underpinning in a busy clinical life, but it is all laid out in this book for our education and illumination.

In fact, my own stroke research was illuminated nearly two decades ago by a rather poor photocopy of Shah Ebrahim's MSc thesis on stroke registers. Luckily we stumbled on it in the early 1980s when we started the Oxfordshire Community Stroke Project. And now, in this scholarly book, he along with Rowan Harwood, continue to illuminate our clinical decisions and our clinical science: why we do what we do, or should do, in the light of the best evidence. This is a splendid book for the shelf of anyone interested in stroke.

Charles Warlow
Department of Clinical Neurosciences
Western General Hospital NHS Trust
Edinburgh

Contents

PART 1 EPIDEMIOLOGY

- Objectives of stroke care

- Risk and risk factors

- Time, places, and people

1 Objectives of stroke care

Are epidemiological ideas and methods of any use to the clinician? Epidemiology is a major tool for public health tasks of monitoring the population's health, assessing needs, prevention, and commissioning services. Such work may seem remote from the day-to-day work of looking after stroke patients, but should provide a broader context within which the effects of clinical activity can be understood. Increasingly, clinicians are expected to be involved in the commissioning and evaluation of services, and to be aware of the wider health and social consequences of their decisions.

Objectives of medical care

Doctors and other health professionals have always wanted to maximize the good they do for their patients. The first task is to identify ways in which medical services can help. Sometimes the patient has already suffered a disease. Sometimes we identify a patient at risk of a disease he or she has not yet acquired. Hypertension is a disease only in so far as it marks someone out at risk of future complications. Sometimes the 'patient' will be a whole population which is the subject of health promotion efforts. If we are to plan and evaluate services for patients at risk of, or having suffered, a stroke, it is desirable to have a framework for thinking about the different functions that medical services offer. A simple classification is shown in Table 1.1.

Stroke care involves all of these functions. There are now several rigorously proven interventions that can decrease the risk of stroke, such as treatment of hypertension, and anticoagulation in patients with atrial fibrillation. Stroke complications such as pressure sores and joint contractures can be prevented with appropriate nursing and physiotherapy interventions. Thrombolytic therapy attempts to 'cure' a stroke that would otherwise have evolved, and a few of the rare causes of stroke, such as infective endocarditis, are curable. High-quality stroke care, such as provided on stroke units, reduces stroke mortality and improves functional outcomes compared with lower-quality care. Stroke patients are prone to pain (for example, in a subluxing shoulder) and depression, which may be relieved by treatment. Many stroke manifestations, such as perceptual impairments, are bewildering and require explanation. Recovery from a stroke is often slower than for many medical conditions, and the risk of recurrence is relatively high, so information on prognosis is required. Finally, the proportion of stroke survivors who remain

Table 1.1   Objectives of medical care

- Prevent disease and its complications
- Cure disease and its complications
- Increase life expectancy
- Alleviate or palliate distressing symptoms
- Maximize physical and social functioning
- Explain unusual phenomena and offer a prognosis
- Support families and other carers

very dependent are often provided with substantial physical and emotional support from their families. Not only is this of great benefit to the patients, but society benefits from not having to pay for professional care. The strains, however, can put the health of the carer at risk, and for all these reasons, support of carers is important.

How epidemiology is useful

Epidemiology informs much of what we can say about all these aspects of stroke care. Prevention is impossible without a knowledge of risk factors. Curing disease, prolonging life, and improving its quality for patients and carers requires knowledge of natural history of stroke and the evaluation of interventions. Developing new treatments and services, to be evaluated in their turn, sometimes hinges on basic scientific advances. We can also get clues from epidemiology, by looking at factors associated with good and bad outcomes.

Doctors often make decisions under circumstances of great uncertainty. Treating and counselling patients was, in some ways, easier when stroke was considered to have a uniformly bad outlook, characterized by Hughlings Jackson's famous assertion that 'you cannot cure a hole in the brain' (Pound *et al.* 1993). Epidemiology can help us to understand, quantify, and manage that uncertainty. The method of medicine itself has come under epidemiological scrutiny and is being refined in the process of evidence-based healthcare. The quality of information we collect in making diagnoses and prognoses, through history taking, examination, and investigation, is often surprisingly poor. However, we often do not use all the information we do have. Some simple statistical methods can improve our performance but are not yet in common use.

A wider view

Medicine does not operate within a vacuum. People have expectations of medical services that go beyond the objectives shown in Table 1.1. Patients', professionals', and carers' goals and views are never the same. Indeed, we have reached a point in society at large where no viewpoint is more valid than another—the patient knows at least as well as the doctor what should be done. While it is necessary to be aware of parallel and often conflicting viewpoints, the role of clinical epidemiology is to bring appropriate evidence to bear on questions of importance to patients, professionals, and carers. For example, there has been a long-running debate about whether patients are best managed at home or in hospital after a stroke. Wade proposed the following reasons for hospital admission: diagnostic doubt, need for nursing care, management of complications, and to start rehabilitation early. Some schemes have attempted to avert hospital admission (Wade *et al.* 1985*a*) and new trials comparing management at home with hospital admission are under way. Interest in keeping patients at home has its roots in reducing burdens on acute hospital care and is largely management and professionally led. By contrast, recent work, looking at hospital admission from patients' and carers' viewpoints, has suggested that patients have great faith in their health services, and value being 'cared about' on admission to hospital when anxious, bewildered, and newly disabled. The corollary is a sense of abandonment when discharged from specialized medical care, usually on the basis that active intervention is unlikely to produce further benefit (Pound *et al.* 1995). How can these potentially conflicting viewpoints be squared? Evidence has to be sought from all the relevant players ('stakeholders', to use the current jargon) in ways that will allow their voices to be heard—tasks for which clinical epidemiology, in conjunction with other health services research disciplines, are well fitted. However, the clinician and his or her managers must strive to provide as much of a service as possible to as many people as possible within a given budget to achieve a utilitarian ethical principle of greatest good for the greatest number. This sometimes sits uneasily with the more traditional ethical principle of doing the best for the individual patient. Current attempts in Britain and elsewhere to blur the distinctions between doctors who practice clinically with patients, and those who practice public health medicine according to utilitarian principles, are exacerbating these tensions.

Health gain

Epidemiology serves two main purposes. First, it aims to discover associations between exposure and outcome variables, and to assess how likely these are to be causal. This is the role in which it is useful to clinical medicine. Secondly, it informs health policy. This requires a quantification of the size of effects, such as the risk associated with a risk factor, or the benefit obtained by one intervention over another. The parallel discipline of health economics draws together information on costs and benefits and, if possible, compares

one intervention with another. There is an understandable tendency to want
to lump together all benefits into a single measurable entity (health gain). The
more ambitious attempt to quantify the 'utility' (value, worth, or desirability)
of states of health so that changes or differences in utility can be costed. This
is a fascinating area of research, but the instruments available remain imprecise and crude. We must be careful that valued tasks such as 'caring about'
patients with stroke, giving explanations and information, and supporting
carers do not get lost amidst the health economists' broad brush strokes of
health-gain measurement. This does not mean that these 'softer' functions
cannot be evaluated. Methods and measurement tools appropriate to the
specific evaluations needed must be used, and services should not be
abandoned for want of proper evidence of how their benefits are obtained—no evidence of benefit is not the same as no benefit.

Compliance

Thinking about 'health gain' also helps us to understand some apparent
ambiguities about stroke care. The evidence that blood pressure reduction
prevents strokes is very strong (MacMahon *et al.* 1990). Effective treatment
is available, yet many strokes attributable to high blood pressure still occur
each year. Why does this occur? Identification of people with hypertension is
poor, and those who are diagnosed are often undertreated (W. C. S. Smith
et al. 1990). Moreover, most people who have a stroke attributable to their
blood pressure are not what is clinically definable as 'hypertensive' (see
Chapter 2, p. 21). The assault on blood pressure would be more effective if it
targeted everyone regardless of their blood pressure, rather than simply
those with a systolic pressure greater than 160 mmHg. This is known as the
'population' or 'mass' approach to prevention, as opposed to the 'high-risk'
approach of simply treating the 'hypertensives'. The problem is that most
people who would have to change their behaviour would not benefit from
doing so. Losing weight, taking more exercise, and eating less salt are all
things most people would rather not do. They are perceived as having an
associated cost which is very much culturally bound. Changes in fashion do
occur, and can be nudged by governments, technology, education, doctors
and others. Such changes may well account for the fall in vascular mortality
in the Western world over recent decades, but are not easy to plan or
implement.

What about people with blood pressure high enough to be diagnosed as
hypertensive? The same principles apply. The intervention, taking drugs, is an
imposition, a nuisance. The drugs may have side-effects (Medical Research
Council Working Party 1985). The benefit for the individual is uncertain,
intangible, and in the future. Indeed, it has been calculated that a mere 1 per

cent decrease in quality of life, on average, associated with taking anti-hypertensive medication, completely obliterates the benefit from avoiding strokes for hypertensive middle-aged men (Fletcher 1992). The cost to the patient of taking treatment can easily outweigh the benefit of avoiding strokes, or can be perceived as doing so, leaving no net 'health gain'.

Health economics

There has always been a tendency for doctors to ignore the costs of their decisions and simply consider doing the best for their patients. Patients would not want it otherwise and would be appalled if they felt that doctors made decisions on the basis of the perceived worth of an individual patient and the costs of treatment. Of course, this is exactly what has happened in health care for years! Perhaps the grossest examples concern age-related rationing of health care, in which elderly people are denied access to coronary care units, renal dialysis, and other expensive treatments on the basis that doctors have valued their lives as not worth saving (Evans 1991). Health economics gets a bad press amongst the medical profession because it attempts to make such decisions transparent and to bring as much objectivity into the process of using health care resources as possible. While there is much to criticize in the methods used by health economists, the alternatives are much less appealing. In the past, those who shouted loudest (teaching hospital consultants) and most dramatically (shroud-waving life-and-death specialities) got the bigger slice of the available cake. Political factors and special pleading by professionals and patient groups will inevitably continue to have an effect on decisions on how health care resources are used. Health economics provides a means of exposing how such decisions are made and provides the framework for a more rational approach.

Health economics has some basic principles:

(1) resources are not unlimited (scarcity);
(2) demand tends to increase owing to ageing of populations, technological advances, and increasing aspirations of people (inflation);
(3) using resources on unproven or inefficient treatments is unethical (utilitarian ethics);
(4) linking costs to outcomes (cost-effectiveness);
(5) choices have to be made between alternative strategies (priority setting);
(6) choices between alternative options should maximize the benefits obtained for society (cost-benefit).

All economic evaluations involve many assumptions which must be made explicitly and their impact on the final analyses must be assessed (sensitivity analysis) (Maynard 1992).

Costs of stroke

Stroke is expensive because so many people end up in hospital for fairly long periods of time. Few published studies have estimated the costs of a stroke. In Scotland, the National Health Service (NHS) costs (i.e. direct costs as opposed to indirect costs of lost economic production) are about 4 per cent of total NHS costs (Isard and Forbes 1992) and if this applied across the UK, would amount to about £1.4 billion in 1996. Direct costs in the USA in 1976 were US$3.2 billion (Adelman 1981) but more recent data are not available; assuming inflation of about 150 per cent over the past 20 years, would mean that current costs are about US$12.4 billion. The direct cost of an individual stroke patient is estimated to be between £4600 in Scotland (1988) and £5900 in Sweden (1983) (Persson *et al.* 1990). Of importance, is that the greatest proportion of first-year costs are spent on the initial hospital admission and in-patient rehabilitation, with only 12 per cent spent on out-of-hospital care (Persson *et al.* 1990).

In considering direct costs, it is important in any chronic disease to examine costs over time and to include long-term care costs, which may be almost as large as acute hospital costs (Raftery 1995). In most costing studies, average costs per stroke have been reported, but it is of great importance to examine factors that determine variation in costs. For example, in Sweden the costs of stroke in women are almost double those for men, independent of age (Persson *et al.* 1990), and are probably explained by the unpaid care provided by women for men with stroke, which is not reciprocated. Indirect costs, particularly those of unpaid carers, may make a major difference to the overall picture, but such work has not been done.

Economic evaluations

There is a range of ways in which the costs of health care can be linked with outcomes. The simplest method does not even consider outcomes but simply compares costs between different options, making the assumption that either approach is equally effective, and is a cost-minimization evaluation. It would be rational to choose the cheapest option if both were equally effective.

Cost-effectiveness studies

These attempt to relate costs to some measure of outcome. This may be some clinical outcome (e.g. reduction in blood pressure or survival). If one intervention results in a greater increase in survival but at higher cost, a cost-effectiveness analysis may help to resolve the best policy. For example, long-term anticoagulation is probably more effective than aspirin in preventing stroke in patients with atrial fibrillation but it costs considerably more and is risky, potentially causing serious bleeding. What is the best option to choose?

Table 1.2 Cost-effectiveness analysis comparing anticoagulation with aspirin in preventing stroke in patients with atrial fibrillation (data from Gustaffason *et al.* 1992). Low and high risk refers to risk of bleeding on anticoagulation

	Anticoagulation only	Anticoagulation or aspirin	Aspirin only
Number eligible for treatment	22 000	75 000	75 000
Annual cost (£) of treatment/patient	500	154	10
Net reduction in stroke, low risk (number/year)	630	1300	910
Net reduction in stroke, high risk (number/year)	260	930	910
Cost (£) per stroke prevented, low risk	17 500	8900	800
Cost (£) per stroke prevented, high risk	42 300	12 400	800

In Sweden, a cost-effectiveness analysis was conducted (Gustafsson *et al.* 1992) and a summary of the findings is shown in Table 1.2.

The most effective treatment is anticoagulation for those who can tolerate it and aspirin for the remainder as this prevents 1300 strokes a year if complications of anticoagulation are kept low, and even if complications are high (intracranial bleeding rate of 2 per cent/year), still prevents more strokes than simply giving everyone aspirin. Therefore, this would be the clinically preferred option if costs are ignored. However, when cost-effectiveness is considered a completely different picture emerges. Aspirin treatment is so cheap (50 times cheaper than anticoagulation) that despite the greater efficacy of anticoagulation, it represents a poor value for money choice. If bleeding complications are high, the cost-effectiveness of anticoagulation becomes even worse. The investigators in this study concluded that prophylactic treatment with anticoagulants in patients with chronic atrial fibrillation saves both strokes and money if bleeding complications are kept low. However, they ignored the greater savings of money obtained from the aspirin-only policy.

Cost-utility studies

These measure the outcomes of treatment options in the same way so that comparisons may be made between different options more easily. The most popular utility used is the quality adjusted life year (QALY) and the cost per QALY has been widely promoted as a yardstick for comparing different interventions. For example, the cost per QALY of GPs giving anti-smoking advice is very low at £170/QALY, as is the cost of treating hypertension to prevent stroke at £600/QALY, whereas breast cancer screening and hospital haemodialysis are expensive at £3500 and £14 000 per QALY respectively (Smith 1990). Very little work on cost-utilities for different stroke care options has been conducted but it is likely that this area will develop in the future. For example, cost-utility analysis comparing the costs of stroke unit care per QALY with other options (e.g. day hospitals, new consultant posts) for investing new resources or redirecting current resources would provide useful information for decision makers.

Cost-benefit studies

In cost-benefit analysis, the outcomes are measured in the same money units as the inputs. This means that lives saved or strokes avoided must be converted into their equivalent cash values. This raises many practical and ethical problems—what is a life worth? Where outcomes can be dealt with in this way, options which result in more overall benefits than costs would logically be chosen. A cost-benefit analysis of comprehensive primary prevention for stroke in Japan compared the current *ad hoc* and inefficient arrangements. A cost : benefit ratio of 1 : 10 supporting the comprehensive care option was found (Sekita 1985).

Discounting

Evaluations of the costs and benefits of treatment are further complicated, where costs come early and benefits late, when a concept called discounting becomes important. The idea is borrowed from accountancy. People want benefits now and costs later. In the example of taking antihypertensive drugs to prevent strokes, the monetary cost, side-effects, and inconvenience of taking medication come early on, and so weigh disproportionately in the cost-benefit equation. We can estimate how much ('the discount rate'), though there is little empirical evidence to go on yet. For the clinician the important message is that we must make antihypertensive medication regimes as simple as possible, and that side-effects should not be tolerated (while being aware that a patient's report of a 'side-effect' is an uncontrolled observation, and the drug may not be the culprit).

Quality in health care

Attempts have been made to define the quality of health services, taking into account broader considerations. Table 1.3 gives a list of desirable attributes (Maxwell 1984). The first two of these, effectiveness and efficiency, are well known, and have been discussed already. The others are less obvious. Artificial ventilation may be effective at prolonging life, for a short while at least, in an unconscious patient after severe stroke, but in the light of what we know about ultimate prognosis for such people, is not appropriate. Humane care will involve many common courtesies and respect for a patient's autonomy and dignity. It will also entail providing care in appropriate settings for disabled and often frail people. Equity calls for equal treatment of people with different characteristics. For instance, are arrangements in place to help the increasing number of people for whom English is not their first

Table 1.3 Quality of health care

- Effective
- Efficient
- Appropriate
- Humane
- Equitable
- Accessible

language, or provision of preventative services amongst socio-economically disadvantaged groups amongst whom there is an excess of stroke deaths? Accessibility is an issue for non-car owners and non-city dwellers, as hospitals are concentrated onto fewer sites. Access to specialist services also needs the co-operation of primary health care and local health care providers, who may ration or underprovide services.

Summary

1. Health care serves a range of purposes—prevention, cure, saving lives, relieving symptoms, relieving disability, explaining health problems, and supporting carers—all of which must be considered in evaluating stroke services.
2. Clinical epidemiology is a major tool for understanding and evaluating health care from a range of equally valid perspectives.
3. The public health and policy imperative to define and measure 'health gain' must be tempered by the crudity of available measurement instruments and a knowledge of the wide range of health care objectives.
4. Econometric concepts such as cost-effectiveness may help in making difficult decisions, and discounting may explain problems with compliance with preventative treatments.
5. The quality of services can be assessed using the categories of effectiveness, efficiency, appropriateness, humanity, equity, and accessibility.

2 Risk and risk factors

Causation

In common with most chronic diseases, strokes do not have a single cause but are due to multiple factors. Even in tuberculosis which does have a single necessary cause—*Mycobacterium tuberculosis*—the risk of being infected, and then of developing tuberculosis, is dependent on a chain of causal factors, some very closely related to the pathogenic process (e.g. inhaling bacilli from a close relative), while others are much further back in the causal chain (e.g. poor childhood nutrition). Epidemiologists are concerned with discovering the characteristics of people and populations that increase or decrease their chances (or risk) of suffering diseases. The mechanisms by which disease occurs in those at increased risk is often suggested by epidemiological enquiry, but working out the detailed pathological pathways is a goal for laboratory scientists.

The question of causation can be answered at several different levels. What genetic, life style, and environmental factors put people at increased risk of a stroke? What pathological processes are going on in the cardiovascular system that impair the cerebral circulation? What are the triggers that cause a high-risk person to have a stroke on a particular day? These questions are concerned with why strokes occur, but at different points along a chain of causality which starts with genes and their products, goes on to the modification of genetic expression by external factors, to produce a person with more or less predisposition to cerebrovascular diseases. The person is then affected by a series of exposures, some of which can be controlled by individuals (e.g. cigarette smoking, diet, inactivity) and some of which cannot (e.g. age, climate, air quality). These fundamental and predisposing causes lead to the occurrence of strokes through pathogenic mechanisms involving blood vessels, blood components, blood pressure, and flow dynamics.

The purpose of studying fundamental causes, rather than pathological processes, is that they lend themselves to attempts at disease prevention. Linking risk of diarrhoeal diseases with water quality can lead to disease control without any need to understand whether a bacterium or virus is responsible for the pathological process. Knowledge of risk factors for HIV infection led to preventive activity before any clear understanding of the mechanism by which the virus affects the immune system. Understanding mechanisms may be rewarded by discovering new treatments for a disease, so enquiry into aetiology and pathogenesis are complementary.

Criteria to establish causality

It is often difficult to be sure that a relationship is causal. Koch's postulates define standard criteria that should be met before a claim of causality may be accepted, and essentially define the specificity of a relationship between a cause (i.e. an organism) and a disease. The cause must be found with the disease and not with any other disease, and the causal factor must be capable of causing the disease in susceptible subjects. Koch's postulates enabled the single necessary and sufficient cause of an infectious disease to be established, but in chronic diseases single necessary and sufficient causes are rare. Perhaps exposure to tobacco and lung cancer comes closest to the infectious disease model of a single cause, but even so many who do smoke will not develop lung cancer and therefore predisposing and protective factors presumably operate to determine its occurrence.

A major problem which has beset stroke epidemiology from the outset is that the pathological damage that leads to a stroke is not a single process but may be due to thrombosis of arteries, platelet emboli from the carotid arteries, fibrin emboli from the atrium of the heart, increased viscosity of blood, or rupture of microaneurysms of intracerebral arteries. Yet the clinical presentation of stroke is remarkably similar whatever the pathogenesis, and until recently accurate discrimination between the major mechanisms, thrombosis and haemorrhage, has not been possible. This has led to much of our understanding of causation being weakened because environmental and personal variables (i.e. risk factors) that increase risk have been measured as if strokes were a single disease. The first prerequisite to establish causality is to ensure that the disease of interest is as homogeneous an entity as is possible given current knowledge about disease mechanisms.

Criteria of aetiological causality were originally framed by Hill (1965) and comprise:

(1) strength of association of a risk factor with the disease;
(2) experiment (changing the risk factor leads to changes in disease occurrence);
(3) dose–response effect (more of a risk factor leads to more disease);
(4) time sequence (a risk factor must exert its effect before disease appears);
(5) consistency (similar associations in other places and times among different people);
(6) biological plausibility;
(7) coherence with other information;

(8) specificity of association (a risk factor is only associated with a particular disease); and

(9) analogy with other examples of cause and effect.

The first five of these criteria are the most powerful in establishing causality, because the others are bound by existing knowledge, and specificity of a relationship may not be a helpful criterion since smoking, for example, is a causal factor of several different diseases. Even strong associations may not be causal (Davey Smith and Phillips 1992; Davey Smith *et al.* 1992), so care must be taken to avoid undue reliance on any single criterion of causality.

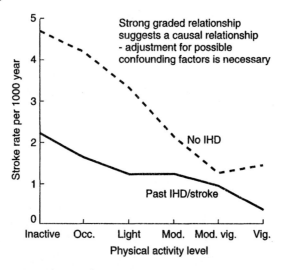

Fig. 2.1 Physical activity and stroke risk: a graded and strong relationship (British Regional Heart Study). IHD, ischaemic heart disease.

Risk

The term 'risk' is widely used as a measure of disease occurrence—incidence or prevalence, depending on the disease. For diseases with an acute onset, such as myocardial infarction and stroke, risk is usually equated with incidence—the number of new cases of disease arising over a defined time period among a defined population at risk of the disease. Epidemiology, like any science, draws inferences from empirical observations, most of which require comparisons. A simple comparison of the *number* of cases of stroke occurring in two places, or at two times, would clearly be subject to the obvious defect that one place may have a greater population and therefore more cases. This basic concept of *a population at risk* is necessary for valid comparisons to be made. To make unbiased comparisons it is necessary to compare like with like and the epidemiological tool for this purpose is the rate. Incidence rate is a proportion comprised of a numerator (the number of new cases in a period of time) and a denominator which is the number of people at risk of the disease over the same time.

When incidence is measured over several years, the population at risk will change as time passes. The most obvious change will be ageing, but some people will leave the area, others will move in, some will die, some will have a stroke and pass from the denominator to the numerator. The denominator can be determined by assuming that the population resident in the area at the mid-point in time of the study is a good-enough approximation to the population at risk over the whole period. For rare diseases this is usually good enough because the numerator is always tiny compared with the denominator and small changes in the denominator will have little impact on the incidence rate. For more common diseases, such as stroke and ischaemic heart disease, it is better to measure the population at risk in terms of person-years at risk. A person followed for 10 years contributes 10 person-years of risk to the denominator, 10 people followed for 1 year also contribute 10 person-years of risk.

Individual risk

The crude incidence of stroke in several collaborating general practices in Oxfordshire in the mid-1980s was 1.60 per 1000 person-years at risk, but varied dramatically with age, more than doubling for every decade from age 55 years (Bamford et al. 1988). Incidence rates give the best approximation available of a person's chances of having a stroke in the absence of any other information about the individual. It is curious that the estimates derived from large numbers of people give the best information we have about individuals. This has long been recognized by insurance companies which base their premiums (their estimates of your risk of dying) on accumulated information about disease incidence at different ages (the major factor), for each sex, in different occupations, and for different body builds, blood pressures, and smoking behaviour.

Consequently, for a woman in Oxford aged 60 years, the risk of having a stroke if nothing else is known about her (e.g. blood pressure, smoking history, presence of heart disease, diabetes, etc.) is 2.35 per 1000 person-years at risk, which is equivalent to an annual risk of 0.00235 for a single woman-year at risk or less than a quarter of 1 per cent a year. At 70 years, the same women will have an annual risk of stroke of 0.00584. This is a still a small risk, less than 1 per cent, but it is a big increase compared with 10 years earlier, a greater than twofold increase.

But do rates derived from Oxfordshire apply elsewhere? In fact, where you live has a major influence on your stroke risk, even within geographically quite close areas (Wolfe *et al.* 1993). From the south to the north of Britain risk of dying of a stroke increases by over twofold, as does the prevalence of stroke (see Fig. 3.4, p. 37). With more information about the individual, a more accurate stroke risk can be calculated (see Chapter 3); it will never be possible to predict with certainty who will and who will not suffer a stroke. The best we can do is give probabilities.

Relative and attributable risk

Comparisons between people with different characteristics requires the incidence in one group to be compared with the incidence in the other. Taking the change in risk of a stroke for the Oxford woman at age 60 and age 70, the risk ratio (which may be called a rate ratio or a relative risk) is simply the ratio of the incidence at 70 to the incidence at 60 years: 0.00584/0.00235 = 2.49, a more than doubling of risk. A risk ratio of 1 would imply that the rates at both ages were the same. The risk ratio disguises the fairly low incidence rates, which can lead to inappropriate alarm if a person considers that simply by living another 10 years they have doubled their risk of having a stroke! Risk ratios are extremely useful when looking for potential causes of stroke because they are good measures of the strength of association between a factor and disease.

Risk ratios are of limited use in clinical practice. The absolute risk is much more relevant to the patient and doctor. The woman of 70 asking about her increased chances of having a stroke should not be told that her risk is now over double of what it was 10 years earlier, but that her annual risk has increased by 0.00584 – 0.00235 = 0.00349, or rather less than half a per cent (this is the *attributable risk* of a 10-year increase in age). Since most people do not think in probabilities, it is usual to express a probability of 0.00349 as the number of events that would occur in a population of 100 or 1000 people. In this case, among a group of 1000 women aged 70, about three more would be expected to have a stroke over the year than would be expected in a comparable group of 60-year-olds. The absolute difference in the two rates is of vital importance in the clinical assessment of risk and gives a baseline perspective that cannot be provided by the relative differences.

Measuring associations

Cohort (or longitudinal) studies are widely used to assess aetiological associations. In a cohort study, the presence or absence of possible risk factors is measured in people free of disease who are then followed up until strokes

Table 2.1 The relationship between the risk ratio and the odds ratio

	Disease occurrence		
Risk factor	Present	Absent	Total
Present	a	b	$a + b$
Absent	c	d	$c + d$
Total	$a + c$	$b + d$	$a + b + c + d$

Risk of disease if risk factor present: $a/(a + b)$ Risk ratio: $\dfrac{a/(a + b)}{c/(c + d)}$

Risk of disease if risk factor absent: $c/(c + d)$

If the disease is rare, i.e. a and c are small compared with b and d:

$a/(a + b) = a/b$; and $c/(c + d) = c/d$;

and the risk ratio simplifies to:

$(a/b)/(c/d) = a \times d/b \times c = $ the odds ratio.

occur. Case-control studies are also used for similar purposes but the starting point are stroke cases and controls who have not suffered a stroke. The presence or absence of possible risk factors are assessed after the onset of the stroke. This means that case-control studies are more prone to bias than cohort studies. For example, controls may not be representative of the population from which the cases were drawn, resulting in selection bias, and cases and controls may recall their exposure to risk factors differently, resulting in information bias.

Cohort studies give direct measures of disease incidence because they follow people over time, whereas case-control studies are frozen at a point in time and cannot measure incidence, as the ratio of cases to controls is fixed by the investigator (e.g. one case to two controls).

Examining the relationship between a risk factor and disease is done in two ways: calculation of the risk ratio or the odds ratio. Table 2.1 illustrates the calculations. For rare diseases, the odds ratio is a good estimate of the true risk (or rate) ratio.

In a cohort study where subjects are classified according to the presence or absence of risk factor(s) at baseline and the occurrence of strokes are then counted as time passes, the true rate ratios can be calculated. In a case-control study, the rate ratios cannot be calculated but the odds ratio provides a fair approximation if the disease is rare. The more common the disease, the less good is the odds ratio as an approximation of the true rate ratio.

For example, a case-control study of the impact of smoking on stroke reported a threefold increased risk of stroke among smokers compared with non-smokers (Bonita et al. 1986). Information from the placebo group of a large longitudinal trial of effects of antihypertensive drugs has also been used to estimate the association between smoking and stroke (Medical Research Council Working Party 1988). We can calculate both the rate ratio and the

Table 2.2 Smoking and risk of stroke: case-control versus longitudinal estimates of risk, data taken from Bonita *et al.* (1986) and MRC Working Party (1988). Note that denominators for the MRC cohort study are approximate, and that the odds ratio estimates are unadjusted and hence do not equal figures reported in the studies

Smoking	Case-control study Stroke		Cohort study Stroke	
	Yes	No	Yes	No
Yes	66	424	48	2420
No	66	1162	60	5970
Odds ratio	$\dfrac{(66 \times 1162)}{(66 \times 424)} = 2.74$		$\dfrac{(48 \times 5970)}{(60 \times 2420)} = 1.97$	
Rate ratio	Not applicable		$\dfrac{(48\,/\,2468)}{(60\,/\,6030)} = 1.95$	

odds ratio from these cohort study data. These data are shown in Table 2.2. The odds ratio tends to overestimate the true rate ratio, but provided the disease frequency is less than about 1 per cent, then this effect is not marked.

Smoking seems to have stronger adverse effects when studied in a case-control study (odds ratio 2.74) than in a cohort design (odds ratio 1.97). This could reflect a real difference between the studies, such as might be produced by the use of different types of cigarette, or different population susceptibility to smoking due to age, sex, or race. More likely, the difference is due to the effects of bias. It is possible that recall bias has led to cases more often giving (or being asked more thoroughly) a history of smoking. Case-control studies can only include survivors, and it is possible that smoking is linked with survival as well as incidence. It is clear, however, that both smoking and hypertension are consistently related to risk of stroke, regardless of the method of study.

Combining risk factors

An advantage of the rate ratio (and odds ratio) compared with absolute differences in risk is that the combined effects of two or more risk factors can be taken into account to give an estimate of the risk of disease. Relative risks usually combine in a multiplicative way. For example, smoking increases the risk of stroke by about 2–3 times, and hypertension increases risk by about 4–5 times. The combined effects of both smoking and hypertension might be estimated to be between eight- and fifteenfold (i.e. 2 × 4 and 3 × 5) increased risk, assuming that the risks multiplied, are independent of each other, and do not interact. The increased risk among hypertensive smokers observed in one case-control study was almost twentyfold (Bonita *et al.* 1986), implying that

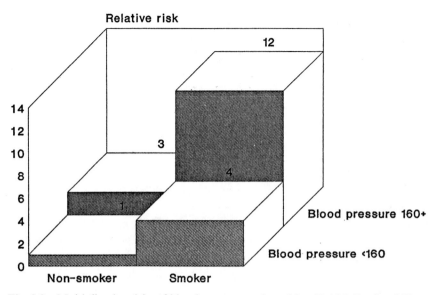

Fig. 2.2 Multiplicative risks of blood pressure and smoking (British Regional Heart Study).

the effects of these two risk factors are multiplicative. This was confirmed in the longitudinal British Regional Heart Study (Fig. 2.2), which demonstrated a relative risk of 12 for hypertensive smokers (Shaper *et al.* 1991). However, another longitudinal study found only a sixfold increased risk among male hypertensive smokers (Salonen *et al.* 1982), raising the possibility of an additive relationship between these risk factors.

A multiplicative relationship between these risk factors implies that each risk factor is operating via a different pathogenic mechanism. Smoking may be having its effects through blood viscosity or platelet function, whereas blood pressure may be causing vessel wall damage. Additive relationships between risk factors suggest that their effects are mediated through the same pathogenic mechanisms.

Population attributable risk fraction

How important are hypertension and smoking compared with other risk factors? The population attributable risk fraction (PARF) gives an estimate of this. It is an important concept because it allows for both the strength with which a risk factor is associated with a disease, and the commonness of the risk factor. A strong risk factor (e.g. acute alcohol intoxication) may only affect a small proportion of the population and therefore be 'responsible for' only a very small number of strokes. The stronger the risk factor and the more commonly it occurs, the larger is its PARF. It is always important to remember that association does not mean causation, and when thinking

Table 2.3 The relationship between risk of stroke among men aged 40–49 and the expected number of cases arising in each blood pressure stratum over 24 years, using data from Framingham study (Dawber 1980)

Systolic BP	Prevalence (%)	Incidence rate/100/24 years	Expected number of cases (%)
<120	16	1.7	27 (4.7)
120-	43	3.6	155 (27.0)
140-	29	5.6	162 (28.3)
160-	8	12.8	102 (17.8)
180 +	4	31.8	127 (22.2)
Total	100		573 (100.0)

about PARF it is easy to fall into the trap of assuming that because a high proportion of a disease may be attributed to a particular risk factor, that removing that risk factor would lead to a commensurate fall in the occurrence of the disease.

Blood pressure provides a good example of the relationship between high relative risk but low PARF. Table 2.3 shows how dramatically the incidence of stroke rises with blood pressure. However, the proportion of people with pressures over 180 mmHg is small, although their relative risk of having a stroke is $31.8/1.7 = 18.7$ times higher than people with pressures below 120 mmHg. The expected number of cases of stroke associated with each blood pressure stratum obviously depends on the numbers at risk. The expected numbers of strokes occurring in each stratum is calculated by multiplying the percentage prevalence of people in a particular blood pressure stratum by the incidence rate for that stratum. People with pressures over 180 mmHg constitute only 22.2 per cent of all the cases that might be expected to occur, and even those who might be considered hypertensive (160 + mmHg) only comprise about 40 per cent of the total cases in this population of men aged 40–49 years. So although hypertension is important in terms of its relative risk, its population attributable risk fraction is not so pronounced.

The implication is that treatment that aims to lower high blood pressure among hypertensives can have only a limited effect in reducing the number of cases of stroke in a whole community. If, for example, treatment of people with systolic blood pressures over 160 mmHg produced a 25 per cent reduction in strokes, or even a 50 per cent reduction, the overall benefits would be quite modest in terms of the reduction in the numbers of strokes. This is shown in Table 2.4. Even on the assumption of a 50 per cent reduction in incidence rates, treatment produces only a 20 per cent reduction in the total numbers of strokes that might be expected. Bonita and Beaglehole (1986) estimated that treatment of high blood pressure could explain only 10 per cent

Table 2.4 The effects of treatment assuming a reduction in incidence of 25 per cent and 50 per cent for people with blood pressures over 160 mmHg, using data from Table 2.3

Systolic BP	Percent prevalence	25% reduction		50% reduction	
		Incidence rate	Expected cases	Incidence rate	Expected cases
<120	16	1.7	27	1.7	27
120-	43	3.6	155	3.6	155
140-	29	5.6	162	5.6	162
160-	8	9.6	77	6.4	51
180 +	4	23.9	96	15.9	64
Total			517		459
	i.e. (573 - 517)/573 × 100 = 10%			(573 - 459)/573 × 100 = 20%	

of the large fall in stroke mortality in New Zealand between 1973 and 1982.

High-risk approaches to disease control (i.e. searching for those with the highest levels of risk factors and treating them as actively as possible), can only contribute a small amount to population control of disease. Rose (1981) has drawn attention to the related prevention paradox: 'a prevention measure that brings large benefits to the community offers little to each participating individual'. Rose estimated that a small downward shift in the population distribution of blood pressure of as little as 2–3 mmHg might be associated with as much reduction in mortality as drug treatment for those at high risk. The effect of shifting the blood pressure distribution downward by 1–2 per cent is shown in Table 2.5. The expected number of cases is about 15 per cent less than that found with the original blood pressure distribution, a greater reduction than achieved by a hypertension treatment that reduces the risk of stroke by 25 per cent, as demonstrated in Table 2.4.

Svanborg's observations (1988) that systolic blood pressures have fallen among successive birth cohorts since the beginning of this century suggest that this downward shift phenomenon is actually happening. Why this has happened and whether further cohorts will be affected remains to be seen.

Calculation of population attributable risk fraction

The PARF can be calculated from either rate ratio or odds ratio estimates of the relative risk, and the proportion of the population exposed to the risk factor. This latter measure can be taken directly from population-based cohort studies where the proportion exposed is known. In case-control studies, the proportion exposed in the control group may not be a good estimate of the true level of exposure in the population, particularly if the controls were selected from hospital admissions (where cigarette smokers will

Table 2.5 The effect of a small downward shift in the distribution of systolic blood pressure—that is per cent prevalence—on the expected number of strokes, using data from Table 2.3

Systolic BP	Percent prevalence	Incidence rate/100/24 years	Expected number of cases
<120	23	1.7	39
120-	43	3.6	155
140-	26	5.6	146
160-	6	12.8	77
180 +	2	31.8	64
Total	100		481 (84%)

be over-represented, for example) or if matching between cases and controls was used in the study design. It may be necessary to make estimates of the proportion of the population exposed from other studies, or routine surveys. The mathematical relationship between attributable risk and relative risk is:

$$\text{Population attributable risk fraction} = P \times (RR - 1)/ [P \times (RR - 1)] + 1$$

where P is the proportion of the population exposed and RR is the relative risk estimate.

Applying this relationship to some of the risk factors for stroke, suggests that some factors such as physical inactivity, despite quite low relative risks, affect so many people that their contribution to the population burden of disease may be substantial. For example, if 60 per cent of the population are inactive, and the relative risk of stroke amongst such people is 2.5-fold, applying the formula:

$$\text{Population attributable risk fraction} = 0.6 \times (2.5 - 1)/[0.6 \times (2.5 - 1)] + 1$$
$$= 47.4 \text{ per cent.}$$

This implies that almost half of all strokes may be attributed to inactivity. The population attributable risk fraction of smoking and high blood pressure were found to be of comparable size (about a third of strokes associated with each) in a New Zealand study (Bonita et al. 1986).

By contrast, a past history of transient ischaemic attack (TIA) affects less than 1 per cent of the population (Sandercock and Warlow 1985), so despite its high relative risk of 5, less than 2 per cent of the stroke burden can be attributed to this cause. Looking for effective treatments for TIAs should therefore be put into some perspective by this information. Even if a remarkable treatment was discovered that prevented every single case of stroke following TIA, it would only lead to a reduction of less than 2 per cent in the overall numbers of strokes. Similar comments apply to the presence of heart failure, diabetes mellitus, and atrial fibrillation, which only affect relatively small proportions of younger people. Among older people, however, the prevalence of heart disease is much higher, with up to 15 per cent with some sort of "heart trouble" (Evans *et al.* 1980). The PARF of some risk factors may become more important with increasing age in terms of their contribution to the overall burden of disease, despite becoming weaker in terms of their relative risk.

The importance of this approach is that it gives an idea of where effort might usefully be made to prevent disease or look for new treatments. So although around half of all strokes may be associated with physical inactivity, this does not mean that increased activity will lead to a reduction in risk of strokes. PARF estimates are not a substitute for trials to estimate the true effects of interventions.

Sources of error

Measuring risk factors

The assumption that participants in an epidemiological study can be divided neatly between those who are 'exposed' to a risk factor and those who are not is an oversimplification. Factors such as age, blood pressure, and number of cigarettes smoked can be further categorized according to the extent and severity of the exposure. Risk of stroke rises progressively with increasing systolic (or diastolic) blood pressure (MacMahon *et al.* 1990; Prospective Studies Collaboration 1995). Classifying subjects as 'hypertensive' or not underestimates the true nature and strength of the association.

There are other difficulties which complicate the interpretation of risk-factor studies. Blood pressure varies from hour to hour and day to day, and may be influenced by threatening experiences (such as having your blood pressure taken). A single reading, or even several readings taken over a short period of time, will only approximately characterize the true 'exposure' to blood pressure. Someone with an uncharacterisitically high measured blood pressure on one visit, will be likely to have a lower one at a subsequent visit. As yet there are no long-term prospective cohort studies that have used mean 24-hour blood pressure from continuous ambulatory blood pressure monitoring to define 'exposure'. The same considerations apply to cigarette smoking, blood cholesterol, physical activity, dietary intake, and psychological stress. If a real association exists between any of these exposures and stroke, the effect of such misclassification will be to underestimate the strength of associations—so-called regression-dilution bias.

Some studies, such as the Framingham cohort, have exposure data re-recorded as time goes by (in the case of Framingham, every 2 years; Dawber

1980). It has been possible to use data such as these to take account of some of the error that is introduced by using imperfect exposure data (MacMahon *et al.* 1990). Another problem is that many risk factors will vary over longer periods of time. The severity of hypertension will change as the individual ages and life-style factors alter. A new risk factor may appear, such as atrial fibrillation, and some may stop, such as smoking, although even then the effects may persist for a period of time.

Left ventricular hypertrophy (LVH), defined either by electrocardiogram, or by echocardiography, has repeatedly been shown to be associated with stroke even after other factors, including blood pressure, have been controlled for (Kannel *et al.* 1983; Shaper *et al.* 1991; Bikkina *et al.* 1994). This may well reflect the fact that in some respects LVH is a better index of 'exposure' to blood pressure than is casually measured blood pressure alone. Studies with repeated assessments of 'exposure' have used complex statistical modelling (Cox proportional hazard regression analysis with time-dependent covariates) to take account of the appearance of new risk factors. A study from the Mayo Clinic with 13 years of follow-up found that the relative risk for 'definite hypertension' increased from 3.3 to 6.8 when a statistical model taking account of changes in hypertension was compared with one which simply classified people as hypertensive or not at baseline (Davis *et al.* 1987). The same was true for history of transient ischaemic attack and a number of other factors.

Current epidemiological practice is to attempt to make adjustments for regression-dilution bias by replicate measurement of exposure variables at least once on a subgroup (say 5–10 per cent) of participants. Measurement imprecision does not just affect exposure variables of interest, but also confounders, for which statistical 'adjustments' are made in multivariate analysis. For such adjustment to be valid, it is assumed that exposure variables are statistically independent, but frequently they are highly correlated with each other, and subject to measurement imprecision. Under these circumstances substantial bias in the estimation of the 'independent' effects of a risk factor is possible (Phillips and Davey Smith 1991). In general, epidemiological studies measure as many participants as possible but only on a single occasion, owing to cost and feasibility considerations. Simulations of the trade-offs between sample size and replicate measurement of exposures suggest that the independent effects of exposure variables would be more accurately assessed by smaller samples with several replicate measurements (Phillips and Davey Smith 1992).

The play of chance

Up to now we have discussed probabilities, risk, and risk ratios as if these can be estimated precisely. Human beings and populations demonstrate variation which results in measurements being affected by the play of chance or random error. For example, in Oxfordshire the incidence of stroke is 1.60 per 1000 per year. However, this is only an estimate of the true incidence based on a sample of cases occurring over a relatively short period of time. If the incidence study had been bigger and carried out for longer, we would be more likely to place greater reliance on the measurements obtained. Our intuitive acceptance of big studies is based on sound statistical theory. As the sample size increases, so do the number of stroke events, and consequently, the precision of our estimate of incidence is greater. Conventionally, we describe the precision of estimates using 95 per cent confidence intervals which represent the boundaries within which we would expect the true value of what we are measuring to lie. By the play of chance, 5 per cent of the time, a fluke will occur and a result more extreme than these 95 per cent confidence intervals will be found. Reducing random error is best done by improving measurement methods, making more measurements, and increasing the numbers of people measured. When measuring incidence of disease, the only means open to reducing random error is increasing the population studied. When measuring risk factors, multiple measurements may be made and better techniques used.

Bias and confounding

In epidemiology, while random errors are acceptable and their size estimated by use of confidence intervals, bias and confounding are more worrying. There are many types of bias—that is deviations from the truth—but the ones that keep epidemiologists awake at night are selection bias and information bias. Selection bias refers to systematic differences in those people who are included in studies from those who are not. For example, in a cohort study, younger and healthier people may choose to take part, resulting in bias in disease incidence rates. Information bias refers to flaws in measurement of exposures or outcomes. For example, in a case-control study, cases may report exposures to health hazards more than controls simply because they make greater efforts to recall the information.

Confounding literally means to 'mix up' and this is precisely what may occur in examining associations between risk factors and disease. For example, having a pet may be associated with a reduced risk of stroke and the hypothesized mechanism of action might be that pet-ownership results in reduced psychological stress and lower blood pressure. But this pet–stroke relationship may be explained by pet-owners being more likely to take part in regular physical activity. Consequently the pet–stroke relationship is confounded by physical activity which is related to both pet-ownership and reduced stroke risk. By contrast, the reported inverse relationship between number of orgasms reported by men and total mortality is not confounded by physical activity as sexual activity is simply another way of measuring general levels of activity and thus may be considered to lie on the same causal pathway (Davey Smith *et al.* 1997). The orgasm–stroke relationship could be confounded by age or by symptoms of angina which would make orgasms less frequent and stroke more likely, and consequently adjustment for these factors would be necessary in evaluating the causal nature of the association.

An example of confounding

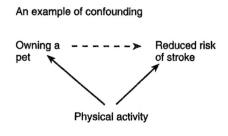

Associations: real or apparent?

In summary, there are five possible explanations for an association between an exposure (or risk factor) and an outcome (such as stroke):

1. Chance: statistical sampling theory tells us that sometimes two variables will appear to be associated simply because of chance variation in the frequency with which risk factors occur in one group compared with another. The probability that an association at least as large as the one measured could have arisen by chance is given by the p-value.

2. Bias: which arises if the chance of ascertaining outcomes is associated with a risk factor (selection bias; for example, if knowing that a man was hypertensive increased the probability of a sudden death being certified as due to stroke), or if collection of risk-factor information is dependent on the outcome event having been experienced (information bias; for example, someone who has had a stroke recalling a head injury shortly beforehand).

3. Confounding: the association is real, but the explanation is that a third variable, not on the same causal pathway, is associated with both the exposure and the outcome (a further example which may be more memorable is of the strong association between ownership of a set of false teeth and stroke which occurs only because age is associated with both the need for false teeth and stroke). Adjustments for confounding factors may lead to biased estimation of associations with disease due to measurement imprecision and correlation between exposure and confounding variables.

4. Causal: the exposure in some way causes the outcome. This is what epidemiologists are most interested in.

5. Reverse causality: the outcome causes the 'exposure'. Physical inactivity is associated with ill-health. But does the inactivity cause the ill-health? Or does the ill-health cause the inactivity?

Summary

1. Criteria for assuming a risk factor is causally related to stroke are: strength of the relationship, the results of experimental changes in the risk factor, graded dose–response relationships, time sequence, and consistency of relationship in different studies. Other criteria are less robust.

2. An individual's risk of stroke varies with age, where they live, and their accompanying stroke risk factors.

3. Risk ratios and odds ratios are used to describe the strength of association between risk factors and stroke. In case-control studies, only odds ratios can be calculated.

4. People with several risk factors are at very high risk of stroke as risk factors tend to multiply together.

5. Population attributable risk fraction describes that proportion of stroke that may be attributed to a specific risk factor. Reducing common risk factors, even if they are only weakly associated with stroke, is likely to result in greater reduction in disease than reducing rare, but strong, risk factors. This is a useful concept for identifying risk factors of great public health importance.

6. Associations between risk factors and stroke may not be causal but may be due to bias, confounding, or random error.

3 Time, places, and people

Variation in time

The decline of stroke

Stroke mortality rates have shown a consistent decline in many countries (Anonymous 1983; Bonita *et al*. 1990; McGovern *et al*. 1992; Wolf *et al*. 1992; Brown *et al*. 1996; Tuomilehto *et al*. 1996*b*; Thorvaldsen *et al*. 1997; Gale and Martyn 1997). In the USA the rate of decline has been about 0.5 per cent/year from 1900 to 1920, 1 per cent/year from 1920 to 1950, about 1.5 per cent/year from 1950 to 1970 and about 4–5 per cent/year from 1974 onwards (Ostfeld 1980; Whisnant 1984). In England and Wales, a similar decline starting in 1900 and affecting all age groups has been seen (Wolfe and Burney, 1992; Charlton *et al*. 1997; Ebrahim, 1998) and is shown in Fig. 3.1. The rise in stroke mortality rates over the war years remains unexplained but affected both men and women and is probably due to coding changes to causes of death that occurred when a new version of the *International Classification of Diseases* was introduced. The pattern is markedly different from that for ischaemic heart disease deaths, which increased from 1929 to the 1950s, and only started to decline in the 1980s.

As the decline in mortality has affected all age groups over this time period, it is termed a period effect, to distinguish it from a cohort effect. Period effects are due to factors operating close to the time of death and consequently tend to affect both men and women and all age groups. Cohort effects are due to influences that depend on the birth cohort a person belongs to and are often (but not always) associated with factors operating around the time of birth. Consequently, changes in mortality are seen at different ages at different times. Mathematical age–period–cohort modelling which attempts to separate out the effects of age, time of birth, and the period of death, confirms that the predominant decline is a period effect. Possible factors might be changes in stroke risk factors such as high blood pressure, or a reduction in case fatality. The decline began long before the main risk factors for stroke had been identified, and long before the introduction of effective and tolerable antihypertensive therapy, suggesting that primary prevention and medical treatment are not the explanations. Mathematical modelling also shows a significant cohort effect, but the pattern is complex. Once the strong downward period effect is removed, cohorts born in the years up to 1880 have an increasing risk of stroke. Cohorts born from 1880 to

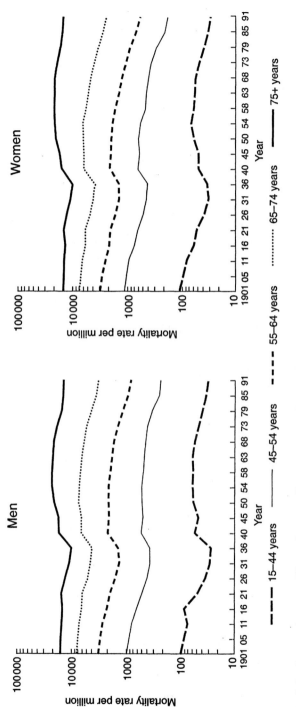

Fig. 3.1 Age- and sex-specific stroke mortality rates per million, England and Wales, 1901–91.

1910 showed successive decreases in mortality, but cohorts born after 1910 have shown successive increases in mortality (Wolfe and Burney 1992). Some of these later cohorts are still relatively young, and at low overall risk of stroke, so the analyses may be misleading, but suggest that we cannot take the continued decline in stroke mortality for granted. Similar patterns have been found in Spanish and other national stroke mortality data (Medrano et al. 1997).

A decline in incidence or in case fatality?

A decrease in mortality can result from a decrease in incidence or a decrease in case fatality. Few studies have used consistent methods over sufficiently long periods of time to allow monitoring of trends in both incidence and case fatality. Improved survival after a stroke has probably contributed a major part of the decline in mortality over this century. From 1955 to 1971 case fatality fell by about 30 per cent in the UK (Haberman et al. 1978). In Framingham, USA, between 1958 and 1978, 1-year case fatality fell from 34 per cent to 13 per cent in men, but not in women (Wolf et al. 1992), and in the Minnesota Heart Study, 28-day case fatality halved between 1970 and 1985 (McGovern et al. 1993), but there was no decrease in Rochester, Minnesota (Brown et al. 1996).

Reductions in case fatality over shorter time periods have been found in Auckland (Bonita et al. 1993), Finland (Numminen et al. 1996; Tuomilehto et al. 1996b), Sweden (Harmsen et al. 1992; Stegmayr and Asplund 1996), and Estonia (Korv et al. 1996). However, negligible changes in stroke case fatality over 5 years have been reported in 17 centres in the World Health Organization Monitoring of Cardiovascular Disease (MONICA) project, where each centre ascertained and defined strokes according to the same protocol (Thorvaldsen et al. 1997).

Falls in hospital case fatality might be due to a trend of less severe stroke patients being admitted to hospital. Another explanation is that the increased use of neuroimaging has led to milder and more equivocal stroke cases being confirmed. One would expect either of these possibilities to be reflected in an increase in incidence, which has not, in fact, been observed. It is also possible that the ratio of cerebral haemorrhage to cerebral thrombo-embolus has declined, resulting in a lower severity of stroke as the latter tend to have a better prognosis.

The only good data on incidence over decades come from Rochester, USA, where the same methods and diagnostic criteria have been used since 1935 (Homer et al. 1987). From 1945 to 1975, a fall of almost 2 per cent/year was found (Garraway et al. 1979; Brown et al. 1996). Similar falls in incidence, over shorter periods, have been reported from Japan (Tanaka et al. 1981; Ueda et al. 1981), and from Finland (Tuomilehto et al. 1986, 1991, 1996b).

In Sweden although mortality has fallen, several studies have failed to detect a parallel decline in incidence (Alfredsson *et al.* 1986; Harmsen *et al.* 1992; Stegmayr and Asplund 1996). The most recent incidence trends in Rochester, USA, have shown an increase (Broderick *et al.* 1989; Brown *et al.* 1996). In 1980–84 the incidence of stroke was 17 per cent higher than in 1975–79. The increased incidence was maintained from 1985 to 1989. Increases have also been reported from Sweden (Terent 1988) and Denmark (Jorgensen *et al.* 1992). In Framingham, incidence has been more or less stable over three decades, although absolute numbers of strokes have been small (Wolf *et al.* 1992). Interestingly, in countries of the former Soviet Union, Central and Eastern Europe, stroke mortality, and probably incidence, rates have increased (Khaw 1996; Leon *et al.* 1997), suggesting that stroke occurrence may be sensitive to general socio-economic conditions.

There are still a number of questions about exactly what is happening to stroke incidence. Various biases might explain some of the trends reported. For example, one study noted a marked improvement in the quality of medical note-keeping over the years, allowing a higher proportion of strokes identified from routine hospital statistics to be classified as 'definite strokes' (McGovern *et al.* 1992). Scrutiny of the data from Rochester reveals that between 1975–79 and 1980–84 the incidence of stroke doubled in women aged 85 and over (Brown *et al.* 1996). A change of this magnitude could only occur through a change in diagnostic practice. The greater availability of neuroradiology may have resulted in an increase in the general level of interest in stroke, and improvements in the recording of physical signs and standard of diagnosis.

Why should incidence of stroke decline?

Examining trends in stroke mortality and incidence is valuable as understanding their causes may help in developing better preventive strategies. In England, government policy has highlighted maintaining the current downward secular trends in stroke mortality as a health target. Without a clear understanding of the factors that determine secular trends it is difficult to develop cogent strategies.

Four main reasons for the downward trend may be put forward: treatment of high blood pressure, reduced exposure to risk factors associated with high blood pressure, reduced exposure to other risk factors for stroke, and the competing risk of ischaemic heart disease (Ebrahim 1997).

Treatment

Treatment of high blood pressure is an implausible explanation for a trend that began in 1900 before any effective antihypertensive therapy was available. Treatment has been put forward as the major explanation and the earlier trends have been discounted because incidence data were not available to 'confirm the mortality trend' (Whisnant 1984). Widespread use of acceptable and effective drugs did not begin until the 1960s (Haberman *et al.* 1978; Acheson and Williams 1980; Ostfeld 1980), and while treatment may be a good explanation for the greater rate of decline observed in the 1970s (Nicholls and Johansen 1983; Tuomilehto *et al.* 1985) it would be necessary to make assumptions about the effectiveness of antihypertensive treatment that are unlikely. Bonita and Beaglehole (1986) estimated that if all hypertensives were treated, and treatment was as effective as in the major published trials, only 10 per cent of the observed reduction in deaths among people aged 30–69 years could be explained by treatment. Similar analyses have been done for the USA (Bonita and Beaglehole 1989; Klag *et al.* 1989; Casper *et al.* 1992). Moreover, older people have experienced just as great a reduction in stroke risk, yet are much less often given antihypertensive treatment.

Changes in risk factors associated with high blood pressure

Reduced salt intake over the past century has been put forward as an explanation for a reduced prevalence of high blood pressure, and hence a lower risk of stroke (Walker 1977; Joosens *et al.* 1979; Simpson 1979; Cummins 1983). A large international study set up to resolve this question (Intersalt) was equivocal, showing strong relationships between urinary sodium output and blood pressure between populations but less clear relationships within populations (Intersalt Cooperative Research Group 1988; Elliott *et al.* 1996). A subsequent meta-analysis of ecological (between population) studies (Law *et al.* 1991a), individual observational studies (Frost *et al.* 1991), and intervention studies using controlled diets (Law *et al.* 1991b), did show a significant and substantial relationship between salt intake and blood pressure, sufficient to account for changes in stroke incidence of the sort of magnitude that has been seen. This study also suggested that the age-related rise in blood pressure was very salt dependent. There is little evidence that salt intake has decreased substantially, although the very high intakes expected in Japan and Portugal were not confirmed in the Intersalt study, and it is possible that large reductions had already taken place. Some recent intervention studies have supported a relationship between blood pressure and salt intake in humans (Cappuccio *et al.* 1997) and chimpanzees (Denton *et al.* 1995), but others have suggested that the effect, although real, is quantitatively small (Trials of Hypertension Prevention Collaborative Research Group 1997). While it remains possible that salt intake is causally related to risk of stroke, this remains unproven. Reaching a firm conclusion is fraught with difficulties, both methodological (Davey Smith and Phillips 1996) and in interpretation (Taubes 1998). In the absence of large-scale, methodologically sound studies unequivocally supporting the salt–blood pressure hypothesis, the role of changes in salt consumption in explaining the time trends in stroke is doubtful. The implications of this for salt restriction as a means of stroke prevention are discussed in Chapter 8.

Various other influences on blood pressure have changed greatly over the years, including obesity, alcohol consumption, exercise, protein, fruit, and vegetable consumption. The shape of the blood pressure curve in populations may have shifted downwards during this century. Svanborg (1988) in a series of cohort studies has shown that the mean systolic pressure of people born in 1901/1902 at age 70 was 168 mmHg, whereas people born 10 years later had mean pressures of 162 mmHg at age 70. A small shift to the left of the population distribution of blood pressure may have a disproportionately great effect on the incidence of stroke (Rose 1981), and is discussed further in Chapter 2 (see Population attributable risk fraction). In Finland mean diastolic blood pressure declined by 9–12 mmHg between 1972 and 1992, enough to account for half the decline in stroke death rate (Vartiainen *et al.* 1995).

Exposure to other risk factors
Major changes in cigarette consumption, physical activity, and diet occurred in the 1970s which may be much more important determinants of the recent reduction in risk of stroke than treatment of high blood pressure (Tuomilehto *et al.* 1991). Among North Americans, who adopted a 'healthy life style' earlier than Britains, ischaemic heart disease risk started to fall sooner than in Britain. It is possible that the shared risk factors between stroke and ischaemic heart disease operate with a different latency; reductions in shared risk factors may have a more immediate effect on stroke than on myocardial infarction. The association between atmospheric pollution and stroke mortality time trends (Knox 1981) may be an important determinant as it would explain variations in stroke risk in the north and south of England, and also social class gradients of risk.

Competing risk of ischaemic heart disease
It has been suggested that stroke-prone individuals have been dying from ischaemic heart disease, because of shared risk factors and an earlier onset of heart disease, and therefore are not surviving to an age when they would have a stroke (Haberman *et al.* 1982). However, stroke mortality rates have fallen more amongst people aged 45–64 years for whom it is more difficult to postulate such an effect on survival.

Variation in place

Studies of geographical variation in stroke incidence have been reviewed (Malmgren *et al.* 1987; Sudlow and Warlow 1996) and major deficiencies in study design highlighted: differing criteria for diagnosis; poor ascertainment of cases, especially those not admitted to hospital; defining the population at

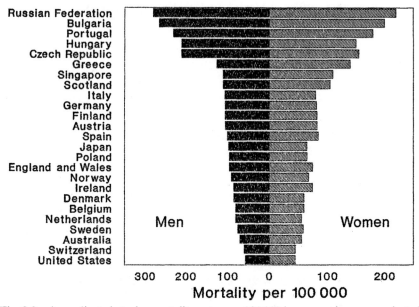

Fig. 3.2 Age-adjusted stroke mortality rates per 100 000 in men and women, selected countries, 1990–92 (from Khaw 1996).

risk; inadequate size of study; study of only a few months rather than complete years; non-standard presentation of rates by age group and sex.

Because of these study defects and other differences between studies it is difficult to decide whether stroke is more or less common in different parts of the world, or whether incidence is truly declining. However, geographical variation is striking, which makes methodological shortcomings less plausible as the sole explanation for these differences. Mortality rates for stroke vary up to eightfold between different countries, being especially high in Eastern European countries and Portugal, and low in USA, France, and Switzerland (Fig. 3.2). Moreover, there are marked variations in mortality trends. Mortality is increasing rapidly in Eastern Europe and decreasing in the rest of the developed world (Fig. 3.3). For much of the world, however, there are no reliable data (Ebrahim 1996, 1998).

The WHO MONICA collaborative study, although designed primarily to monitor time tends, also demonstrates geographical variation in both incidence and mortality amongst the (mainly European) centres taking part. The MONICA study uses standardized and validated ascertainment methods, but unfortunately has variable coverage of strokes not admitted to hospital. Variation is a little less than suggested by routine mortality statistics, but is still at least threefold (Thorvaldsen *et al.* 1995).

The best quality data come from a collaborative re-analysis of incidence studies which have fulfilled the most stringent quality criteria (Sudlow and

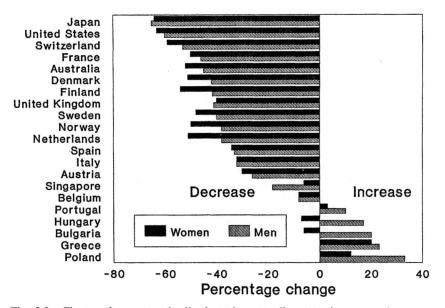

Fig. 3.3 Changes in age-standardized stroke mortality rates in men and women, selected countries, 1960–64 and 1985–89 (from Khaw 1996).

Warlow 1997). As a minimum, these studies had good ascertainment of non-hospitalized strokes, including those occurring in residential and nursing homes, used consistent clinical definitions, recorded first-ever strokes, and had accurate denominator population data. Most had sufficient rates of neuroimaging or autopsy to permit comparison of pathological types of stroke. Eleven such studies were identified. They represent a limited range of different population types, being mainly of White, European populations. Age-standardized incidence varied from 238/100 000 in Dijon, France to 627/100 000 in Novosibirsk, Russia. However, between these extremes there was little variation, either in overall incidence or in distribution of pathological types of stroke.

In Britain, the prevalence of stroke in 24 towns shows marked variation, as shown in Fig. 3.4. Since prevalence is related to incidence by duration of disease, if stroke patients in the different towns in the British Regional Heart Study had different survival prospects (perhaps through variation in quality of health care), this might explain the variation. However, it is more probable that the differences reflect the north–south variation in incidence of stroke.

Studies of migrants show that they tend to acquire the risk of the country they migrate to, rather than retain the risk of the country they come from. This supports the idea that stroke risk is modifiable by life style or environmental means (Marmot *et al.* 1975; Kagan *et al.* 1979; Bonita *et al.* 1984).

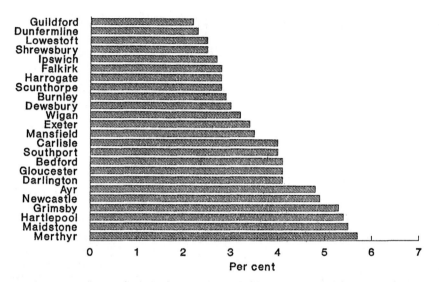

Fig. 3.4 Prevalence of stroke in men in 24 British towns (British Regional Heart Study).

The use of information about variation in place is that it may give clues to aetiology, and the means of and scope for prevention (Khaw 1996). It may be especially useful when trying to detect differences in stroke risk due to potential risk factors that are so ubiquitous in a single population (e.g. air pollution, salt intake) that contrasting groups for comparison cannot be found.

People: variation within populations

Risk factors can be classified as *inherent biological traits* such as genes, age and sex, *physiological characteristics* such as blood pressure, *manifestations of arterial disease* such as transient ischaemic attack, *behaviours* such as smoking, *social characteristics* such as social class, and *environmental characteristics* such as temperature (Marmot and Poulter 1992). Some studies of risk factors have used fatal strokes as the outcome variable, whereas others have used all strokes. Results will be similar unless the risk factor is associated only with case fatality and not incidence. Studies using incident strokes will have more power and greater precision in their estimates of the strength of associations.

A genetic predisposition to stroke

Family history
Do strokes run in the family? In the British Regional Heart Study, a large prospective cohort of British men, having either or both parents die of a stroke

or a heart attack increases a man's risk of stroke independently of other risk factors by 30–40 per cent (Wannamethee *et al.* 1996). Strokes are common and share risk factors with the major cause of death in Western countries, ischaemic heart disease, and therein lies the problem of trying to estimate whether a family history of stroke indicates a specific predisposition or chance. In general, family studies are a weak method of assessing genetic predisposition because families share more than genetic material (Gurling 1984).

Other prospective studies have shown inconsistent associations between parental history and stroke risk (Khaw and Barrett-Connor, 1986; Welin *et al.* 1987; Boysen *et al.* 1988; Harmsen *et al.* 1990; Jousilahti *et al.* 1997). One reason for inconsistent findings is the relatively low power of even large cohorts to detect real associations as the numbers of strokes that occur are relatively small. In addition, classification of parental cause of death may be inaccurate. If misclassification is evenly spread between those with and without strokes, this will tend to reduce the strength of any observed association. However, if those at high risk of stroke are more likely to report that their parents died of stroke, this would lead to an information bias; a spurious association between stroke and parental history would result. The effect of inaccurate information has been examined in the Framingham study, where the parents of 178 members of the cohort were themselves also cohort members. All were asked their parents' cause of death. Cause of death was carefully verified for cohort members, and when reported and verified caused of death were compared, only 77 per cent of reported stroke deaths were confirmed. No association was found between risk of stroke and reported parental stroke, but amongst the cohort's offspring (for whom parental cause of death was known) a strong relationship emerged (Kiely *et al.* 1993).

Family history of stroke is associated with an increase of systolic blood pressure of up to 10 mmHg (Miall *et al.* 1967; Sigurdsson *et al.* 1983), but the association of family history with stroke is independent of its effect on blood pressure and other risk factors. It is probable that a substantial familial effect exists, but it is not clear whether the family effect operates through other unknown risk factors for stroke, which were not allowed for in these studies, or through a genetic component of increased susceptibility to stroke.

Twin studies

Studies of the occurrence of disease among identical and dissimilar twins provide the strongest evidence of genetic predisposition. Case reports of association of a stroke between identical twins are of limited value in assessing the true genetic component of increased risk of stroke, partly because strokes are common and may occur in both twins by chance, and partly because of the bias produced by selecting twins for study because one of them has the disease of interest. The only sound methodology for studying common diseases amongst twins is to use twin registers and to examine the concordance of stroke in identical (monozygotic, MZ) and non-identical (dizygotic, DZ) twins. This avoids selection bias and allowance can be made for the expected chance association. An American twin-registry study suggested a fourfold increase in concordance amongst MZ compared with DZ twins (Brass *et al.* 1992), but only achieved a 60 per cent response rate, and used self-reported prevalent, rather than incident or fatal, strokes in the comparison. A more robust twin study has been reported using data from the Swedish Twin Registry (de Faire *et al.* 1975). Ischaemic heart disease deaths were twice as likely among MZ as DZ male twins with a similar but less pronounced pattern in female twins. The concordance rates for stroke deaths (ascertained from death certificates) were similar among both MZ and DZ twins for both male and female twins. However, stroke deaths were up to 20 times as common as expected in both types of twins, which implies that a shared uterine or family environment are strong risk factor for stroke.

A twin study has demonstrated that multi-infarct dementia affecting both twin pairs is associated with a much higher chance of a parental history of stroke (Jarvik and Matsuyama 1983). It is therefore possible that a genetic effect is operating to make strokes more likely but not sufficiently severe to cause death.

Further twin studies might examine the concordance in strokes between twins brought up together and apart, examining in addition the time of separation. This sort of analysis is becoming feasible as cohorts of twins separated during the Second World War get older and suffer strokes. This will help distinguish whether very early environmental or intrauterine influences are affecting subsequent stroke risk.

Early life influences: the 'Barker hypothesis'
The influence of the intrauterine environment or early family life on subsequent risk of stroke was suggested by an ecological study that demonstrated a strong association between geographical variation in maternal mortality in 1911–14 and the stroke death rates among the cohort born at that time (Barker and Osmond 1987). Retrospective cohort studies (following up subjects on whom there were existing records of birth weight) demonstrate an association between birth weight and risk of ischaemic heart disease and stroke (Barker 1992; Martyn *et al.* 1996).The association might be mediated via blood pressure, which is related to birth weight (Gennser *et al.* 1988; Barker *et al.* 1990; Taylor *et al.* 1997) and tends to show a familial relationship (Miall and Oldham 1963; Havlik *et al.* 1979). In a large cohort of American nurses who self-reported their birth weights, however, the relationship between risk of stroke and birth weight remained after adjustment for blood pressure and multiple other cardiovascular risk factors.The association was quite weak across the range of normal birth weights (2.5–4.5 kg), but was more pronounced amongst the 13 per cent of

participants with more extreme birth weights (Rich-Edwards *et al.* 1997). The hypothesis has been further tested in special historical groups. Adults exposed to starvation as fetuses during the 1941 seige of Leningrad or the winter of 1944 in The Netherlands show inconsistent patterns of cardiovascular risk despite marked reductions in their average birth weights (Stanner *et al.* 1997).

Maheswaran and colleagues (1997) have demonstrated that the general downward secular trend in stroke mortality rates has occurred at a slower rate in Greater London than in the rest of south-east England. Furthermore, they have found that a cross-over in age-specific mortality rates for Greater London and the south-east of England has occurred at different periods and is consistent with a cohort effect, with similar rates in Greater London and south-east England in people born around 1916–21. They have then used this cohort effect to test the early life hypothesis by examining trends in maternal and neonatal mortality which might be expected to show a similar cross-over in rates in 1916–21 if early life factors were important in explaining the cohort effect. This was not the case; if anything the trends were in the opposite direction.

It seems likely that while early life influences, in particular birth weight, play a part in the risk of adult disease, other variables operating in adult life interact with early life factors to determine risk of chronic diseases in late life (Kuh and Ben-Shlomo 1997). For example, impaired *in utero* development (as indicated by a low birth weight) is modified by adiposity in later life in its effect on risk of coronary heart disease (Frankel *et al.* 1996; Leon *et al.* 1996). The interpretation and practical implications of this work are still far from clear.

Homocystinuria and homocystinaemia
Homocystinuria is an autosomal recessively inherited inborn error of metabolism which causes skeletal defects (similar to Marfan's syndrome), lens dislocation, and mental retardation. It also causes a tendency to both venous and thrombotic complications, such as deep vein thrombosis and cerebral infarction. More recently much milder forms of the disease have become apparent, presenting with vascular disease at times of stress to the metabolic pathway involved, which is folate and vitamin B6 dependent, for example, during pregnancy (Newman and Mitchell 1984).

Numerous observational studies have reported associations between serum homocysteine concentration and stroke. In the British Regional Heart Study, men in the top quarter of the distribution of homocysteine concentrations were four times as likely to suffer a stroke as men in the lowest quarter, with a progressive increase in risk across the four quarters. This association remained as strong after adjustment for multiple other risk factors (Perry *et al.* 1995). Serum samples in this study were non-fasting, so a degree of misclassification will have been introduced in assigning the exposure variable (some men will have had a higher, and others a lower, homocysteine than 'usual' depending on their recent diet). In a case-control study in which exposure was measured using a more sophisticated test—the methionine loading test—to identify subjects with hyperhomocysteinaemia and cases were aged under 55 years, a much stronger fortyfold increased risk was found among those with hyperhomocysteinaemia (Clarke *et al.* 1991). A meta-analysis of all the published observational data indicated that a prolonged reduction of homocysteine by 1 µmol/l was associated with about a 10 per cent reduction in risk of vascular disease (Boushey *et al.* 1995).

Raised blood homocysteine may be a very important risk factor as the heterozygous state is common, affecting about 1 in 70 of the population. A dose–response relationship between blood homocysteine and supplementation with folic acid, pyridoxine, and vitamin B_{12} has been reported (Homocysteine Lowering Triallists Collaboration 1998; Malinow *et al.* 1998), and a number of randomized trials are under way to test the hypothesis that supplementation reduces the incidence of vascular disease, including stroke.

Major risk factors for stroke

Many factors appear to influence the chance of having a stroke: male sex, increased age, high blood pressure, smoking, race, body build, alcohol, ischaemic heart disease and atrial fibrillation, previous transient ischaemic attacks, diabetes, lower social class, raised lipids, polycythemia, physical inactivity, various medications (antihypertensives, aspirin, oestrogens), diet, place of residence, climate, and air quality. The magnitude of some of these associations is shown in Table 3.1 and Fig. 3.5.

Apart from age, the strongest factor associated with stroke is blood pressure. Risk increases continuously over the whole range of blood pressures measured, and holds for systolic, diastolic, and mean blood pressure (MacMahon *et al.* 1990). A single casual blood pressure reading underestimates stroke risk considerably, compared with repeated measures (Keli *et al.* 1992). A 10 mmHg rise in diastolic blood pressure increases stroke risk by 2.3. The strength of association between blood pressure and stroke declines with increasing age: the relative risk between the highest and lowest fifths of blood pressure being ten-, five-, and twofold at ages less than 45, 45–64, and greater than 65 years, respectively (Prospective Studies Collaboration 1995). Raised systolic blood pressure is probably more important than diastolic, especially in elderly people, even in the absence of a raised diastolic pressure (isolated systolic hypertension) (Rutan *et al.* 1988; Keli *et al.* 1992).

Early studies appeared to have underestimated the effects of smoking on risk of stroke (Dawber 1980). Further analysis of the Framingham and other data has found a twofold increased risk associated with smoking, with a dose–response relationship, after allowing for other major risk factors (Wolf

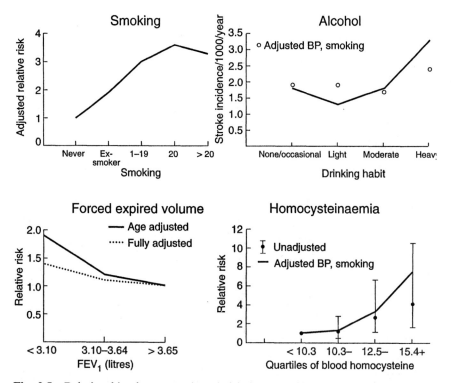

Fig. 3.5 Relationships between selected risk factors and stroke risk in the British Regional Heart Study.

et al. 1988; Shinton and Beevers 1989). Several subsequent prospective studies have confirmed the finding (Kuller *et al.* 1991; Shaper *et al.* 1991; Robbins *et al.* 1994; Haheim *et al.* 1996). The role of alcohol has also only recently been recognized despite its known relationship with blood pressure (Klatsky *et al.* 1977; Saunders 1987). The risks of acute intoxication appear to have a direct effect on risk of stroke, but long-term intake may also have an effect independent of blood pressure (Gill *et al.* 1986; Camargo 1989; Gorelick 1989). The pattern is complex. 'Moderate' consumption appears to be protective for ischaemic stroke (Stampfer *et al.* 1988*b*; Gill *et al.* 1991; Palomaki and Kaste 1993), whereas increasing alcohol consumption may be associated with increasing risk of haemorrhagic stroke. Some authors have suggested that the pattern of the association between alcohol consumption and stroke risk is not consistent with a causal relationship (Hansagi *et al.* 1995; Wannamethee and Shaper 1996).

Curiously, and in marked contrast to coronary artery disease epidemiology, blood cholesterol concentration does not seem to be a risk factor for stroke (Prospective Studies Collaboration 1995). The lack of association overall may conceal an increased risk of ischaemic stroke with a decreasing risk of

Table 3.1 Stroke risk factors

Factor	Relative risk	References
Inherent traits		
Age, per decade	2.2	Bamford et al. (1988), Bonita (1993), Brown et al. (1996)
Race	Up to 2	Marmot et al. (1984), Balarajan (1991), Caplan (1991b), Yatsu (1991), Broderick et al. (1992)
Genetic		
Homocysteinaemia (top versus bottom quarter)	5–7	Boers et al. (1985), Clarke et al. (1991), Verhoef et al. (1994), Berwanger et al. (1995), Boushey et al. (1995), Perry et al. (1995)
Family history	1.4–2	Khaw and Barrett-Connor (1986), Welin et al. (1987), Thompson et al. (1989), Kiely et al. (1993), Graffagnino et al. (1994), Wannamethee et al. (1996)
Stroke in monozygotic twin	1–5	de Faire et al. (1975), Brass et al. (1992)
Physiological characteristics		
Blood pressure per 10 mmHg diastolic	2.3	MacMahon et al. (1990), Prospective Studies Collaboration (1995)
Forced expiratory volume	2	Welin et al. (1987), Strachan (1991), Wannamethee et al. (1995a)
Blood cholesterol	–	Iso et al. (1989), Lindenstrom et al. (1994), Prospective Studies Collaboration (1995)
Lp(a)	–	Woo et al. (1991), Shintani et al. (1993)
Fibrinogen (top versus bottom quarter)	2.5	Wilhelmsen et al. (1984), Kannel et al. (1987), Welin et al. (1987), Qizilbash et al. (1991)
Haematocrit	–	Gagnon et al. (1994)
Endogenous tPA (top 5% versus rest)	3.5	Ridker et al. (1994)
Obesity	1–2	Larsson et al. (1984), Folsom et al. (1990), Abbott et al. (1994a), DiPietro et al. (1994)
Diabetes mellitus	2–3	Abbott et al. (1987), Manson et al. (1991), Burchfiel et al. (1994), Tuomilehto et al. (1996a)
Snoring	2	Koskenvuo et al. (1987), Palomaki et al. (1989), Palomaki (1991)
Behaviours		
Alcohol consumption (30+ units/week)	2.5–4	Gill et al. (1986, 1991), Shaper et al. (1991), Kiyohara et al. (1995), Lee et al. (1995)
Smoking	2	Bonita and Beaglehole (1986), Iso et al. (1989), Shinton and Beevers (1989), Thompson et al. (1989), Robbins et al. (1994)
Dietary vitamin C (top versus bottom third)	2	Acheson and Williams (1983), Gale et al. (1995), Gillman et al. (1995)
Dietary potassium (bottom third versus rest)	2–5	Khaw and Barrett-Connor (1987)

Factor	Relative risk	References
Exercise	0.3–0.5	Paffenbarger et al. (1970), Lapidus and Bengtsson (1986), Wannamethee and Shaper (1992), Lindenstrom et al. (1993), Shinton and Sagar (1993), Abbott et al. (1994b), Gillum et al. (1996a)
Life events	2	House et al. (1990a)
HRT	0.5–2	Wilson et al. (1985), Paganini-Hill et al. (1988), Stampfer et al. (1991), Falkeborn et al. (1993), Lindenstrom et al. (1993), Hulley et al. (1998)
Combined oral contraceptive	2.5–3	Hannaford et al. (1994), WHO Collaborative Study (1996a,b)
Environmental factors		
Temperature	–	Pan et al. (1995)
Air pollution	–	Knox (1981), Zhang et al. (1988)
Social characteristics		
Social class	1.6–3.5	Acheson and Sanderson (1978), Marmot and McDowall (1986), Hannaford et al. (1994), Howard et al. (1995)
Other factors		
Birth weight (per 454 g increase)	0.9	Martyn et al. (1996), Rich-Edwards et al. (1997)
Heart failure	2.5–4.4	Kannel et al. (1983), Wolf et al. (1991b)
Ischaemic heart disease	2.5	Herman et al. (1982b), Shaper et al. (1991), Wolf et al. (1991b)
Atrial fibrillation	5	Wolf et al. (1987, 1991a), van Merwijk et al. (1990)
Carotid bruit	2–3	Wolf et al. (1981), Van Ruiswyk et al. (1990), Wiebers et al. (1990)
Aortic arch atheroma	5	Amarenco et al. (1994), Mitusch et al. (1997)
TIA	7	Dennis et al. (1990)
Previous stroke	9–15	Burn et al. (1994)
Peripheral vascular disease	2	Ogren et al. (1995)
Acute infections	5	Grau et al. (1995)
Warfarin treatment	7–10	Hart et al. (1995)
Migraine	1.3–1.8	Tzourio et al. (1993), Buring et al. (1995), Merikangas et al. (1997)
Postpartum	8.7	Kittner et al. (1996)

No estimate is given when the publication did not calculate a relative risk.

HRT, hormone replacement therapy; Lp(a), lipoprotein (a); TIA, transient ischaemic attack; tPA, tissue plasminogen activator.

haemorrhagic stroke with increasing cholesterol concentration (Iso *et al.* 1989). An increase in risk may be confined to the extremes of the cholesterol distribution (Yano *et al.* 1989; Neaton *et al.* 1992; Lindenstrom *et al.* 1994). Care is required in interpreting risk associated with low cholesterol, however, as this group is characterized by a wide range of co-morbid health conditions (Iribarren *et al.* 1995).

Oral contraceptive use is associated with risk of cerebral thrombosis (odds ratio 2.5 for current users, 1–1.3 for former users), but not with haemorrhage. Risk increases with dose of progestogen, dose of oestrogen, and is greater in current smokers (odds ratio 5–7). Low-oestrogen pills are associated with negligible risk in non-smoking women with normal blood pressure (Hannaford *et al.* 1994; Heinemann *et al.* 1996; WHO Collaborative Study 1996*a*). Early studies linked oral contraceptive use with subarachnoid haemorrhage, but this was probably due to a link between oral contraceptives and raised blood pressure. If blood pressure is controlled, the association between oral contraceptives and haemorrhagic stroke is weak (odds ratio 1.4; 95 per cent confidence interval (CI), 0.8–2.3), although the risk is increased 10–15-fold in hypertensive women, and threefold in smokers (Stampfer *et al.* 1988*a*; Vessey *et al.* 1989; Thorogood *et al.* 1992; WHO Collaborative Study 1996*b*). All the risks are somewhat higher in women living in developing countries, where the drugs used and quality of follow-up care may be poor.

Hormone replacement therapy (HRT) has been associated with reduced odds of stroke in several observational cohort studies and would appear to be a logical treatment option to prevent stroke in postmenopausal women. However, in a randomized trial of HRT (oestrogen plus progestogen), in women with ischaemic heart disease, no protective effects on either cardio-vascular events or mortality were found (Hulley *et al.* 1998). Women treated with HRT had an excess of strokes over those receiving placebo. These findings suggest that the apparent benefits of HRT found in observational cohort studies are due to a selection bias, resulting in women who are perhaps more 'health conscious', and therefore at intrinsically lower risk of stroke, opting to take HRT. Presumably, statistical control for potential confounding factors (such as smoking, blood pressure, and cholesterol) fails to make adequate adjustment for these, and other factors, that tend to lower risk in 'health conscious' women. The findings emphasize the importance of testing the effects of interventions in randomized controlled trials.

Risk factors for stroke subtypes

Most studies have only considered the risk factors for all types of stroke combined, or for clinically classified thrombotic stroke. In general, case-control studies tend to comprise patients with cerebral thrombosis or embolism because of survival bias (those with cerebral haemorrhage are more likely to die), and because in most countries cerebral thrombosis is more common than cerebral haemorrhage, relative risk estimates are weighted towards describing the risk factors of thrombo-embolic events.

Several studies have examined the aetiology of haemorrhagic and occlusive subtypes of stroke. In general, raised blood pressure (Tanaka *et al.* 1982; Lin *et al.* 1984; Stemmermann *et al.* 1984; Brott *et al.* 1986; Calandre *et al.* 1986; Harmsen *et al.* 1990; Juvela *et al.* 1995), smoking (Tanaka *et al.* 1982; Stemmermann *et al.* 1984; Abbott *et al.* 1986; Gill *et al.* 1989; Robbins *et al.* 1994; Lee *et al.* 1995), and alcohol consumption (Tanaka *et al.* 1982; Stemmermann *et al.* 1984; Calandre *et al.* 1986; Gill *et al.* 1991; Kiyohara *et al.* 1995) are associated with both haemorrhagic and occlusive stroke. Diabetes mellitus is not associated with haemorrhagic stroke (Burchfiel *et al.* 1994; Jamrozik *et al.* 1994). Atrial fibrillation is associated with risk of cortical but not lacunar (Lodder *et al.* 1990) or primary haemorrhagic stroke (van Merwijk *et al.* 1990). Minor ischaemic stroke, lacunar stroke, and transient ischaemic attack (TIA) share many risk factors in common (Dennis *et al.* 1989*a*; Lodder *et al.* 1990).

Other risk factors

Diet

A number of nutrients have been suggested to be important, including flavonoids, carotene (Keli *et al.* 1996), magnesium, calcium, protein (Abbott *et al.* 1996; Appel *et al.* 1997; McCarron 1998), fish (Keli *et al.* 1994; Morris *et al.* 1995; Gillum *et al.* 1996*b*; Orencia *et al.* 1996), and folic acid. An association has been found between a high dietary intake of potassium (derived from 24-hour dietary recall reports) and subsequent deaths from stroke in a longitudinal study of people aged 50–79 and followed for 12 years (Khaw and Barrett-Connor 1987). In this study a 10 mmol daily increase in dietary potassium was associated with a 40 per cent reduction in risk of stroke death. This association held up when adjustment was made for hypertension (in itself associated with a low potassium intake), age, sex, obesity, smoking, and blood glucose.

Consumption of foods containing vitamin C, which are also usually potassium-rich, is associated with a lower risk of stroke (Acheson and Williams 1983). A correlation exists between regional stroke mortality rates in the UK and regional consumption of vitamin C-containing green vegetables and fruit (data obtained from the National Food Survey). There are plausible pathogenic mechanisms (capillary fragility, reduced platelet adhesiveness) that might explain an effect on haemorrhagic stroke, and the effect of potassium on hypertension might explain a lowered thrombotic tendency. The correlations observed were high but, as the authors acknowledged, this sort of information is a weak method of detecting and testing causal relationships.

This association between vitamin C in the diet and stroke might be an example of an ecological fallacy. Whenever a disease varies in time or between places it is obvious to look for factors that also vary between times or places. Such factors may have nothing to do with the risk of disease and to assume that they do is to make an false presumption—an ecological fallacy. In this case the difference in stroke mortality follows a north–south pattern in the UK, with the highest rates in the north. Unfortunately many other factors also follow this same north–south distribution, and to find an association between one such factor (consumption of fresh green vegetables and fruit) and stroke does not imply causation. Similar correlations might be found between low stroke mortality and a high rate of car ownership, or some other indicator of socio-economic advantage. It is necessary to confirm the relationship among individuals as well as populations before the association can be suspected of being causal.

Our own attempts to test this hypothesis among patients using a case-control method, and measuring vitamin C levels by dietary recall and white cell vitamin C assay, did not show an association between vitamin C and risk of stroke (Barer *et al.* 1989). In part, this may have been because of difficulty in measuring usual vitamin C levels and intake after a stroke has occurred. Observations using a longitudinal design are a much more powerful method of testing the hypothesis.

Prospective studies have subsequently confirmed the association, although the evidence still falls short of establishing causality. In the Framingham study, an increase in intake of three servings of fruit or vegetables per day was associated with a relative risk of 0.78, independent of blood pressure and other risk factors (Gillman *et al.* 1995). A 20-year follow-up of a cohort who took part in a nutritional survey found that both vitamin C intake (determined by a 7-day diet record) and plasma ascorbate levels were associated with risk of death from stroke. The third of participants with the highest vitamin C levels had a risk of stroke death of 0.5 (95 per cent CI, 0.3–0.8) compared with the lowest third, after taking account of other cardiovascular risk factors, social class, and other dietary variables (Gale *et al.* 1995). A meta-analysis of observational studies suggests that vitamins C and E and β-carotene are each associated with reduced cardiovascular events, but randomized trials have not confirmed a benefit of increased intake (see Chapter 8). These trials have not so far been designed to detect a decrease in stroke incidence (they were largely cancer prevention trials), so the question remains open, and a number of large trials are in progress (Jha *et al.* 1995).

Febrile illness

Febrile illness (respiratory infection in 80 per cent of cases) in the month prior to onset was associated with a ninefold increased risk of ischaemic stroke among patients under 50 years old in a case-control study (Syrjanen *et al.*

1988). A case-control study of patients of all ages reported a history of infection in the previous week to have an odds ratio of 4.5 for stroke, increasing to 7.0 for patients reporting fever, and independent of other risk factors (Grau *et al.* 1995). A prospective study found that men in the top quarter of the distribution of the inflammatory marker, C-reactive protein (CRP), were at double the risk of stroke as men in the bottom quarter. The effect was independent of smoking and other thrombotic markers (including fibrinogen and homocysteine) (Ridker *et al.* 1997).

The mechanism for this association is not clear, but was not due to bacterial endocarditis and septic emboli. It is possible to speculate on several immune or blood coagulability hypotheses. One possibility is that patients were predisposed to thrombosis through hyperhomocystinaemia and the infection was sufficient stimulus for a thrombosis to occur. Another possibility is that the association is mediated via plasma fibrinogen, which is associated with risk of stroke (Wilhelmsen *et al.* 1984; Qizilbash *et al.* 1991) and which varies by season (Stout and Crawford 1991). Khaw and colleagues (Woodhouse *et al.* 1994; Khaw and Woodhouse 1995) measured vitamin C, fibrinogen, factor VIIc, and acute-phase proteins, and correlated them with respiratory symptoms amongst 97 elderly people seen every 2 months for a year. Dietary vitamin C and plasma ascorbate levels were low in winter, and were strongly inversely associated with the haemostatic factors and acute-phase proteins. They proposed a mechanism whereby low levels of vitamin C altered the biological response to infection, increasing fibrinogen (itself an acute-phase protein, associated with the inflammatory response), and thereby increasing the incidence of stroke. This mechanism could explain some of the excess winter mortality from vascular diseases seen in the UK, social class differences in stroke incidence, and the relationship between lung function and risk of stroke (as people with damaged lungs are more prone to infection) (Strachan 1991; Wannamethee *et al.* 1995*a*). An alternative explanation akin to the ecological fallacy (a 'temporal fallacy') must also be considered. Anything that changes with the seasons might be implicated in stroke aetiology (Bulpitt 1995), but the data are still intriguing.

Cold stress

Seasonal variation in risk of dying from stroke has been reported (Sakamoto-Momiyama 1978; Haberman *et al.* 1981; Jakovljevic *et al.* 1996) which may be due to an effect on survival after suffering a stroke or a direct effect on incidence. In Australia, stroke incidence has been shown to closely parallel ambient temperature (Christie 1981), and in Nottingham a significant negative correlation between air temperature and numbers of patients admitted to hospital with an acute stroke 2 days later was found (Barer *et al.* 1984). No seasonal variation in incidence was observed in Oxford or Framingham (Wroe *et al.* 1992; Kelly-Hayes *et al.* 1995). Paradoxically, admissions to hospital in Carlisle, UK, peaked in the summer months (Chin *et al.* 1980), although the differences reported could be explained by chance variation, or differences in the age structure of the population at risk during the summer, or a tendency for older people having strokes to be admitted to hospital because relatives are away on holiday during the summer. Seasonal variation in infection, fibrinogen, or dietary intake might also be responsible (Khaw and Woodhouse 1995).

Cold causes both a rise in blood pressure (Brennan *et al.* 1982) and an increase in blood viscosity (Keatinge *et al.* 1984), which together might explain the increased risk of stroke associated with cold weather. Body temperature in the hours after stroke is related to outcome. A quarter of stroke patients have a raised temperature, although only half of these have evidence of infection, and they do worse than patients with low body temperature (Reith *et al.* 1996). Temperature may merely be a marker for tissue damage, but a neuroprotective effect of cooling is plausible, if untested. An antipyretic effect might explain some of the benefit from early aspirin administration (International Stroke Trial Collaborative Group 1997). Unfortunately, the simple measure of central heating for old people at greatest risk does not produce any change in their seasonal mortality pattern (Keatinge 1986), nor their risk of stroke (Shinton 1992).

Risk in particular circumstances

Transient ischaemic attack

Considerable effort is put into identifying and investigating patients with transient ischaemic attacks (TIAs). These are arbitrarily defined as episodes of focal neurological disturbance of vascular origin lasting less than 24 hours, although the vast majority last less than an hour. Moreover, prognosis is no different from that of longer-lasting transient episodes, or 'completed' strokes with minor persisting impairments (Dennis *et al.* 1989*a*).

In the Oxfordshire community stroke project, 184 people presented to medical attention with a TIA (Dennis *et al.* 1989*b*). Following registration, the risk of stroke was 4.4 per cent in the first month (relative risk 80), 8.8 per cent in the first 6 months, and 11.6 per cent over the first year (relative risk 13). Risk of stroke was 5.9 per cent/year over 5 years (relative risk 7), risk of death was 6.3 per cent/year, and the combined risk of heart attack, stroke, or death was 8.4 per cent/year. Only 60 per cent of the strokes were in the same vascular territory as the TIA (Dennis *et al.* 1990).

The reported prognosis of TIA varies greatly according to how the patients are selected. In a hospital-referred series, the stroke risk was 6.6 per cent in the first year, and 3.4 per cent/year over 5 years (Hankey *et al.* 1991, 1993*a*). Age, sex, number of TIAs in the preceding 3 months, peripheral vascular disease, left ventricular hypertrophy, residual neurological signs, experience of both

Table 3.2 Risk of stroke in patients with atrial fibrillation

Age	Number of risk factors	Annual stroke risk (%)
<65 years	None	1.0
	One or more	4.9
65–75 years	None	4.3
	One or more	5.7
>75 years	None	3.5
	One or more	8.1

carotid and vertebrobasilar TIAs, and amaurosis fugax were all important independent risk factors for subsequent stroke. On the basis of these, prognostic models have been created (Hankey et al. 1992; Dutch TIA Trial Study Group 1993). Unfortunately, the validity of these models was found to be only modest when they were tested against actual outcome in an independent patient series, and insufficiently good to permit their sole use in selecting patients for interventions such as carotid endarterectomy (Hankey et al. 1993b). One of the problems is that most strokes occur in patients with few adverse prognostic features (Dippel and Koudstaal 1997). Severity of stenosis is a strong prognostic factor (Hankey et al. 1992; Streifler et al. 1995; European Carotid Surgery Triallists 1998). Risk with asymptomatic stenosis is low (about 1–3 per cent/year) (Norris et al. 1991; European Carotid Surgery Triallists 1995; Ogren et al. 1995). Ulceration of the stenotic plaque increases risk further amongst patients with severe stenoses, but it is unclear whether ulceration of a less severe stenosis is of importance (Eliasziw et al. 1994). TIA (or asymptomatic carotid stenosis) is as strong a risk factor for subsequent heart attack as is a history of angina, emphasizing that management of cardiac risk is as important as management of cerebrovascular risk in these patients.

Atrial fibrillation

Age, history of hypertension, and previous stroke or TIA all contribute to risk of stroke for patients with atrial fibrillation. Table 3.2 shows the annual stroke risk for patients with and without any of these factors (Atrial Fibrillation Investigators 1994).

The Stroke Prevention in Atrial Fibrillation (SPAF) study identified recent heart failure, hypertension and previous thrombo-embolism as risks, with risk estimates of 2.5 per cent/year if none of the factors was present, 7.2 per cent/year for one factor, 17.6 per cent/year for two or three factors (Stroke Prevention in Atrial Fibrillation Investigators 1993a). In addition to these clinical features, echocardiographic global left ventricular dysfunction and left atrial size greater than 4.7 cm were independent risk factors, with annual risks for none, 1 or 2, and three or more factors of 1.0 per cent, 6 per cent, and 18.6 per cent (Stroke Prevention in Atrial Fibrillation Investigators 1993*b*).

Older people

Many of the studies quoted did not study the people most at risk of stroke—those over 75 years. The importance of some risk factors seems to decline with age, in particular hypertension (Evans *et al.* 1980; Evans 1987; Mattilla *et al.* 1988). In a pooling of a large number of cohort studies, the relative risk of stroke for people with a diastolic blood pressure of 102 mmHg compared with 75 mmHg was 10 for those aged less than 45, 5 for people aged 45–64, and only 2 for those aged over 65 years (Prospective Studies Collaboration 1995). Evans' study of the population of Newcastle is surprising because although only 16 per cent of the population were over 80 years no relationship between blood pressure and risk of stroke was found. Despite the weakening of the association between hypertension and stroke among elderly people, the trials of antihypertensives in older people showed a positive benefit of treating old people (Mulrow *et al.* 1995). The benefits (if any) of treatment in very old age (over 80 years) remain unclear.

In the Framingham study the relative risks associated with hypertension, ischaemic heart disease, heart failure, and atrial fibrillation all decreased progressively from age 50 to age 90. The relative risks associated with smoking and diabetes also decrease with age (Boysen *et al.* 1988; Shinton and Beevers 1989). The risk difference (attributable risk) for these groups was largely maintained, or, in the case of atrial fibrillation, increased, with age, underlining their continuing importance as public health targets in older people (Wolf *et al.* 1991*a*). The relationships between other risk factors and stroke in the high seventies and eighties remain unanswered.

Estimating individual risk

In Chapter 2, we saw that an individual's risk of stroke is best estimated by considering the experience of large populations of similar people. People are generally interested in their own risk of stroke rather than the 'average' risk for all other people. In particular they may want to know how much they stand to benefit from an intervention to reduce their risk. Can we use information about risk factors to tailor advice to individuals?

The risk of stroke more than doubles with each decade increase in age. But is this simply all due to ageing? Blood pressure, obesity, physical inactivity, heart disease, and glucose intolerance all increase with age. Moreover, there is a tendency for stroke risk factors to cluster together. Smokers are less active, drink more, and have higher blood pressure. We can try to separate out the 'independent' effects of many different factors using mathematical models, but the process is beset with uncertainties. Individual studies are rarely large enough to estimate relative risk with sufficient precision. Many studies have recorded fatal strokes only, rather than all strokes. The importance of factors which are difficult to quantify exactly (such as cigarette smoking) or which vary from day to day (such as blood pressure) tends to be underestimated compared with more easily defined factors such as age, sex, or the presence of atrial fibrillation. Rare problems (such as mitral stenosis) are unlikely to figure in any mathematical model as they have too few strokes associated with them, although they may dominate the risk of an individual suffering with them. Finally, most people are as interested in avoiding a heart attack as a stroke and scores which use all bad cardiovascular disease events that might happen are likely to be better accepted, understood, and used than those that focus on either heart disease or stroke.

Simple scores can be useful, however, in training and increasing awareness of stroke, which is frequently overlooked in preventive health programmes. To target prevention activity, a score comprising age, blood pressure, smoking, and anginal symptoms can be computed which identifies the highest-risk fifth of the population who will go on to experience 80 per cent of the strokes over the next 5 years (Coppola *et al.* 1995). Data from the Framingham study have been published combining the risks associated with age, systolic blood pressure (treated or untreated), cigarette smoking, diabetes, atrial fibrillation, other cardiovascular disease (history of myocardial infarction, angina, heart failure, or intermittent claudication), and ECG-defined left ventricular hypertrophy, to give an estimated 10-year probability of stroke and other cardiovascular diseases (see Appendix 3.A). Models such as these can be easily entered onto a computer spreadsheet program, and used during consultations for information, education, and to promote compliance with advice (Wolf *et al.* 1991*b*; D'Agostino *et al.* 1994; Vallance and Martin 1997). This approach offers considerably more sophistication than is currently used by the majority of physicians. However, caution is required since scores estimating individual risk never work as well in other populations from the one in which the data were originally derived. Further validation of such individual risk prediction equations is required before they can be used with confidence in clinical management.

Summary

1. The decline in stroke mortality is due to a decline in incidence and case fatality, and the factors responsible may include a downward shift in the population distribution of blood pressure, and changes in other factors that may influence the frequency of stroke, such as atmospheric pollution and diet. Treatment of high blood pressure may explain only about 10 per cent of the decline.

2. Family and twin studies, and the 'Barker hypothesis', suggest that early influences in life (intrauterine or within the family environment) may have an impact on subsequent risk of stroke. Such influences may be mediated through blood pressure, although an independent family effect is probable and subsequent exposures in adult life may be equally important in determining risk.

3. Age, blood pressure, smoking, physical inactivity, acute alcohol intoxication, and pre-existing cardiovascular disease all increase the relative risk of stroke by several fold. With increasing age, relative risks of these factors tend to decline but their attributable risk remains high because of the strong association between stroke incidence and age.

4. The importance of risk factors is best assessed by considering not only the size of the relative risk, but also the proportion of the population exposed to the risk factor, using the population attributable risk fraction. Risk factors with high population attributable risk fractions are primary targets for trials of prevention and treatment.

5. A more precise estimate of an individual's risk can be made by combining the effects of several risk factors. Risk factor scores may have a place in improving the detection and management of people at high risk of suffering a stroke.

6. Patients with transient ischaemic attack and atrial fibrillation are often offered risky preventative therapies, which could be avoided if low-risk groups could be defined reliably. This can be done for atrial fibrillation but not TIA.

Appendix 3.A Framingham risk scores for stroke among men and women

Risk score for men aged 55–85 years

Risk score	0	+1	+2	+3	+4	+5	+6	+7	+8	+9	+10
						Points					
Age (years)	54–56	57–59	60–62	63–65	66–68	69–72	73–75	76–78	79–81	82–84	85
Untreated SBP (mmHg)	97–105	106–115	116–125	126–135	136–145	146–155	156–165	166–175	176–185	186–195	196–205
Treated SBP (mmHg)	97–105	106–112	113–117	118–123	124–129	130–135	136–142	143–150	151–161	162–176	177–205
Diabetes	No		Yes								
Cigarettes	No			Yes							
CVD	No				Yes						
AF	No				Yes						
LVH	No					Yes					

SBP, systolic blood pressure; CVD, cardiovascular disease (history of myocardial infarction, angina, intermittent claudication, heart failure); AF, atrial fibrillation; LVH, left ventricular hypertrophy on ECG.

Risk score for women aged 55–85 years

Risk score		Points										
	0	+1	+2	+3	+4	+5	+6	+7	+8	+9	+10
Age (years)	54–56	57–59	60–62	63–64	65–67	68–70	71–73	74–76	77–78	79–81	82–84
Untreated SBP (mmHg)		95–106	107–118	119–130	131–143	144–155	156–167	168–180	181–192	193–204	205–216
Treated SBP (mmHg)		95–106	107–113	114–119	120–125	126–131	132–139	140–148	149–160	161–204	205–216
Diabetes	No			Yes							
Cigarettes	No			Yes							
CVD	No		Yes								
AF	No						Yes				
LVH	No				Yes						

SBP, systolic blood pressure; CVD, cardiovascular disease (history of myocardial infarction; angina, intermittent claudication, heart failure); AF, atrial fibrillation; LVH, left ventricular hypertrophy on ECG.

Conversion of points derived from risk factor profiles to probability of stroke over 10 years

Points	10-year probability, men (%)	10-year probability, women (%)	Points	10-year probability, men (%)	10-year probability, women (%)	Points	10-year probability, men (%)	10-year probability, women (%)
1	3	1	11	11	8	21	42	43
2	3	1	12	13	9	22	47	50
3	4	2	13	15	11	23	52	57
4	4	2	14	14	13	24	57	64
5	5	2	15	20	16	25	63	71
6	5	3	16	22	19	26	68	78
7	6	4	17	26	23	27	74	84
8	7	4	18	29	27	28	79	
9	8	5	19	33	32	29	84	
10	10	6	20	37	37	30	88	

PART 2 DIAGNOSIS

- Diagnosis

- Clinical disagreement

- Investigation

- Severity

4 Diagnosis

Diagnoses provide medical explanations for health problems and define specific curative, palliative, and preventative treatments and enable prognoses to be given. Diagnosis gives both the patient and the doctor a certain security associated with this knowledge, and a means of communicating the nature of the problem succinctly.

The use of 'stroke' as a diagnostic term is not straightforward. Strokes are caused by thrombosis, embolus, or haemorrhage. Not all patients who present with signs and symptoms of hemiplegia have had a stroke, however. The nomenclature used to describe patients can lead to problems, in particular, calling strokes 'cerebrovascular accidents' or CVAs. The implication is that, given hemiplegia, a stroke has occurred and no other pathological processes need to be ruled out. The terms 'right' or 'left' CVA can also cause confusion because they may refer to the side of the lesion or the side of the signs.

Strokes must be separated from other diseases that mimic stroke because the treatment and prognosis are often different. Within the category of stroke, it is important to distinguish haemorrhage from thrombosis and emboli because antiplatelet agents are routinely used in the latter, but may be hazardous for the former group. Furthermore, exclusion of haemorrhage is even more important where thrombolytic therapy is being contemplated. In so far as different types of infarct or haemorrhage have different implications for therapy or prognosis, it may be worthwhile making efforts at further subdivision. For example, it may be beneficial to identify cardio-embolic stroke, as it is usual to consider anticoagulation in these cases, although the evidence supporting such treatment is limited.

For research purposes it is desirable to deal with homogeneous pathological entities so that potentially useful information about variation in natural history or treatment effects in patients who have suffered haemorrhagic or lacunar stroke is not lost in the majority with thromboses.

Accuracy of diagnosis

A stroke is a focal or global neurological impairment of sudden onset, and lasting more than 24 hours (or leading to death) and of presumed vascular aetiology (World Health Organization 1978). This definition has served well for most clinical and research purposes, although of course it will not distinguish cerebral infarcts from haemorrhages. The definition also includes subarachnoid haemorrhage, which for most purposes behaves, and is managed, as a separate entity (van Gijn 1992; Kopitnik and Samson 1993). Furthermore, 'cerebrovascular disease' may present without a hemiplegia or other recognized neurological signs. In older people epileptic seizures presenting for the first time are most often a manifestation of 'silent' cerebral infarction. Another important presentation is vascular dementia which, for all practical purposes, is clinically indistinguishable from other types of dementia. These presentations differ from hemiplegic stroke in the number, location, and severity of the thrombo-embolic events.

The commonness of stroke may encourage diagnostic laziness, but it is important to remember that the stroke syndrome may have many causes. Some of these causes may lead to an increased predisposition to thrombosis, embolism, or haemorrhage; others may produce a hemiplegic stroke syndrome, but not through a vascular pathogenic mechanism. The doctor's first task when seeing a patient with a focal or global neurological impairment is to decide whether or not the symptoms and signs are caused by a vascular lesion. It is wrong to assume that if a patient has a typical history and signs of hemiplegia then the probability of the diagnosis being vascular stroke is certain.

The accuracy of clinical diagnosis is measured by comparison with some 'gold standard' and calculation of the sensitivity (i.e. ability to detect disease when it is present) and specificity (i.e. ability to rule out disease when it is absent) are necessary (Table 4.1). Autopsy evidence is often taken to be the best indicator of the presence or absence of a pathological lesion, and comparisons with clinical diagnosis have been made by Heasman and Lipworth (1966). These authors attempted to examine the accuracy of diagnosis in as unselected a series of cases as possible, and the autopsy rates were substantially higher than usual during the period of their study. A total of 9501 autopsy diagnoses were compared with the final clinical diagnoses, from which it is possible to calculate the sensitivity and specificity (that is, the accuracy or 'validity') of a clinical diagnosis of stroke (Table 4.2).

These estimates of accuracy may be inflated because they are only relevant to those patients who died and therefore had severe and probably more obvious symptoms and signs. It is possible that clinical diagnosis is less accurate when the symptoms and signs are less severe.

Sensitivity and specificity are not indicators of accuracy of diagnosis that appeal to clinicians' intuition. Clinicians do not know what the autopsy result is or will be, but only their own diagnosis. In other words, their experience of accuracy is derived from the rows of tables such as 4.2 and not from the columns (i.e. sensitivity and specificity). Clinicians are rightly interested in the extent to which they will be correct if they say the patient has a stroke (i.e. positive predictive value), and the opposite of this, how often they will be wrong when they think a patient does not have a stroke (i.e. negative

Table 4.1 Calculation of sensitivity and specificity of a test by comparison with a gold standard

Diagnostic test	Gold standard	
	Disease present	Disease absent
Positive	a, true positive	b, false positive
Negative	c, false negative	d, true negative
Sensitivity $a/(a + c)$		
Specificity $d/(b + d)$		

Table 4.2 The accuracy of final clinical diagnosis of stroke from 'not stroke' using autopsy findings as the diagnostic standard (from Heasman and Lipworth 1966)

Final clinical diagnosis	Autopsy diagnosis		
	Stroke	Not stroke	Total
Stroke	820	276	1096
Not stroke	92	8313	8405
Totals	912	8589	9501

Sensitivity of clinical diagnosis $820/912 = 0.90 \times 100 = 90\%$
Specificity of clinical diagnosis $8313/8589 = 0.97 \times 100 = 97\%$

predictive value). Using Heasman and Lipworth's data, the clinician will be correct in the diagnosis of stroke 75 per cent of the time (i.e. 820/1096), and correct in not diagnosing a stroke 99 per cent of the time (i.e. 8313/8405). This fits with intuition: doctors do not often miss a stroke because the signs are so obvious, but there are other causes of these signs which may lead to a false positive diagnosis, hence a less than perfect positive predictive value.

Elderly people are most likely to suffer from misdiagnosis of stroke. This may be because non-specific presentation is more common when they are acutely ill (e.g. confusion, incontinence, immobility) and when there is multiple pathology. These factors make it harder to distinguish, for example, whether an exacerbation of bronchitis has led to increased weakness from an old stroke, or whether a new stroke has occurred. The accuracy of clinical diagnosis might be improved by training, relating the clinical signs detected with neuroradiolgical and autopsy examinations, by increased monitoring of progress of patients, and by better knowledge of the natural history of stroke.

Table 4.3   Accuracy of diagnosis of stroke from other causes of neurological impairment

	Gold standard	Sensitivity (%)	Specificity (%)
Heasman and Lipworth (1966)	Autopsy	80	–
Hatano et al. (1976)	Autopsy	99	69
Weisberg and Nice (1977)	CT scan	72	76
Norris and Hachinski (1982)	CT scan + autopsy	100	22–76
Allen (1983)	CT scan + autopsy	67	91
Sotaniemi et al. (1990)	Final diagnosis + CT	77	89

Differentiating stroke from other diseases

More typically the problem for doctors is to distinguish non-vascular from vascular (i.e. thrombosis, haemorrhage, or embolism) causes of neurological impairment. Several studies have examined this question and are summarized in Table 4.3.

The variability of these estimates of diagnostic accuracy are surprising at first sight. Part of the explanation may be the type of patients studied. Older patients may have a higher risk of non-vascular pathology (e.g. subdural haematoma, cerebral abscess, cerebral metastases, iatrogenic hypoglycaemia, etc.) which will lead to more false-positive diagnoses of stroke, and thus a lower specificity of clinical diagnosis. For example, Allen (1983) excluded any patient over 75 years, which may explain why the specificity found in this study was so high.

Another explanation is the skill of the clinician. Norris and Hachinski (1982) examined the effect of the doctor's experience is some detail. They asked junior emergency-room doctors, neurology residents, and neurology consultants to assess 93 subsequently autopsy-proven stroke patients for four items of information—stroke present or not, ischaemic or haemorrhagic pathogenesis, right- or left-sided lesion, hemisphere or brainstem lesion. From this they derived an 'accuracy' score by adding up correct answers so that the maximum score a doctor could get was 372 (i.e. 93 × 4). They demonstrated that consultants were the most accurate (89 per cent), neurology residents still had something to learn (77 per cent accuracy), and that junior emergency-room doctors had the most to learn (38 per cent accuracy).

Norris and Hachinski (1982) also looked at the question of the specificity of clinical diagnosis, that is how often doctors were correct when they ruled out a diagnosis of a stroke clinically. They examined the diagnoses of the same groups of doctors among a consecutive series of 50 patients admitted to their unit as stroke patients who subsequently turned out not to have had a stroke. The junior emergency-room doctors gave a correct diagnosis of not stroke in 22 per cent, neurology residents in 32 per cent, and consultants in 76 per cent of cases.

Table 4.4 The relationship between frequency of non-vascular pathology causing neurological impairment and predictive value of clinical diagnosis

1. A low frequency of non-vascular pathology: 1% (e.g. primary care or non-specialist setting). Sensitivity 90%; Specificity 90%.

Clinical diagnosis	True diagnosis		
	Stroke	Not stroke	total
Stroke	99	9	108
Not stroke	891	1	892
Total	990	10	1000

Positive predictive value of a clinical diagnosis of stroke: 99/108, i.e. 92%

2. A high frequency of non-vascular pathology: 10% (e.g. specialist or referral setting). Sensitivity 90%; Specificity 90%.

Clinical diagnosis	True diagnosis		
	Stroke	Not stroke	total
Stroke	90	90	180
Not stroke	810	10	820
Total	900	100	1000

Positive predictive value of a clinical diagnosis of CVA: 90/180, i.e. 50%

The frequency of misdiagnosis, or the predictive value of a positive diagnosis (i.e. 1 – misdiagnosis rate) of stroke is often reported (Heasman and Lipworth 1966; Norris and Hachinski 1982; Allen 1983; Sandercock *et al.* 1985a; Libman *et al.* 1995) but is not a very useful figure because it depends on the frequency of other non-stroke diagnoses among the patients studied. Reference to Table 4.4 may help to explain this. Although accuracy of diagnosis remains the same, altering the proportion of strokes to non-strokes will have a major effect on the positive and negative predictive values. For example, Norris and Hachinski found that 108 (13 per cent) out of 821 consecutive patients initially thought to have a stroke turned out to have some other pathology. The Oxford Community Stroke study (Sandercock *et al.* 1985a) only found 5 (1.5 per cent) out of 325 first strokes with unsuspected non-vascular pathology. Since the most common reason for misdiagnosis in Norris and Hachinski's study was generalized seizures occurring in patients who had had a previous stroke, it is not surprising that their estimate of misdiagnosis was so much higher than the Oxford group who only considered first events, excluding those with previous strokes.

The mode of onset of a stroke is thought to be an indicator of non-vascular pathology and Allen (1983) demonstrated that a stuttering or progressively evolving onset of the stroke was more often associated with a 'mass' lesion (i.e. tumour or subdural haematoma). The sensitivity and specificity of a stuttering onset for mass lesions were 56 per cent and 80 per cent, respectively, but this onset was associated with only a 14 per cent predictive value; that is, for every 100 patients suspected of having a mass lesion rather than a stroke because of a stuttering onset, the doctor would be wrong in 86 cases and correct in 14 cases. This level of detection would probably cause a neuroradiologist performing CT brain scans to question the clinical skills of the referring physician. Weisberg and Nice (1977) found very similar results in a comparison of patients suffering a sudden onset with those whose onset was not sudden. Allen (1983) drew attention to the sensitivity of a poor history as an indicator of a mass lesion, but in this case too, the predictive value was low—13 per cent.

It is quite possible that two doctors can be equally accurate (i.e. same sensitivity and specificity) in their clinical diagnosis of stroke but have very different 'misdiagnosis' rates (or predictive values). Table 4.4 shows how this can happen. The low frequency of non-vascular pathology might represent the practice of a primary health care or emergency-room doctor. The high frequency of non-vascular pathology might be seen by a neurologist in a tertiary referral hospital specializing in difficult cases. In both high- and low-frequency situations the accuracy of diagnosis is assumed to be the same: sensitivity 90 per cent, specificity 90 per cent.

This relationship between predictive value and prevalence of the disease of interest makes predictive value an unstable and therefore less useful measure of misdiagnosis or diagnostic accuracy.

Diagnosis of cerebral haemorrhage and infarction

Very high specificity of diagnosis (a very low misdiagnosis rate) is required by some of the emerging therapies for acute stroke treatment. If in the early hours after stroke onset, a computed tomography (CT) scan shows no evidence of haemorrhage or any other abnormality, the decision to administer a potentially dangerous thrombolytic agent will rest entirely on the doctor's ability to exclude non-vascular pathology. A misdiagnosis rate of 10 per cent or more would not be acceptable in these circumstances.

More generally, the need to distinguish haemorrhage from thrombo-embolic mechanisms of stroke has gained in importance with increased use of antiplatelet drugs, anticoagulation (Chapters 9 and 11), and thrombolytic agents. Within the infarction category, a case has been made for separating lacunar strokes from other types of infarction, as they form a distinct clinical group, with a different prognosis and response to treatment (Bamford and Warlow 1988; Bamford et al. 1991). In many countries much effort is put into

Table 4.5 Calculation of the likelihood ratio

Clinical diagnosis	True diagnosis	
	Haemorrhage	Infarction
Haemorrhage	a	b
Infarction	c	d

Likelihood ratio: Proportion with diagnosis and positive clinical diagnosis (i.e. $a/(a + c)$, i.e. sensitivity) to proportion without diagnosis but with a positive clinical diagnosis (i.e. $b/(b + d)$, i.e. 1 – specificity)

i.e.$[a/(a + c)] / [b/(b + d)]$

i.e. sensitivity/(1 – specificity)

identifying potential cardio-embolic sources, with a view to anticoagulation therapy.

The predictive value of such clinical diagnosis (i.e. how often a diagnosis is correct) is determined largely by the frequency of haemorrhage among the patients studied, in the same way that the ability of doctors to pick out non-vascular pathology is more dependent on its frequency than on the clinical accuracy of the doctors (Table 4.4).

The likelihood ratio

A method of summarizing the accuracy of a diagnosis (or of an investigation or test) is to calculate the likelihood ratio, that is the ratio of the proportion of patients who truly have the diagnosis and have a positive clinical diagnosis to the proportion of patients who do not really have the diagnosis but have an erroneous positive clinical diagnosis. This is shown in Table 4.5. The likelihood ratio has some virtues. First it is a single number, but more importantly it can be used to calculate easily the predictive value of diagnostic skill (or of an investigation or test) for different frequencies of the disease of interest. This is because of the simple relationship between the initial probability (or frequency) of the disease of interest (before any attempt at diagnosis has been made), the likelihood ratio, and the final probability of the true diagnosis after clinical diagnosis has been made (which is, of course, the predictive value of clinical diagnosis).

For example, if the true probability of cerebral haemorrhage in a series of stroke patients is 20 per cent (a 'prior' probability—in the sense of before use of any diagnostic test—of 0.20 to use the jargon of Bayes's theorem), the pre-test odds of haemorrhage are $0.20/(1 - 0.20)$ which is 0.25. The relationship between probability and odds is:

$$\text{odds} = \text{probability}/(1 - \text{probability}).$$

Table 4.6 Comparison between clinical and autopsy diagnosis of type of stroke (from Heasman and Lipworth 1966)

Clinical diagnosis	Autopsy diagnosis					
	Haemorrhage	Thrombosis/ embolism	Subarachnoid	Ill-defined	Other causes	Total
Haemorrhage	257	65	40	2	175	539
Thrombosis/embolism	36	159	3	8	145	351
Subarachnoid	34	2	112	–	17	165
Ill-defined	5	8	–	9	19	41
Other causes	45	76	16	9	–	146
Totals	377	310	171	28	356	1242

Multiplying the pre-test odds by the likelihood ratio gives the 'posterior' odds (in the sense of after attempts at diagnosis) of haemorrhage being truly present. The probability of haemorrhage is then calculated from the relationship:

$$\text{probability} = \text{odds}/(1 + \text{odds}).$$

A full discussion of the calculation of odds, likelihood ratios, and probabilities is given by Sackett *et al.* (1985).

There is doubt about the ability of clinicians to diagnose the type of pathology causing a stroke. An early study (Aring and Merritt 1935) relating autopsy findings with clinical symptoms and signs found that headache at onset, vomiting, neck stiffness, fits, depressed consciousness, high blood pressure at presentation, signs of tentorial herniation and blood in the cerebrospinal fluid (CSF) were all much more common in patients who had suffered a cerebral haemorrhage than an infarct.

Heasman and Lipworth's study (1966) looked at this problem in detail. Their comparison between clinical and autopsy diagnoses as shown in Table 4.6. They reported their results in terms of predictive values, such as only 257 (48 per cent) out of 539 clinical diagnoses of cerebral haemorrhage were confirmed at autopsy. It is possible to calculate the sensitivity and specificity of clinical diagnosis as a means of discriminating between haemorrhage and infarction from their data. The sensitivity is 257/377 (i.e. 68 per cent) and the specificity is 583/865 (i.e. 67 per cent). (The closeness of the two figures is simply a fluke and has no significance.)

The likelihood ratio (sensitivity/(1 − specificity)) derived from Heasman and Lipworth's data is $0.67/(1 − 0.67) = 2.03$. The pre-test probability (or prevalence) of haemorrhage in their series was $377/1242 = 0.30$, which is equivalent to pre-test odds of 0.436. Multiplying the pre-test odds by the likelihood ratio gives the post-test odds, which are: $0.436 \times 2.03 = 0.88$.

Table 4.7 Accuracy of clinical information and tests to diagnose haemorrhage from infarction as the cause of a stroke

Source	Diagnosis of haemorrhage		
	Sensitivity (%)	Specificity (%)	Likelihood ratio
Allen (1983)			
Overall clinical	48	91	5.3
Guy's score method (14+)	52	98	26.0
Bloodstained CSF	50	98	25.0
Von Arbin et al. (1981)			
Overall	33	93	4.7
Impaired consciousness	72	80	3.6
Neck stiffness	28	97	9.3
Britton et al. (1983)			
CSF protein >1g/litre	89	92	11.1
Xanthochromic CSF	70	95	14.0
Harrison (1980)			
Headache	56	57	1.3
Vomiting	45	93	6.4
Fits at onset	6	91	0.7
Neck stiffness	48	89	4.4
Bloodstained CSF	90	100	infinity
Lee et al. (1975)			
Bloody/xanthochromic CSF	75	96	18.8

The post-test odds can then be converted back to a proportion (or percentage), which gives 0.88/(1 + 0.88) = 0.47 or 47 per cent.

In other words, the diagnostic ability of doctors studied in this series was sufficient to increase the probability of a haemorrhage from 30 to 47 per cent. This is (and should be) almost the same as the predictive value of a diagnosis of haemorrhage shown in Table 4.4, 257/539 = 47.7 per cent (the difference is due to rounding errors in the calculations).

All this effort may seem unnecessary when the predictive value could have been easily calculated in the first place. Likelihood ratios really come into their own when different diagnostic tests are compared, when a series of investigations are used, and strategies for use of invasive or risky investigations have to be planned. The higher the likelihood ratio, the more discriminating is the diagnostic method or test, and hence the more useful. Moreover, the work of converting probabilities to odds can be avoided if a nomogram is used (see Sackett et al. 1985).

Likelihood ratios of clinical signs and tests

Other estimates of clinical and test accuracy in diagnosing haemorrhage from infarction have been reported and are summarized in Table 4.7, together with

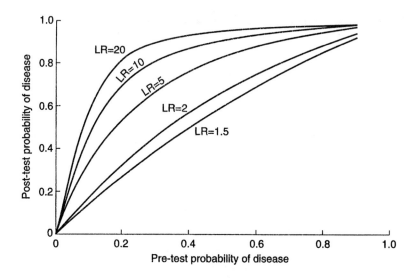

Fig. 4.1 Post-test probabilities of disease following a positive test result for a range of likelihood ratios (LRs) and pre-test disease probabilities.

likelihood ratios. In each of these studies the frequency of cerebral haemorrhage varied from half to less than a fifth affected, which would have led to very different estimates of the predictive value of tests or of clinical symptoms and signs. For example, in the study carried out by von Arbin *et al.*, the predictive value of bedside clinical diagnosis was 6/20 = 30 per cent; whereas Allen (1983) found that his clinical skills in diagnosing haemorrhage gave a predictive value of 14/26 = 53 per cent, which appears much better. It would be tempting to assume that Allen had superior clinical skills but this would be overlooking the fact that this difference in predictive value is due to the fact that haemorrhage was twice as common in the series of cases of Allen (18 per cent) as in that of von Arbin *et al.* (9 per cent), despite both being consecutively selected. However, the likelihood ratios show that there is little to choose between them.

Another feature of these likelihood ratios for cerebral haemorrhage is that a high value is usually obtained because of a high specificity (i.e. a low false-positive rate). A sign or test that is pathognomonic for a disease must be 100 per cent specific, in other words it must never occur when the disease is not present. This will give a predictive value of 100 per cent because there are no false positives, and a likelihood ratio of infinity. So the higher the likelihood ratio the more probably the diagnosis (e.g. of cerebral haemorrhage) can be ruled in. A range of post-test probabilities for different likelihood ratios and pre-test probabilities of disease are shown in Fig. 4.1.

The figure demonstrates how at high pre-test probabilities, even very accurate tests are not able to increase the probability of disease by a great

Table 4.8 The Guy's Hospital score for discriminating haemorrhagic from thrombotic stroke (from Allen 1983)

	Clinical feature	Score
Onset		
Loss of consciousness	One or none	0
Headache within 2 hours	Two or more	+21.9
Vomiting		
Neck stiffness		
Level of consciousness at 24 hours	Alert	0
	Drowsy	+7.3
	Unconscious	+14.6
Plantar responses	Both flexor/single extensor	0
	Both extensor	+7.1
Diastolic blood pressure at 24 hours	BP (mmHg)	+ (BP × 0.17)
History or atheroma markers		
Angina	None	0
Claudication	One or more	−3.7
Diabetes		
History of hypertension	Not present	0
	Present	−4.1
Previous TIA or stroke	None	0
	Previous event(s)	−6.7
Heart disease	None	0
Aortic/mitral murmur		−4.3
Cardiac failure		−4.3
Cardiomyopathy		−4.3
Atrial fibrillation		−4.3
Cardiomegaly (X-ray)		−4.3
Myocardial infarction within 6 months		−4.3
Constant		−12.6

margin. When disease is rare (i.e. at low disease pre-test probabilities) tests with high likelihood ratios are most useful. However, tests with relatively modest likelihood ratios (in the range 4–10) may be extremely helpful in cases where the chances of disease being present are higher (for example, around 50 per cent).

Guy's Hospital score

This score (see Table 4.8) depends on obtaining good-quality information about the onset of the stroke, the state of the patient at 24 hours, and past medical history. For many patients it may be difficult to do this reliably (see Chapter 5). The score is quite simple to use, the presence or absence of symptoms, signs, and history are added up (except for diastolic blood pressure, for which the phase and arm taken in were not reported, which is multiplied by a constant and then added to the score). As can be seen,

Table 4.9 Use of the Guy's Hospital score among the Oxford Community Stroke Project patients and London teaching hospital patients

Score threshold	Oxford patients			London teaching hospitals		
	Haemorrhage			Haemorrhage		
	Present	Absent	LR[a]	Present	Absent	LR[a]
25+	9	5	8.0	43	2	50.9
14 to 24	13	9	6.4	15	4	8.9
4 to 13	12	27	2.0	20	38	1.2
−5 to 3	7	78	0.4	9	89	0.2
Less than −5	1	67	0.07	0	74	0
Totals	42	186		87	206	

[a]LR, likelihood ratio.

persisting impaired consciousness level adds a large component to the score. The extra diagnostic accuracy obtained by use of a scoring method was not considered very impressive (Allen 1983) but its likelihood ratio shows that it is five times better than conventional clinical diagnosis in increasing the probability that a patient truly has a diagnosis of stroke due to cerebral haemorrhage (see Table 4.7).

The extra diagnostic power of the score can be demonstrated by applying the likelihood ratios of conventional diagnosis and the Guy's Hospital score to the same pre-test odds. Assuming that the true frequency of haemorrhage is 0.20 (i.e. 20 per cent), this is equivalent to pre-test odds of 0.25.

Conventional clinical diagnosis (likelihood ratio 5.3):

$$0.25 \times 5.3 = 1.325 \text{ (posterior odds)} = 0.57 \text{ probability}$$

i.e. 57 per cent predictive value.

Guy's Hospital score method (likelihood ratio 26):

$$0.25 \times 26 = 6.5 \text{ (posterior odds)} = 0.87 \text{ probability}$$

i.e. 87 per cent predictive value.

The Guy's Hospital score has been tested in several studies: the Oxford Community Stroke Project, a series of patients from a London teaching hospital (Sandercock et al. 1985b), three Italian hospitals (Celani et al. 1994), and an Acute Stroke Unit in Glasgow (Weir et al. 1994). Sandercock and colleagues concluded that a cut-off of 4 would maximize the accuracy of the score (i.e. achieve the highest sensitivity and specificity). In practice, however, the task is to either rule out or rule in a diagnosis. To use a single cut-off point does not permit all the information to be used. In general, highly abnormal values are more useful than borderline abnormalities in diagnosis. The data presented by Sandercock and colleagues is recast in Table 4.9 to show the diagnostic importance of different thresholds of the score.

It is evident from describing the score in this way that very high and very low scores have much greater diagnostic importance. The suggested threshold of 4 will achieve a predictive value of 45 per cent for cerebral haemorrhage in Oxford, whereas a threshold of 25+ has a predictive value of 64 per cent, and a threshold of less than −5 has a predictive value for cerebral infarction of about 98 per cent.

A clinical example

An example may clarify the use of the score. A man of 73 presented with sudden onset of left hemiplegia which was associated with loss of consciousness for at least 2 hours. He had a frontal headache when seen by a doctor 6 hours later. He was drowsy throughout the first day of hospital admission. He had a left extensor plantar, a diastolic (phase V) blood pressure of 100 mm Hg and was complaining of anginal chest pain when initially seen. He had had a myocardial infarction 10 years earlier but no rhythm disturbance or heart failure. He had had no previous neurological symptoms or past history of hypertension and his chest X-ray was normal. His Guy's Hospital score was:

$$21.9 + 7.3 + 0 + [100 \times 0.17] - 3.7 + 0 + 0 + 0 - 12.6 = 29.9.$$

The prior odds of cerebral haemorrhage might be as low as 0.11 (i.e. 10 per cent probability). The Oxford likelihood ratio for this score is 8.0. This gives a posterior (i.e. after application of the score) probability that this man has had a cerebral haemorrhage of 47 per cent. The same man admitted to a London Teaching Hospital would have a posterior probability of haemorrhage of 85 per cent. The greater posterior probability of haemorrhage using the London Hospital data is probably explained by the higher prevalence of haemorrhage in the London series of patients, yielding higher likelihood ratios at higher scores. Such a high probability of haemorrhage is sufficient to rule out use of anticoagulants or antiplatelet agents, without further investigation with CT scanning to exclude cerebral haemorrhage more certainly.

The Guy's score has been criticized because the information for some of the variables is difficult to collect, and because the scoring is complex enough to make it difficult without a calculator. The validation study of Weir et al. (1994) had 'complete' data on only 32 per cent of their 991 stroke patients, despite the fact that they also deleted four items from the scale.

Another clinical score, the Siriraj score, was developed in Thailand where the prior probability of haemorrhage is much greater, and contains only five items (level of consciousness, history of headache within 2 hours of onset,

Table 4.10 Use of the Siriraj score among the Thai and Glasgow hospital patients

| Score threshold | Thai patients | | | Glasgow patients | | |
| | Haemorrhage | | | Haemorrhage | | |
	Present	Absent	LR	Present	Absent	LR
6+	51	1	23.0	3	4	6.3
2 to 5	69	8	3.9	15	8	15.8
−1 to 1	19	20	0.4	15	99	1.3
Less than −1	3	35	0.04	18	320	0.5
Total	142	64		51	431	

LR, likelihood ratio.

vomiting after onset, diastolic blood pressure, and the presence of three 'atheroma markers': diabetes, angina, and intermittent claudication) (Poungvarin et al. 1991). As with the Guy's score, a weighted sum of these items is calculated. Despite its simplicity, it performs at least as well as the Guy's score. Three validation studies have been carried out (Poungvarin et al. 1991; Celani et al. 1994; Weir et al. 1994). Table 4.10 presents likelihood ratios for various Siriraj score thresholds.

The Glasgow likelihood ratios do not increase with increasing score thresholds as expected, but this is probably due to the small numbers suffering haemorrhages compared with the Thai data. Despite the simplicity of the Siriraj score, data were missing from half the Glasgow patients (Weir et al. 1994). However, it is apparent from both the Glasgow series and an Italian study (Celani et al. 1994) that scores greater than 1 were associated with a high likelihood ratio (between 10 and 14) suggesting reasonable validity for diagnosing cerebral haemorrhage.

An eight-item score, developed in France and much less extensively evaluated, claims an interesting and potentially useful property. In the validation series studied, 36 per cent of patients had a score below a cut-off of + 1, and all these patients had infarcts (Besson et al. 1995). In these patients the positive predictive value for infarct was 100 per cent (95 per cent CI, 93–100 per cent), implying an infinite likelihood ratio. If this were replicated in other series, this would obviate the need to scan these patients, as the diagnosis would be certain.

Such diagnostic scores might be thought unnecessary as most hospitals have CT scanners and access is much easier than in the past. However, many patients continue to be managed at home, without access to neuroradiology. In poorer countries, where stroke is common but resources are scarce, such methods of diagnosis of haemorrhage may be of help in deciding whether to institute immediate treatment with antiplatelet drugs. In the future, if effective drugs are found for acute stroke, pre-hospital treatment may require making an assessment of the probability of haemorrhage prior to starting treatment.

Promising diagnostic tests

A further advantage of likelihood ratios is that promising diagnostic methods are less likely to be overlooked. At present there is (rightly) little enthusiasm for lumbar puncture to diagnose haemorrhagic from thrombotic stroke (Consensus Conference 1988). Yet the estimates of its likelihood ratio range from infinity (Harrison 1980) to 11 (Britton *et al.* 1983). To illustrate how using two diagnostic methods may improve ability to distinguish haemorrhage from thrombosis, the combinations of clinical scoring methods and lumbar puncture could produce predictive values of 97–99 per cent, which would mean that in only 1 case in 100 would a diagnosis of haemorrhage be wrong.

For example, if the pre-test odds of haemorrhagic stroke are 0.25 (i.e. 20 per cent, odds $= 0.2/(1 - 0.2)$), using a Guy's Hospital score (threshold of $14+$), which has a likelihood ratio of 26:

$$0.25 \times 26 = \text{post-test odds} = 6.5.$$

The post-test odds may then be used as the pre-test odds for the application of another test, assuming independence between the tests; in this case, lumbar puncture which has a likelihood ratio of 11:

$$6.5 \times 11 = \text{post-test odds} = 71.5.$$

This is equivalent to a predictive value of:

$$71.5/(1 + 71.5) = 98.6 \text{ per cent.}$$

If the probability of haemorrhagic stroke is lower than 20 per cent, say only 10 per cent, then use of the Guy's Hospital score and lumbar puncture gives a predictive value of 96.9 per cent. This strategy is not to be recommended in clinical practice as lumbar puncture may be hazardous in patients with raised intracerebral pressure associated with very large infarcts or haemorrhages. The strategy is presented to illustrate the potential value of combining two approaches to diagnosis. In practice, such diagnostic strategies should be tested in an unselected series of patients to examine their true predictive value, as it is quite possible that the likelihood ratios of new diagnostic methods will not operate independently, that both methods will fail in a proportion of cases, and that their use may not be associated with such high predictive value as reported in initial studies.

For some clinical decisions of relatively low risk (e.g. giving aspirin), the use of a clinical score may be good enough, but for others of higher risk (e.g. giving thrombolytics), this may not be accurate enough and a CT scan must be considered mandatory. For epidemiological purposes, such as describing trends or differences in occurrence between places, or times, or characteristics of individuals (e.g. smoking, blood pressure, etc.), the level of diagnostic accuracy achieved by clinical scoring is more than adequate.

Clinical stroke syndromes

One neurological textbook famously suggests that stroke should not be diagnosed unless the doctor can name the artery involved (Patten 1977). This is not the case for most practical purposes. However, attempts have been made to identify subgroups of stroke with distinctive characteristics.

Oxford Community Stroke Project (OCSP) classification

This classification applies to cerebral infarction only, and relies on only clinical data, requiring no information from investigations (Bamford *et al.* 1991). Four patterns of neurological impairment were described: total anterior circulation infarcts (TACI), partial anterior circulation infarcts (PACI), lacunar infarcts (LACI), and posterior circulation infarcts (POCI). Presumed underlying pathology was determined from the neurological literature.

Total anterior circulation infarcts
TACIs have a combination of:
(1) new higher cerebral dysfunction (dysphasia, dyscalculia, visuo-spatial disorders);
(2) homonymous hemianopia; and
(3) ipsilateral motor and/or sensory deficits in at least two of the face, arm, and leg.

Impaired consciousness rendering testing impossible is interpreted as a deficit. These symptoms are consistent with occlusion of the proximal middle cerebral artery, in isolation, or associated with internal carotid artery occlusion. Two-thirds of these infarcts are embolic, the rest thrombotic.

Partial anterior circulation infarcts
PACIs comprise two of the three elements of a TACI, higher cerebral dysfunction alone, or a motor/sensory deficit more limited than that defining a TACI (i.e. one limb alone, or hand and face but not whole arm). These are presumed to be due to embolic occlusion of one of the two divisions of the middle cerebral artery, or a smaller branch.

Table 4.11   Accuracy of OCSP classification for predicting the location of cerebral infarction on CT scan

Syndrome (proportion in series)	Sensitivity	Specificity
TACI (31%)	0.97	0.96
PACI (40%)	0.94–0.95	0.82–0.90
LACI (18%)	0.71–0.77	0.92–0.98
POCI (12%)	0.73–0.81	0.95–1.00

Lacunar infarcts

LACIs present with pure motor or sensory stroke, sensori-motor stroke, ataxic-hemiparesis (cerebellar-type ataxia with ipsilateral pyramidal signs), dysarthria–clumsy hand syndrome, or acute focal movement disorders. Motor/sensory signs must involve at least two of the face, arm, and leg. These represent thrombotic occlusion of the deep perforating branches of the middle cerebral artery, supplying the internal capsule or pons.

Posterior circulation infarcts

POCIs present with ipsilateral cranial nerve palsy plus contralateral motor/sensory deficit, bilateral motor/sensory deficit, disorder of conjugate eye movement, isolated cerebellar dysfunction, or isolated homonymous hemianopia. These infarcts are in the vertebrobasilar arterial territory, one-fifth being embolic, the rest thrombotic.

This classification has been shown to have reasonable inter-rater reliability ($\kappa = 0.54$–0.89) (Lindley et al. 1993; Lindgren et al. 1994a). The validity with which it predicts the vascular territory involved, as demonstrated by CT scanning, has been demonstrated in a consecutive series of 108 cerebral infarcts admitted to hospital (Wardlaw et al. 1996). Eighty of 91 patients whose CT scan showed a definite new infarct were classified correctly. Most discrepancies involved probable clinical misclassification, in particular, distinguishing PACI and LACI. Sensitivities and specificities, shown in Table 4.11, were calculated under both the assumptions that the 17 scans without a visible infarct were, or were not, correctly classified. Validity of clinical diagnosis is reasonable, but by no means perfect. Similar findings were reported from two earlier studies (Anderson et al. 1994b; Lindgren et al. 1994a).

The relationship between clinically identified lacunar strokes and finding an associated 'lacune' or small, deep infarct on neuroimaging is variable. The sensitivity of clinical diagnosis in different case series ranges from less than 35 per cent to 77 per cent, with false positive rates between 7 and 14 per cent (Bamford and Warlow, 1988).

Table 4.12   Accuracy of pathological diagnosis using the TOAST classification

Syndrome (proportion in series)	Sensitivity	Specificity
Athero-thrombo-embolic (35%)	0.68	0.81
Cardio-embolic (15%)	0.52	0.94
Small-vessel thrombotic (38%)	0.81	0.81
Other (1%)	0.18	1.0
Undetermined (11%)	0.29	0.92

These accuracy figures are very dependent on the performance of the 'gold standard' neuroimaging technique. The older figures were based on early CT technology. Newer scanners and the advent of magnetic resonance imaging (MRI), with much better resolution (especially for the pons), improve the sensitivity up to about 70 per cent (Boiten and Lodder 1991; Toni *et al.* 1994; Wardlaw *et al.* 1996).

Pathological classifications

A number of classification schemes have been developed which rely on clinical and investigational data to make presumptions about pathology (Bamford 1992). One such example, the TOAST classification, was formulated as part of a trial of an anticoagulant (ORG10172) in acute stroke treatment (hence 'TOAST'). Categories of athero-thrombo-embolic, cardio-embolic, small-vessel thrombotic, other pathology, and undetermined pathology (including multiple potential causes) were defined (Adams *et al.* 1993). The rationale behind pathological classifications is that both management and prognosis depend on knowledge of pathology, and a more precise formulation than is provided by purely clinical systems (such as the TACI, PACI, LACI, POCI scheme) is both desirable and feasible.

Reaching a TOAST diagnosis requires a CT scan, carotid duplex scan, and echocardiography (preferably trans-oesophageal) in all cases, with investigations being instrumental in making the classification in about one-third of cases. In Europe this is rarely achieved (Beech *et al.* 1996).

A validation study compared initial TOAST classification based on clinical and initial CT results with 'final' diagnosis based on extensive investigation, including repeat CT scan (Madden *et al.* 1995). Sixty-two per cent of initial diagnoses were 'correct', although the 'gold standard' diagnosis will have been subject to some error. The sensitivity of the initial diagnosis (compared with the final diagnosis) was modest, and, if the scheme were to be used to guide judgements such as the use of thrombolytic therapy, probably inadequate (Table 4.12). Moreover, some series have reported that up to 40 per cent of strokes have 'undetermined pathology' despite extensive work-up, which undermines the rationale somewhat (Sacco *et al.* 1989). Inter-observer agreement on reaching diagnoses has been shown to be reasonable (Adams *et al.* 1993; Gordon *et al.* 1993).

Cardiac embolism

The estimated proportion of strokes which are cardio-embolic is 15–20 per cent (Cerebral Embolism Task Force 1986, 1989; Bogousslavsky *et al.* 1988). A case-series from the Oxfordshire Community Stroke Project reported that only 20 per cent had a major, and 11 per cent a minor, potential cardio-embolic source (Sandercock *et al.* 1989). There is good evidence that atrial fibrillation (AF) is causally related to stroke, from cohort, case-control, and intervention (anticoagulation) studies (see Chapters 2 and 3). Using arteriography and trans-cranial Doppler studies, direct evidence of embolism was found in only 26 per cent of patients with atrial fibrillation and stroke, although after exhaustive investigation it has been estimated that 62 per cent of the strokes were caused by emboli related to atrial fibrillation and a further 14 per cent were from other, co-morbid, heart problems (Bogousslavsky *et al.* 1990).

A diagnosis of cardiac embolism relies on documenting a likely cardiac source of emboli, and excluding a severe carotid stenosis or other causes of stroke (Adams *et al.* 1993). Some radiological features are also taken to indicate embolism, but these cannot always differentiate cardiac from aortic arch or artery-to-artery embolism. There is no system for determining the primacy of competing potential pathologies. Thus a lot of investigative effort is currently expended in 'working up' stroke patients without any corresponding increase in diagnostic certainty. The 'gold standard' for diagnosing embolism, acute cerebral arteriography, is risky and difficult or inappropriate to apply routinely or in large research series. Therefore, we do not know the true incidence of embolism, our ability to diagnose it accurately, or, in many cases, what to do once it is diagnosed. Technological advances, including magnetic resonance and CT angiography, and real-time imaging with carotid and trans-cranial Doppler to detect emboli, may provide answers to these problems.

Silent infarction

A silent stroke is one diagnosed on CT or MRI scanning without corresponding symptoms or signs. A lesion may be silent because of its location, or because symptoms are not reported, signs not elicited, or because either are transient. To an extent, therefore, the definition of a silent stroke depends on how thoroughly appropriate features are sought. As with any asymptomatic condition, the importance of silent infarction depends on its prognostic implications.

Silent infarction has been demonstrated in stroke-free subjects by autopsy (prevalence 13 per cent; Shinkawa *et al.* 1995) and MRI (prevalence 9–13 per cent; Kobayashi *et al.* 1991; Lindgren *et al.* 1994*b*). Silent infarction identified by CT scanning was present in 26 per cent of stroke-free subjects with atrial fibrillation (Feinberg *et al.* 1990). In patients with TIA or completed stroke, silent infarction is detectable in between 11 and 38 per cent of cases (Chodosh *et al.* 1988; Herderschee *et al.* 1992; Ricci *et al.* 1993; Boon *et al.* 1994; Jorgensen *et al.* 1994). The majority (about 80 per cent) of these are small, deep infarcts (lacunes), even in cases with atrial fibrillation, raising the question of the underlying pathology of the lesions seen on CT.

Prevalence of silent infarction increases with age and this probably explains much of the reported variation between studies. In general, risk factors for silent infarction are no different from those for symptomatic stroke. In patients presenting with stroke, silent infarction appears not to alter short-term prognosis. Data on long-term prognosis, prognosis in the absence of symptomatic stroke, and implications for cognitive function are lacking. There is no evidence to suggest that an asymptomatic carotid stenosis should be considered 'symptomatic' in the presence of a silent infarct.

Vascular dementia

Dementia is a global impairment of higher metal functions, including orientation, memory, concentration, intellect and reasoning, in the absence of impaired consciousness (Cooper 1991). Between 10 and 30 per cent of cases have multiple cerebral infarcts as their predominant pathology, and as many cases again have mixed vascular and Alzheimer's disease pathology. Infarcts may be cortical or subcortical. Site of infarction is more important than absolute volume of brain tissue lost. A history of stroke increases the risk of dementia ninefold (Amar and Wilcock 1996).

Differentiating vascular dementia from other causes is difficult clinically. There are various published scores and criteria (Verhey *et al.* 1996), including the Hachinski scale (Hachinski *et al.* 1975), the Californian Alzheimer's Disease Diagnostic and Treatment Center criteria (ADDTC) (Chui *et al.* 1992), the DSM-IV (American Psychiatric Association 1993), ICD-10 (World Health Organization 1993), and NINDS-AIREN criteria (Roman *et al.* 1993). These are all essentially clinical tools, with provision for inclusion of neuroimaging data whenever these are available. Agreement between these criteria is poor. In one study 51 of 167 demented patients fulfilled at least one set of guidelines for vascular dementia, but only five fulfilled them all (Wetterling *et al.* 1996).

Table 4.13 Accuracy of proposed diagnostic criteria for vascular dementia

	Sensitivity for VD versus others	Specificity for VD versus others	Sensitivity for VD/mixed versus AD	Specificity for VD/mixed versus AD
Hachinski score	0.43	0.88	0.30	0.97
NINDS-AIREN	0.58	0.80	0.43	0.91
ADDTC	0.63	0.64	0.58	0.88

VD, vascular dementia; AD, Alzheimer's disease.

Using a neuropathological gold standard, the validity of some of these have been compared (Table 4.13) (Gold *et al.* 1997). There was good agreement between diagnoses made by the ADDTC and NINDS-AIREN criteria (κ = 0.76). Low sensitivity and poor specificity in excluding mixed dementia are the main problems. For epidemiological and clinical-trial purposes, a high specificity is required to ensure homogeneity in the study group, and the Hachinski score performs best. For clinical practice, the best trade-off between sensitivity and specificity represents the optimal 'accuracy'. Identifying as many patients as possible with a vascular component, who might benefit from risk-factor control or aspirin treatment, requires a high sensitivity for the combined group of vascular and mixed dementia (best achieved by the ADDTC criteria).

From the point of view of stroke epidemiology, it is reasonable to consider vascular dementia as a presentation of stroke, and, where technically feasible and clinically appropriate, to reduce remediable vascular risk factors. Two caveats are that vascular dementia will share the same mixed pathology as other stroke, and that strategies for prevention, or the retarding of progression, are as yet unproven by randomized trial.

Summary

1. The accuracy with which doctors distinguish vascular strokes (i.e. infarcts, emboli, haemorrhages) from other non-vascular pathology ranges from a sensitivity of 67 per cent to 100 per cent, and a specificity of 22 per cent to 91 per cent. Variation is due to the clinical skill of the doctor, the age range of patients studied, and the clinical setting (e.g. hospital, specialist stroke unit).

2. Up to 13 per cent of patients thought initially to have had a vascular stroke turn out to have some other pathology. The most common causes of diagnostic error are epilepsy, including Todd's paresis, delirium and loss of consciousness (drugs, alcohol, metabolic, intercurrent illness,

orthostatic syncope), mass lesions (subdural haematomas, tumours), depression, and dementia syndromes.

3. Clinical methods may be used to distinguish haemorrhagic from thrombo-embolic stroke with sufficient accuracy (predictive value up to 99 per cent) for epidemiological purposes, and probably for use of antiplatelet agents for patients with thrombo-embolic stroke. Further work is needed to define the accuracy of this approach.

4. The clinical diagnosis of stroke syndromes with similar characteristics, including lacunar stroke, is reasonably accurate.

5. Cardiac embolism is probably important, but is of unknown incidence, and is difficult to diagnose with certainty.

6. Silent infarcts are relatively common, affecting about 10 per cent of the series of patients studied at autopsy or by neuroimaging and between 10 and 40 per cent of patients who have already suffered a TIA or stroke.

7. Criteria available for the diagnosis of vascular dementia are very variable in their accuracy and show poor agreement with each other.

5 Clinical disagreement

Clinicians often disagree

Whenever two or more doctors are asked to assess the same patient it is unlikely that they will agree completely on their clinical findings. This phenomenon is well recognized in several fields of medicine, ranging from taking a history (Cochrane *et al.* 1951), examination of the pedal pulses (Meade *et al.* 1968), chest examination (Spiteri *et al.* 1988), to interpretation of exercise electrocardiograms (Blackburn *et al.* 1968). It is not surprising, therefore, that in the assessment of stroke patients, agreement is not absolute. Information on which doctors disagree can be considered in terms of its importance in diagnosis, management, and prognosis. If the information is crucial, every effort must be made to reduce disagreements; if the information is of little value, there is no point in wasting time collecting it, much less trying to improve its reliability. Disagreements may matter. For example, if two clinicians disagree on the presence of a carotid bruit, the patient may or may not be exposed to the risk of investigation or denied the benefits of treatment. Disagreements on factors that determine rehabilitation potential (e.g. mental state, severity of stroke, pre-stroke ability) may lead to patients being denied access to therapy and discharged to nursing homes inappropriately or before their full potential has been achieved.

In one study, four consultants examined 12 patients, looking for seven impairments that might be caused by an acute stroke (Garraway *et al.* 1976). The overall agreement between the four doctors was only 34 (41 per cent) out of a total of 84 (i.e. 12 × 7) possible agreements. Agreements for assessment of mental function, proprioception, posture, and motor function were low, whereas spatial neglect, comprehension, and expression showed reasonable agreement.

Disagreements are also found in taking a history, as demonstrated by an Italian study (Tomasello *et al.* 1982), where the question of observer variation was important as a multi-centre study was being undertaken. Agreement between eight examiners of 55 patients who had suffered recurrent transient ischaemic attacks or minor strokes was measured using an 'index of agreement' (the ratio of the number of subjects with agreement in responses to the total number of patients). Using this index, around 50 per cent agreement was found for both the frequency and number of transient ischaemic attacks. Agreement on neurological symptoms was higher, with 66 per cent agreement on the presence of visual, sensory, or speech impairments, and higher agreement (76 per cent) on motor impairments. The examiners did better on neurological signs, with high agreement for visual field defects (92 per cent), but agreement on cerebellar signs (38 per cent), sensory signs (25 per cent), and plantar responses (21 per cent) were all low.

It is perhaps even more surprising that agreement was low since a standardized data record was used by all examiners. The authors concluded that disagreements may have been due to differences in the interests of the examiners, the motivation of the patients, imperfect recall of short-lived symptoms, and differences in dialect, education, and social status between examiners and patients.

Chance levels of agreement

In fact, the level of agreement in this Italian study was overestimated by the index of agreement used. The index used is affected by the frequency of a particular abnormality. If a sign is rare (e.g. cranial bruit) or very common (e.g. motor weakness), then even when there is little agreement between examiners, a high level of chance agreement will be found. For example, if observer 1 thinks that 10 per cent of stroke patients have sensory impairments and 90 per cent do not, and observer 2 thinks that the proportions are 20 per cent and 80 per cent respectively, then the probability that both observers will agree on the absence of sensory impairment, without even examining the patient, is:

$$0.90 \times 0.80 = 0.72, \text{ i.e. 72 per cent.}$$

This is because the rules of probability require independent probabilities to be multiplied together to produce the probability of two events occurring. In this case the events are observers 1 and 2 agreeing on the absence of a sign. The probability that both observers will agree on the presence of sensory impairment, again without examining the patient is:

$$0.10 \times 0.20 = 0.02, \text{ i.e. 2 per cent.}$$

This adds up to an overall agreement of 74 per cent, as shown in Table 5.1.

The chance association between their findings (the numbers in the body of Table 5.1) is obtained in the same way as calculating the expected values for a chi-square (χ^2) 2 x 2 table. The crude percentage agreement looks quite acceptable—74 per cent, but this 'agreement' was of course produced entirely by using expected chance levels of association. Note also that this chance level of agreement is higher than many of the levels of agreement reported in the Italian study! In other words, many of the observed agreements could easily have been due to chance rather than any consistency between examiners.

Table 5.1 Chance association in agreement between two observers, where observer 1 decides the prevalence of abnormality is 10 per cent and observer 2 uses a prevalence of 20 per cent abnormality

	Observer 1		
Observer 2	No sensory impairment	Sensory impairment	Totals
No sensory impairment	72	8	80
Sensory impairment	18	2	20
Totals	90	10	100

Crude percentage agreement 72 + 2 / 100 = 74%

With more common or rarer findings (e.g. weakness or neck rigidity) the percentage crude agreement becomes an even less good estimate of the true level of agreement, as shown in Table 5.2. This level of agreement—97 per cent—looks very impressive when reported as an observed level of agreement, but once again it is entirely the result of chance.

Adjusting for chance agreement

The Cohen's kappa statistic (Cohen 1960) allows for this chance variation by subtracting the chance agreement from the observed agreement, and expressing this chance-adjusted agreement as a proportion of the potential real agreement possible (i.e. 100 per cent minus the chance agreement):

$$\text{kappa} = \kappa = (P_o - P_c)/(1 - P_c)$$

where P_o is the observed proportion of agreement and P_c is the expected chance proportion of agreement. It is usual to express these proportions as

Table 5.2 Chance agreement between two observers when observer 1 thinks that 1 per cent of patients have neck rigidity and observer 2 thinks that 2 per cent have the sign

	Observer 1		
Observer 2	Neck rigidity	No neck rigidity	Totals
Neck rigidity	0.02	1.98	2.00
No neck rigidity	0.98	97.02	98.00
Totals	1.00	99.00	100.00

Crude percentage chance agreement (97.02 + 0.02) / 100 = 97%

Table 5.3   Observed and chance agreement between two observers on a prior history of stroke, assumed to be present in 33 per cent. Numbers in brackets are numbers expected by chance

	Observer 1		
Observer 2	Past history	No past history	Totals
Past history	20 (10.9)	7 (22.1)	33
No past history	13 (22.1)	60 (44.9)	67
Totals	33	67	100

Observed agreement = 80 per cent
Chance agreement = 55.8 per cent

numbers between 0 and 1 rather than as percentages. Consequently kappa will range from +1 for complete agreement to –1 for complete disagreement, and a value of 0 will indicate only chance agreement. The χ^2 statistic can be used to give a significance level to the kappa value.

The observed agreement with this hypothetical data (Table 5.3) is:

$$(20 + 60)/100 = 80 \text{ per cent or } 0.80,$$

which seems quite acceptable, and the χ^2 value is 28.22, which suggests that it is highly unlikely to have arisen by chance. The numbers in brackets are the expected or chance values, which are calculated in the usual way (i.e. (33 × 33)/100 = 10.9). These expected values give a chance agreement of:

$$(10.9 + 44.9)/100 = 55.8 \text{ per cent or } 0.558.$$

The kappa statistic is:

$$\kappa = (0.80 - 0.558)/(1 - 0.558) = 0.55$$

which indicates only moderate agreement once the effects of chance have been taken into account. Levels over 0.75 are usually taken to indicate excellent agreement (Landis and Koch 1977). In this example, to exceed this kappa value, the crude percentage agreement would have to be at least 90 per cent.

Relative and absolute measures of agreement

When continuous variables such as blood pressure are measured repeatedly, it is conventional to present two measures of agreement: the within-subject variance and the ratio of the between-subject variance to total variance, the interclass correlation coefficient. The former is an absolute measure of agreement between measurements and the latter is a relative measure. The crude percentage agreement is an absolute measure of agreement and the kappa statistic can be considered as a relative measure (Chinn and Burney 1987). While the crude percentage agreement is criticized for its dependence on the prevalence of the condition studied, kappa is also biased by prevalence, producing spuriously low levels of agreement at low prevalence (Goggenmoos-Holzmann 1993).

Whenever data on agreement are presented, it is essential that both the raw data and the kappa statistics are presented to give the reader a fuller impression of both the absolute and the relative levels of agreement. This also allows readers to calculate alternative measures of agreement, such as the average correct classification rate (Chinn and Burney 1987). In situations where a variable is ordered into more than two categories (e.g. small, medium, large), kappa values tend to be lower than for two-category variables (e.g. small, big). Weighted kappas tend to hide the true levels of agreement for individual variables (or items within a scale, for example) and should be avoided in preference to providing kappas for each variable or scale component (MacClure and Willett 1987).

A further confusion with measures to assess agreement is the issue of who is really right. This concern relates to whether there is a correct value that is estimated by each of the clinicians (or methods of assessment). In many circumstances, there is no reasonable 'gold standard' with which to make comparisons. Even if there is a gold standard, it is essential to bear in mind that the 'correctness' or accuracy of a method or observer is best assessed by measures of sensitivity and specificity (see Chapter 4).

Clinical disagreements in stroke

Patients' recall and medical records

Data obtained from the British Regional Heart Study have been examined to determine whether patients' recall of a stroke agrees with information obtained from medical records (Walker *et al.* 1998). This information is presented in Table 5.4. The initial medical record showed crude agreement of 97.7 per cent and a kappa of 0.54, indicating moderate agreement.

However, these summary statistics hide the true picture, which is only revealed by careful examination of the 2 × 2 table. According to initial medical record review, patients tended to over-recall stroke, with a 'false positive' recall of $118/201 = 59$ per cent. With knowledge of patient recall, further review of the medical records shows a quite different pattern: 29 additional strokes were found on careful scrutiny of the records; 51 of the medical records described a transient ischaemic attack which would, most likely, have been described to the patient as a small stroke, thus reducing the

Table 5.4   Agreement between patient recall of stroke and medical records (data derived from Walker et al. 1998)

	Initial medical record review		Supplementary record review	
Patient recall	Stroke	No stroke	Stroke	No stroke
Stroke	83	118	163	38
No stroke	19	5687	14	5692
Totals	102	5805	177	5730

false positive recall rate to 38/201, 19 per cent. The other side of the coin, 'false negative' recall, is a much smaller problem, with only 19 medical records describing a stroke in people claiming not to have suffered from one. Of these 19 medical reports, five were errors of fact due to poor writing and transcription errors, and in the remaining 14 cases, the patient suffered with multiple co-morbidities, including cardiovascular diseases.

Since patient recall is the predominant mode of enquiry used in clinical practice to define past medical history, the tendency to over-recall may have important consequences if investigation or therapy is based solely on this information. In research, where accurate data are required, very careful scrutiny of medical records, in addition to patient recall, is essential to ascertain, with reasonable accuracy, all strokes occurring. Unfortunately, many large epidemiological studies are not able to adopt this methodology as they use only routine clinical information systems (Asplund *et al.* 1988, 1995).

Clinical symptoms and signs

An American study measured the agreement between six neurologists who examined 17 stroke patients over the course of 3 days, using a balanced design in which each patient was seen by four of the doctors (Shinar *et al.* 1985). Since each patient was seen four times, a total of 68 possible agreements were available for each piece of information. Answers to apparently straightforward questions were subject to disagreement. The history of a previous stroke was agreed upon on 45 (66 per cent) of the 68 occasions, with similar levels of agreement for presence of headache at onset and past history of a transient ischaemic attack. Perfect agreement by all four doctors was achieved much less often: past history of stroke, 35 per cent; headache at onset, 41 per cent; transient ischaemic attack in the past, 29 per cent. These authors also used the kappa statistic to adjust for the level of chance agreement. Surprisingly, only two items of history achieved good agreement: alcohol ingestion within 24 hours of stroke ($\kappa = 0.65$), and time of last meal ($\kappa = 0.46$). Other important information such as level of consciousness, seizure at onset, headache, vomiting, and the course of the illness over the first 24 hours only achieved modest agreement (κ values from 0.32 to 0.39). Presence of a focal deficit at onset, previous transient ischaemic attack, deficit present on waking, and use of anticoagulants or antiplatelet agents all showed levels of only chance agreement, with kappa values from 0.15 to 0.08.

The crude percentage agreements of neurological signs were shown to be quite misleading. Kappa values showed excellent agreement for the following: swallowing, deviation of eyes, articulation and speech impairment, side of hemiplegia. Only chance levels of agreement were found for the following: tongue weakness, depressed mood, neck stiffness, cervical bruits, and pure motor syndrome.

By contrast with these findings, a reliability study of the National Institutes of Health Stroke Scale, using videotaped patient examinations, demonstrated extremely high levels of agreement (intraclass correlation coefficients 0.92–0.95; Goldstein and Samsa 1997). However, the findings are presented in such a way that it is impossible to calculate kappas for the individual items making up the stroke scale, and inappropriate reliance is placed on an analysis of correlations between mean scores. It is possible that the excellent agreement, as shown by the intraclass correlations, is due to the study design using videos, which avoided any variation attributable to performance of the clinical examination. If the observers were expected to conduct their own neurological examinations, it would be more appropriate to examine observer variation under these clinical circumstances rather than use video assessments. It is essential that the method used to estimate repeatability of examinations is appropriate for the setting in which the test or method will be used.

Stroke subtype

Observer variation in the type of stroke (i.e. haemorrhagic, embolic, lacunar, thrombotic) has also been studied. Using the same study design and patients as referred to above (Shinar et al. 1985), each of the four doctors seeing the 17 patients was asked to give a provisional diagnosis after taking a history and examining the patient (Gross et al. 1986). Complete agreement on diagnosis was achieved for only 7 (41 per cent; κ, 0.38) of the 17 when the categories of infarction were combined into a single group, otherwise there was no case in which each neurologist agreed on the specific diagnosis. Further diagnostic work-up, which included CT scans for every patient, improved agreement: 10 (59 per cent) perfect agreements (κ, 0.69) when infarction was a single category, and six (35 per cent) perfect agreements (κ, 0.61) when subcategories of infarction were considered. Similar findings were reported from the Physicians' Health Study (Berger et al. 1996) with larger kappa values for a simple haemorrhage, ischaemic versus undetermined classification (κ, 0.81), but much lower kappa values were found for classification by subtypes of ischaemic and haemorrhagic stroke, despite the majority of patients having had a CT scan.

The Oxfordshire Community Stroke Project produced an alternative pathophysiological classification of stroke (see Chapter 4). The between-clinician agreement in its use in a consecutive series of 85 patients was reasonable (Lindley *et al.* 1993). Much of the disagreement was traced to differences in the assessment of common neurological signs (e.g. poor agreement on sensory loss and confusion, modest agreement on hemianopia).

Disability and quality of life

The Barthel activities of daily living (ADL) index is widely used as a measure of outcome in rehabilitation trials and in descriptive studies of stroke patients. Tests of reliability can be misleading and an early evaluation of the Barthel scale concluded that 'the Barthel ADL index is a reasonable, robust and reliable clinical measure' (Collin *et al.* 1988) but chance levels of agreement were not considered, kappa statistics were not calculated, and the disagreements, calculated from data provided in the paper, varied from 1 to 9 points out of 20. Correlation coefficients are inadequate guides to reliability of such scales and the method of calculating mean differences and standard deviations provides a better way of describing between observer variation for continuous or scale measures (Bland and Altman 1986).

A study of the test–retest repeatability on postal surveys of several commonly used disability and quality of life measures found that the Barthel and Nottingham ADL scale (Nouri and Lincoln 1987) had kappa agreements in the range 0.6–1.0 for the majority of individual scale items, indicating good to excellent agreement between occasions 2 weeks apart (Gompertz *et al.* 1993). By contrast, the Nottingham Health Profile and the Geriatric Depression Scale were much less repeatable. This poor performance probably reflects the intrinsically subjective and variable nature of the responses made to the questions included in scales of this type.

When data are presented as mean and standard deviations of differences between test and retest scores, the amount of variation is surprisingly large and of a size usually considered to be clinically important. Table 5.5 shows the mean difference and the limits of agreement for several scales when used to assess test–retest repeatability to two postal questionnaires sent out 2 weeks apart to 22 stroke patients. The mean difference should be zero if the responses were identical on both occasions, thus positive or negative differences will indicate bias on repeat testing. The limits of agreement should be related to both the range of the scale (so that the measurement error with respect to maximum and minimum scores can be assessed) and to the clinically important difference that would be worth detecting—for example, 2 points on the Barthel scale may mean the difference between being able to walk independently or not. As shown in Table 5.5, the Barthel index has little evidence of bias with a very small mean difference between test and retest. The

Table 5.5 Repeatability of stroke outcome scales in a repeated postal survey

	Mean difference	Limits of agreement (scale range)
Barthel	−0.5	4.2 (0–20)
Nottingham ADL	−0.7	2.8 (0–22)
Geriatric Depression Scale	−0.4	5.6 (0–15)
Nottingham Health Profile		
Energy	14	60 (0–100)
Pain	2.5	36 (0–100)
Emotion	1.0	46 (0–100)
Sleep	4.0	32 (0–100)
Social isolation	−9.2	56 (0–100)
Physical mobility	2.9	42 (0–100)

limits of agreement are 4.2. This means that a score of 10 could be as low as 5.8 and as high as 14.2 out of 20, simply due to measurement error. When groups of patients are compared, this degree of measurement error is overcome by increasing sample sizes. In an individual patient, such changes would prompt urgent clinical re-assessment to 'explain' the deterioration or improvement. Consequently, such scales cannot be recommended for clinical use in the management of individual patients.

More recent measures of quality of life, such as the EuroQol (EuroQol Group 1990) and the Medical Outcomes Study Short Form-36 (SF-36) (Ware *et al.* 1993), have also been used in stroke patients and show similarly large limits of agreement (Dorman *et al.* 1998), which is not surprising as they comprise similar items to the older Nottingham Health Profile.

It is clear that despite a considerable industry devoted to disability and quality of life measurement, the problems of measurement error have not been overcome and indicators that can provide reliable information on changes in individuals or small groups of patients are not available. In circumstances where individual change is important to document, it is likely that measures of impairment (e.g. muscle power) or closely defined disability tasks (e.g. timed walking tests, dexterity) may be more precisely measured and provide a better index of progress.

Improving clinical agreement

Definition, standardization, and explanation

We must therefore accept that disagreement exists and that it is sufficiently undesirable that something should be done about it. Only one study has attempted to measure the impact of strategies to improve agreement

(Garraway *et al.* 1976). The method used was to define categories more closely, and to standardize the method of examination. This led to improvements in the agreement on motor function, spatial neglect, proprioception, comprehension/expression, and mental function. Postural function (i.e. balance and posture) remained difficult to agree on. Despite improvements, side of hemiplegia was inaccurately recorded on 6 out of 12 patients by one or more of the examining doctors. This was probably the result of using 'CVA' as a diagnostic label with inevitable confusion between the side of hemisphere damage and the side of the hemiplegia. As well as defining categories more carefully and standardization of examination techniques, doctors need to be more careful about the terms used to describe strokes.

Further explanation and discussion with the doctors, and increased standardization of terms and recording methods led to further improvements in agreement. With considerable effort it was possible to improve overall agreement from 41 to 68 per cent of all items measured and to reduce between-observer differences in function scores to a quarter of the differences observed before training. This study also demonstrated that not only do doctors disagree with each other, they are not terribly consistent from one week to the next in their own opinions. Inconsistency ranged from 17 to 31 per cent of all items assessed, with the biggest differences in mental function, proprioception, and motor function.

This study was undertaken because several different doctors were to assess patients in a trial of the effects of a stroke unit. Agreement between doctors was essential to ensure comparability between those assessed in the stroke unit and those managed on medical wards. Despite the training, it is quite possible that, with time, doctors would drift back to their usual practice and disagreements would recur. In long-term studies it is usually necessary to ensure that observers have regular training sessions to ensure that standards of agreement are maintained. In clinical practice this should be a routine part of continuing education.

Information value

Defining the information that is essential for diagnosis, management, and prognosis is a useful starting point. There is little point in refining the techniques of measurement for information of little practical value. Table 5.6 attempts to classify information about stroke patients according to its potential value in each of these three areas. Only side of weakness, speech impairment, orientation, swallowing, and gaze paresis have reasonable levels of clinical agreement (Shinar *et al.* 1985; Lindley *et al.* 1993; Gompertz *et al.* 1994*a*).

Perceptual impairment requires training to improve agreement, and some important information, such as continence of urine, pre-stroke ability,

Table 5.6 A classification of information for its use in diagnosis, management, and prognosis, together with the level of clinical agreement

Diagnosis	Management	Prognosis
Side of weakness*	Side of weakness*	
Speech impairment*	Speech impairment*	Speech impairment*
Previous stroke*	Swallowing*	Swallowing*
Mode of onset	Perceptual loss**	Perceptual loss**
Stroke risk factors*	Orientation**	Orientation**
Headache	Degree of weakness	Gaze paresis*
Vomiting	Conscious level*	Conscious level*
Photophobia	Mood	Mood
Neck stiffness	Balance/gait	Balance/gait
	Continence −	Continence −
	Visual field loss	Visual field loss
	Pre-stroke ability +	Pre-stroke ability +
	Type of stroke	Type of stroke

* Good clinical agreement, ** good agreement after training, + moderate agreement, − fair agreement. All others show only poor to chance levels of agreement.

presence of stroke risk factors (e.g. high blood pressure, diabetes, smoking), has not been assessed for clinical agreement. All the other information listed has been shown to have low levels of clinical agreement.

The next step to improve agreement is to consider the reasons for disagreement and to decide what (if anything) can be done about them. The McMaster group (Sackett *et al.* 1985) have classified sources of variation as due to the examiner, the examined, and the examination.

The examiner

Tiredness of the examiner is likely to be a major cause of disagreement. It has been shown that tired doctors make more mistakes when interpreting ECGs (Friedman *et al.* 1971). Traditionally, the neurological part of the clinical examination is left until last and by this time, particularly if the patient is deaf or delirious, a reliable examination is unlikely. Some doctors record a diagnosis of 'right CVA' when they mean that the patient has a left hemiplegia (or right hemisphere damage). The short hand leads to much confusion because it is not clear whether the 'right' refers to the brain or the body. It is better to record observations and not inferences from observations. Elderly patients suffer strokes most commonly, and are not easy to examine. Consequently doctors may fail to record information that is essential to diagnosis, management, or prognosis because of a technically poor examination. This may be because of ignorance (several medical schools in the UK still do not have academic departments of geriatric medicine to teach such skills), disinterest, or an assumption that, having diagnosed a stroke, not much can (or should) be done for the patient.

The examined

Dysphasia, cognitive impairments, depressed conscious level, and associated problems will all make history taking and physical signs more prone to variability, especially in the acute phase. As symptoms and signs improve (or deteriorate) quite rapidly in the early phase, and extra items of information are discovered (from helpful relatives, neighbours, family doctors, etc.), it is sensible to consider the initial examination as just the beginning of the data collection and interpretation process.

The examination

The hospital ward or emergency room environment is not usually conducive to testing higher cognitive function or enquiring about sensitive issues such as urinary continence, because of noise and the urge to get onto the next patient. This may also lead to a poor doctor–patient interaction, especially if a patient's hearing aid, spectacles, and false teeth are not used appropriately and if the patient is lying uncomfortably on an examination trolley. The situation is not helped if the doctor is simultaneously interrogating the patient, answering a telephone call, and trying to find a bed for the patient.

Solutions

Some solutions are obvious but not often implemented. Doctors should do an examination appropriate to the task in hand. In the emergency room the aim is to assess the urgency of the clinical condition of the patient and the need for admission. The admitting physician's job is to ensure that the diagnosis of a vascular stroke is reasonably likely, that other causes of neurological impairment (e.g. hypoglycaemia, meningitis, mass lesions, etc.) have been excluded, and that information for immediate management has been obtained (e.g. swallowing, medication, need for pressure sore prevention). The subsequent tasks are to collect and interpret information to aid subsequent management and give a prognosis. This needs to be done using multiple sources (e.g. the patient, ward staff, old records, home support services, friends, etc.), and may require a series of small focused examinations of the patient in a quiet environment. These tasks are easy to neglect.

Sackett and colleagues (1985) recommend repeating key findings, and asking colleagues to examine the patient unguided by prior knowledge of the findings, which is part of the tradition of bedside teaching. It does, of course, imply that doctors have sufficient knowledge to elicit signs in the first place.

Sackett suggests that serious faults in medical education exist when it is possible for doctors to reach advanced stages of training without ever having their technique of interviewing or examining watched and criticized by another colleague or teacher. Certainly the standard examination of stroke patients in the UK might lead one to believe that patients do not have any higher cortical function, apart from the motor cortex, and comprise merely of cranial nerves (usually reported as intact, although smell is seldom, if ever, tested) and spinal reflex arcs.

Another approach to improve agreement is to replace the traditional blank page upon which doctors write their findings with a more systematic pre-printed record of essential information to be collected. Routine use of mental test scores (mainly concerned with memory and orientation) is common in geriatric medical practice, and this approach might be extended to include standardized assessments of other useful information, such as mood, perceptual impairment, and pre-stroke ability.

The use of standardized proformas, such as one produced by the Royal College of Physicians, may prove helpful in improving the quality of information collected (Davenport et al. 1995). This approach resulted in substantially higher kappa values than previously reported (Shinar et al. 1985; Lindley et al. 1993) for a range of important data, but did not improve the moderate agreement previously found for many aspects of neurological examination (Gompertz et al. 1994a). However, information collected using a stroke audit proforma from case record review, in a comparison of stroke unit and general ward care, demonstrated low levels of recording of information usually considered to be essential for adequate care of stroke patients (Gompertz et al. 1995). Furthermore, the standardized assessment scales recommended by the Royal College of Physicians and British Geriatrics Society are not widely used in Britain (Dunn and Lewis 1993) and randomized controlled trial evidence from the USA suggests that routine use of functional assessment scales is not associated with any benefits for patients, but that 43 per cent of doctors used such information to change treatment (Rubenstein et al. 1989).

Development and testing of better means of obtaining important information about stroke patients, and evaluation of the impact of this information on clinical outcomes and decision making, is essential but still remains to be done.

Summary

1. Disagreement in clinical findings between even well-trained clinicians is common.

2. The usual methods of reporting agreement as a crude percentage of observed to total possible agreements does not allow for chance

association, and tends to overestimate the degree of agreement. Kappa values are chance adjusted and give a more reliable measure of agreement.

3. In reporting agreement of categorical data, raw 2 × 2 data should be presented, in addition to kappa statistics. For continuous variables, while intraclass correlation coefficients and within- and between-subject variances are of value, presentation of mean differences between observers and limits of agreement provide clinically relevant information.

4. Agreement about historical information (such as history of a previous stroke, use of antiplatelet drugs) and physical signs (carotid bruits, neck stiffness, side of stroke) is poor and often no better than chance agreement.

5. It is necessary to define which information is necessary for diagnosis, management, and prognosis and to attempt to improve the reliability of the collection of this information. Other information of questionable reliability and value should be discarded.

6. Improved standardization of examination methods, record keeping, and appropriate task-orientated examination, together with more direct observation of clinical technique, may lead to improved clinical agreement. Evaluations of improved methods of information collection are required.

6 Investigation

How good is a test?

A test is commonly considered to be of value if it alters management. This is an oversimplification of the way most doctors use investigations. The value of any investigation can be thought of at any one of six levels (shown in Table 6.1). These range from technical efficacy (how good are the pictures?) through to patient outcome and health policy considerations.

The further up the hierarchy that a test is evaluated, the more relevant it is to the patient and society as a whole. In most cases considerations of patient outcome and societal benefits will be technically and logistically difficult to demonstrate. To be of value in improving overall 'health gain' a test must have demonstrable efficacy at the lower levels of technical, diagnostic, and therapeutic efficacy. For example, if a CT scan is degraded by movement artefact, interpreted inaccurately, or fails to influence clinical management, it is unlikely to have any effect on patient outcomes. Evaluations of the effects of tests on patient outcomes or overall societal benefits may be difficult to interpret because the whole chain must be complete for an effect to be seen, culminating in the test influencing the use of an effective treatment (or avoiding harmful treatment). Factors other than the performance of the test may therefore have a more direct influence on outcomes. Diagnostic efficacy is also of value in its own right. Diagnostic certainty is useful both to patients and their doctors, and avoidance of further tests ('diagnostic thinking efficacy') is certainly desirable (Thornbury 1994).

There has been an explosion in the number of investigations used in imaging the location and nature of strokes, and in investigating their aetiology. In a survey of nine hospitals in six European countries, the proportion of stroke patients receiving brain imaging varied from 30 to 98 per cent. Angiography was used in 0–30 per cent of cases, carotid Doppler in 0–97 per cent, and echocardiography in 0–44 per cent. Such variation in utilization is common where the indications for, and the value of, investigations are unclear. It may represent overuse of tests in academic centres where they are readily available, but might equally indicate a lack of access to appropriate care for some patients (Beech *et al.* 1996).

Developments in the technical efficacy of imaging has outpaced evaluative studies demonstrating diagnostic, work-up, therapeutic, outcome, and

Table 6.1 Definition of levels of efficacy for investigation

Level of efficacy	Examples
Technical	Failure to complete test, image resolution
Diagnostic	Yield of abnormal tests, diagnostic accuracy (sensitivity, specificity)
Diagnostic thinking (work-up)	'Helpfulness of test', ruling in and ruling out diagnoses, ordering or avoidance of further tests
Therapeutic	Changed management or management options
Patient outcome	Prevention, cure, morbidity, or mortality reduction as a result of test (e.g. QALYs gained), cost-effectiveness analyses
Societal	Cost-utility in comparison with other (healthcare) options

societal efficacy. This has made it hard to identify the place of many tests in routine practice.

Computed tomographic (CT) scanning

Who needs a CT scan?

The question of which patients merit a CT scan does not arise for many stroke patients, particularly in poorer countries and for the 25–50 per cent of stroke patients who are not admitted to hospital (Barer *et al.* 1984; Oxfordshire Community Stroke Project 1985; Wolfe *et al.* 1993). The Oxfordshire study showed that it is certainly possible to arrange a CT scan for those patients remaining at home—a creditable 80 per cent of all stroke patients were scanned. There were delays, however, with only 62 per cent of both hospital and community patients getting a scan within 3 weeks of onset of the stroke. After this time it is quite possible that small haemorrhages will have resolved and will be no longer visible on CT scans (Dennis *et al.* 1987).

The Oxford group defined patients who require a CT scan as those who have an atypical clinical course; are young (although age was not defined); those in whom treatment with antiplatelet or anticoagulant drugs might be used; and those where there is diagnostic doubt (Sandercock *et al.* 1985a; Warlow 1996). Although these criteria seem sensible, it is difficult to find evidence to support them.

Atypical clinical course
Evidence that an atypical, stuttering, or prolonged onset of symptoms and signs is relatively more common among patients with a non-vascular cause

for their neurological impairment is equivocal (Weisberg and Nice 1977; Allen 1983; Sandercock *et al.* 1985a). In those studies that found such an association, the predictive value of this information is quite low (see Chapter 4). In a large series of patients with confirmed stroke admitted to hospital in Lausanne, neurological deficit progressed over 24 hours or more in 10 per cent, and fluctuated in a further 7 per cent (Bogousslavsky *et al.* 1988). If a CT scan was done for every patient with an atypical onset of stroke, from 1.3 per cent (Sandercock *et al.* 1985a) to 14 per cent (Allen 1983) of patients would turn out to have a non-vascular lesion. The majority would have a stroke, and around four-fifths (Sandercock *et al.* 1985a) to half (Allen 1983) of non-vascular lesions would be missed because they did not present with an unusual onset.

Younger patients
The rationale for an age criterion is that some rare causes of stroke (e.g. arterio-venous malformations, aneurysms, angiomas) are more common and more often treatable. The difficulty is in deciding on an age threshold. Some fairly common non-vascular lesions become more common with increasing age and are just as treatable as in younger patients—in particular subdural haematomas and meningiomas. Up to the age of 75 it is likely that many neurosurgeons will consider evacuating a subdural haematoma. After this age, the overall condition of the patient may determine the feasibility and likely prognosis of surgery. If an age criterion is to be used, then it seems illogical to set it much below 75 years of age if the purpose is to detect clinically unrecognized but surgically treatable pathology.

Diagnostic doubt
A clinical diagnosis of vascular stroke can never be absolutely certain. Doctors differ in the degree of uncertainty that they can tolerate, and if a CT scan is done merely to check that a highly probable diagnosis is true, then this is wasteful of resources. It is quite possible that time is the most useful clinical tool for distinguishing strokes from non-vascular disease, watching the course of the patient's illness over a few days to weeks. No systematic studies of this strategy have been carried out, so it is not possible to compare the sensitivity and specificity of 'watchful waiting' with CT scanning in diagnosing non-vascular problems. It would be sensible to monitor not just neurological signs, but also functional ability (sitting balance, transfers, walking, feeding, dressing, etc.), and cognitive state (using the Mini-Mental State Examination, for example; Folstein *et al.* 1975). Patients with a deteriorating or static course or with disproportionate impairment of consciousness might be the right ones to investigate with CT scanning. Another approach is to ask the question 'what caused this stroke?'. A full diagnostic formulation must distinguish infarct from haemorrhage, and include a consideration of arterial disease,

potential cardiac embolic sources, and the possibility of rarer causes than thrombo-embolism (such as arterial dissection, arteritis, or metabolic syndromes). If the patient has risk factors for stroke (other than age) then it might be thought less necessary to consider non-vascular pathology. Risk factors are neither necessary nor sufficient for stroke diagnosis, however. A CT scan will rarely give direct answers to any of these questions, but the location, size, and number of infarcts will give some clues about aetiology. This, in turn, may guide further investigation and management.

There are some other reasons for confirming diagnoses. Many doctors will want a scan to 'rule out' rare but important diagnoses, such as tumour or subdural haematoma. Patients may welcome this information also. In the case of stroke, this has never been put to the test, but in an experiment performed by Sox and colleagues, the extent of reassurance afforded to patients with non-cardiac sounding chest pain was greater if they were investigated by electrocardiography than if they were not (Sox *et al.* 1981). A final (possibly fanciful) reason given for wanting (repeated) CT scanning is to document the extent of infarction as an aid to evaluation should a recurrent stroke occur in the future (Schneider *et al.* 1996).

Use of antiplatelet agents or anticoagulants

Antiplatelet agents are of established benefit in preventing fatal and non-fatal vascular events among patients with mild strokes and TIAs (Antiplatelet Trialists Collaboration 1994*b*). It is reasonable to expect that they should be prescribed for almost all stroke survivors. Anticoagulants are indicated in cases of atrial fibrillation (European Atrial Fibrillation Trial Study Group 1993) and will commonly be used in other cases where emboli from the heart are suspected (Cerebral Embolism Task Force 1989). One trial has demonstrated benefit from thrombolysis by tissue plasminogen activator (tPA) given within 3 hours of stroke onset (NINDS rt-PA Stroke Study Group 1995). In all these cases it is sensible to ensure that the stroke was not caused by a haemorrhage. Moreover, if haemorrhage occurs while the patient is being treated by antiplatelet or anticoagulant agents, stopping or reversing therapy may be beneficial. Thrombolytic therapy is certainly complicated by cerebral bleeds, and no one would contemplate such therapy if haemorrhage had not been ruled out. There is evidence from prevention and acute treatment trials that the incidence of cerebral haemorrhage is increased by aspirin, heparin, or warfarin therapy, but there is no direct epidemiological evidence supporting their avoidance in acute haemorrhagic stroke (nor is there likely to be). Low-dose heparin probably does not cause any increase in haemorrhagic transformation of infarcts (International Stroke Trial Collaborative Group 1997), but there are few data on its safety in primary intracerebral haemorrhage, nor whether a CT scan is required before instituting this treatment.

CT scanning would therefore appear to have diagnostic efficacy, and in most cases the results of the scan will influence treatment (therapeutic efficacy), but evidence is lacking on outcomes (are mortality and morbidity reduced by scanning?) and social efficacy (is it worth health services investing in scanners?). In this case, in most parts of the developed world and latterly in the UK, the need to ensure that secondary prevention is 'safe' by excluding patients with haemorrhage, has been sufficient to move towards a policy of CT scanning all acute stroke patients.

Accuracy of CT scans

The accuracy of a CT scan in diagnosing a stroke is given by its sensitivity and specificity, but a difficulty arises because, apart from an autopsy, the only suitable standard for comparison, cerebral angiography, is risky. Comparisons have been made with magnetic resonance imaging (MRI), but as this was developed after CT, studies have been aimed at validating MRI rather than CT. If a clinician diagnoses a stroke on history and examination, but nothing is seen on the CT scan, an estimate of the sensitivity (or false negative rate) can be made. In practice, false negative scans are common—around 20–40 per cent of all scans (Wade et al. 1985b)—and these are usually interpreted as representing cerebral infarcts (Oxfordshire Community Stroke Project 1985).

It is less likely that patients thought clinically not to have a stroke will be CT scanned, so reliable estimates of the specificity (or false positive rate) are difficult to obtain. Comparison with autopsy diagnosis has been tried (Toghi et al. 1981), but patients undergoing both a CT scan and an autopsy are hardly typical of most patients suffering a stroke. The major determinant of whether the CT scan will pick up a stroke is the size of the lesion. Small lesions are more often missed, leading to the low observed sensitivity, and it is easy to overinterpret a CT scan, leading to a false-positive diagnosis of stroke when nothing is found at autopsy (Toghi et al. 1981). Timing of the CT scan is critical, and unless the CT scan and autopsy are performed within a few days of each other, it is quite possible that a small CT lesion will have resolved, or be missed quite easily at autopsy, meaning that the autopsy is perhaps not as accurate as CT scanning in some cases.

Another approach has been to consider the 'final diagnosis' (based on clinical evidence, investigations, and clinical course) as the 'gold standard'. A Finnish study evaluated the diagnosis of stroke in 1191 patients who had CT scans (for any reason) over the course of 1 year. This group included patients with other neurological diseases, so there was the opportunity to estimate specificity. Sensitivity was 0.77 and specificity was 0.97, with a likelihood ratio of 26 (Sotaniemi et al. 1990). Scanners have improved technically over time, and can achieve greater resolution than they once could. It is likely that sensitivity has increased correspondingly.

Variations in interpretation

Variation in the interpretation of CT scans has been reported among patients with brain tumours (Swets *et al.* 1979) and stroke (Shinar *et al.* 1987). Although CT scans are often considered to be the 'gold standard' against which clinical and other investigations should be compared, it is worth remembering that interpretation of an image is subjective and consequently liable to observer variation. Variation should be less marked for examination of CT scans than for clinical history and examination (see Chapter 5) because two major sources of variation do not exist—the CT scans cannot vary, neither can the way in which the examination is performed.

When six neurologists were asked to report the CT scans of 17 patients, excellent agreement was achieved when the categories were grouped as 'normal', 'haemorrhage', 'infarct', and 'other'; all six agreed on 13 out of 17 scans, and five out of six neurologists agreed on three of the remaining four patients, with a kappa coefficient of 0.90, indicating a very high level of agreement (Shinar *et al.* 1987). However serious disagreement occurred on one scan, reported normal by five neurologists but the other saw a deep, large infarct. A further scan was also subject to disagreement, reported normal by four neurologists but two found deep, small infarcts. Aneurysms and arteriovenous malformations were detected on several occasions in the presence of both haemorrhages and infarcts.

When the neurologists were asked to describe the location of lesions, perhaps surprisingly they found on average two lesions per CT scan, which made working out agreement on location of lesion rather complicated. They could distinguish reasonably well whether a lesion was superficial, deep, in the cerebellum or extracerebral space, but more particular locations such as thalamus, operculum, and insula were not agreed upon at all well. The side of the main lesion, lesion density, mass effect, oedema, and lesion size were subject to moderate to poor agreement ($\kappa = 0.65$–0.34) (Shinar *et al.* 1987).

These neurologists tended to overinterpret the CT scans and this led to a glut of diagnoses, which in some cases might have resulted in more invasive investigations. It is clearly unwise to expect much agreement on the precise location of lesions, their size, and their effects (i.e. oedema, mass effect). The implication of this is that attempts to use such information for correlation with clinical presentation, symptoms, signs, and progress requires that either a single observer is used (and there is no published information on within-observer variation), or that more standardized criteria are used when reporting CT scans.

Wardlaw and Sellars (1993) tried to improve matters by introducing a structured reporting system for infarcts on CT scans, and then tested its reliability. Two experienced neuroradiologists achieved reliability which was good ($\kappa = 0.78$) for site and size (but better for large than small infarcts), excellent (κ = 0.80) for swelling, and fair (κ = 0.30) for haemorrhagic transformation (better for haematomas than petechial haemorrhage). This was reasonably well replicated when six junior general radiologists' opinions were compared with those of their consultants.

The value of CT scanning

The value of any investigation can be assessed in three main ways: the proportion of altered diagnoses; the proportion of patients whose management is changed; and finally the number of lives saved or disability prevented. Since a major emphasis in medicine is the art of diagnosis, it is possible to overvalue the importance of altered diagnoses. CT scanning makes a relatively small contribution to diagnosis of stroke from other conditions that mimic it. Its main use is in characterizing mass lesions such as subdural haematoma, primary and secondary neoplasms, and abscesses.

Altered diagnoses

The Oxfordshire Community Stroke Project (Sandercock *et al.* 1985a) has provided some of the best data on the diagnostic changes produced by a policy of universal CT scanning of stroke patients. Only patients with a first stroke were included in this study, and 89 per cent were seen by a neurologist early in the course of the illness. Only 5 (1.5 per cent) out of 325 patients turned out to have unsuspected non-vascular pathology. In two patients this was a subdural haematoma, but only one was treated surgically and the other was not because of her age (86 years) and general condition. Two patients with gliomas both died.

The amount of unsuspected non-vascular pathology found may in part reflect the clinical skills of doctors, and the source of the patients studied. In the Oxford study, primary-care doctors referred 736 patients as suitable for the study, of whom only 325 (44 per cent) were considered to have suffered a first stroke by the neurologist, who was able to pick out clinically 16 of the 21 patients with space-occupying lesions. Allen's series of patients (1983) included 9 (5 per cent) out of 174 found to have non-vascular pathology. An early American series (Weisberg and Nice 1977) found that 18 (20 per cent) out of 90 patients had tumours or subdural haematomas. Older patients might be expected to have a higher risk of non-vascular pathology, but among 79 patients aged 65 to 97 years, admitted to hospital, only one astrocytoma was detected (O'Brien *et al.* 1987). Clinical history taking and examination are of value in distinguishing strokes from non-vascular pathology.

Altered management

Clinicians might value knowing the 'true' diagnosis, or ruling out a particular diagnosis. The value of this increased certainty can be measured in terms of its impact on changes in management. For example, if a CT scan shows a massive cerebral infarct in a patient with impaired consciousness then further investigations to establish the cause of unconsciousness will not be necessary and intensive treatment, such as ventilation, might not be started. The effects on management can considered under several headings: antiplatelet agents, anticoagulants, surgery, palliative treatments (e.g. dexamethasone, radio-therapy, hospice care).

Antiplatelet agents   In the Oxford study 11 (3 per cent) of 325 patients were on aspirin at the time of their stroke (Sandercock *et al.* 1985a). One patient had had a cerebral haemorrhage and aspirin was therefore stopped, and seven had no evidence of haemorrhage and treatment was continued. The remaining three were not scanned and it is not clear what happened to their treatment. Presumably most of the 119 patients (37 per cent) with CT-scan-proven cerebral infarcts would be eligible for treatment with aspirin and could be started on it safely (provided they survived the stroke and had no contraindication to its use). The 106 (33 per cent) patients with a CT scan that showed no lesion or only atrophy may be classified as thrombo-embolic strokes (as the Oxford group did), but this prejudges the issue. It is possible that they may have suffered small haemorrhages which had resolved by the time a CT scan was performed. The safety of giving aspirin to such patients remains in some doubt. The 29 patients who had a haemorrhage can be assumed to have benefited by not being prescribed aspirin.

Two more recent series are worth citing for comparison. Both were hospital-based, but in countries where a high proportion of stroke patients are admitted. A Swedish study CT scanned all their patients, twice if possible, and half also had MRI. Twenty-eight of 228 patients (12 per cent) had an intra-cerebral haemorrhage. Within 2 weeks, a scan showed an infarct in 82 per cent of patients with total anterior circulation stroke, 74 per cent with partial anterior circulation stroke, 70 per cent of lacunar strokes, and 50 per cent of posterior circulation strokes. MRI increased these figures by 5–10 per cent (Lindgren *et al.* 1994a). The Lausanne Study identified a symptomatic infarct in 82 per cent of their patients, and haemorrhages in 11 per cent (Bogousslavsky *et al.* 1988). The greater proportion of scans with positive diagnoses reflects the newer equipment used compared with the Oxford study, and the use of repeated scans when the first scan was normal. Management of the great majority of patients in these studies can be assumed to have been influenced by their scans on the basis of use or avoidance of antiplatelet drugs.

Anticoagulants   Anticoagulants are now well established as secondary prevention for patients who have suffered a stroke and have atrial fibrillation, and no contraindication to long-term anticoagulation. CT scanning is required to exclude haemorrhage. The Oxford study found that 46 patients

(14 per cent) had atrial fibrillation; two had cerebral haemorrhages and one a haemorrhagic infarct, 11 were not investigated, and haemorrhagic lesions were found at autopsy in a further three patients. CT scanning thus showed that anticoagulant treatment was potentially unsafe in 3–14 patients (i.e. 6–30 per cent) in atrial fibrillation.

Surgery   Evacuation of a cerebellar haematoma can be considered provided an early diagnosis is made. The Oxford study detected only one patient with a cerebellar haematoma during life out of five that occurred in their series. This patient was not offered surgery.

Carotid endarterectomy is of benefit in patients with minor stroke or TIA with an ipsilateral severe carotid stenosis (see Chapter 11). The Oxford study found 19 (6 per cent) patients that were potentially eligible for this operation. CT scanning showed that two of them had had cerebral haemorrhages and they were not therefore investigated as a prelude to surgery.

Evacuation of subdural haematomas and excision of accessible meningiomas are of benefit to some patients. Although the Oxford study detected two patients with subdural haematomas, only one was operated on, with a successful outcome. The results of surgery for subdural haematoma are probably age dependent with a trend for 'conservative' management to be given to patients in their 80s, thus reducing the value of making this diagnosis, especially in very old and frail patients.

Palliative treatment   Only two patients (0.6 per cent) with unsuspected primary brain tumours were discovered in the Oxford study. The CT scan led to a change in their management in that they were given dexamethasone, and presumably attempts at rehabilitation were stopped. Both died.

Lives saved and disability prevented

On this measure of the value of CT scanning, the following might be included: the patient with a successfully treated subdural haematoma; the three patients with atrial fibrillation and cerebral haemorrhage who might have died or got worse if they had been anticoagulated; the two patients with cerebral haemorrhage who might have had a risky angiogram to define their suitability for carotid endarterectomy; and the 29 patients who avoided antiplatelet drugs because of cerebral haemorrhage. So up to 35 patients out of 325 (11 per cent) considered in the Oxford study benefited from CT scanning in terms of either lives saved or disability prevented, or possible risks avoided.

Clinical decision tree analysis

Since evaluating all this information is difficult to do in your head, an alternative approach to working out how to use an investigation is to construct a clinical decision tree. The usefulness of a test depends on its accuracy (i.e. sensitivity and specificity), the frequency of outcomes of interest, and also on the value placed on the information obtained. Figure 6.1 shows a simple decision tree for use of a CT scan to detect non-vascular pathology. The first step is to describe the possible outcomes of doing a CT scan: diagnosis of stroke made; diagnosis of non-vascular pathology, untreatable; diagnosis of non-vascular pathology, treatable. The possible consequences of not doing a CT scan must also be defined: definite stroke diagnosis not made; untreatable non-vascular pathology missed; treatable non-vascular pathology missed. Each of these outcomes must be assigned some value or, technically speaking, a 'utility'. Each outcome of investigation with CT scanning has a different value; but what value? Readers might care to rank the outcomes from worst to best in an effort to decide on their own values. In general, to miss a potentially treatable diagnosis is bad, and in the example shown has been given a score (or utility) of zero. The best outcome might be to make a diagnosis where there is at least a possibility of surgery leading to complete recovery; this has been given a value of 1.0. From the point of view of detecting and treating non-vascular pathology the other outcomes seem to have little to choose between them and have been given a utility of 0.5. Note that utilities, like probabilities, take values from 0 to 1. Readers may disagree with the values given and can try out the effect of substituting different values for the utility of each outcome.

It is then necessary to use the information on the occurrence of non-vascular pathology to work out the probability of the different outcomes occurring. For example, there is a 98 per cent probability that a stroke will be found on CT scanning and an approximately 2 per cent chance that non-vascular pathology will be found, half of which may be treatable. Similarly, the same probabilities of non-vascular pathology will apply to those stroke patients who do not have a CT scan. Let us assume that the sensitivity and specificity for detection of non-vascular pathology scan by CT are both 100 per cent, which avoids complicating the issue by false positives and negatives which will occur in practice.

The overall value (or utility) of doing a CT scan is then calculated by working backwards from the utilities applied to the different outcomes, which are multiplied by their frequency of occurrence. Thus, making a diagnosis of stroke is useful and has been given a utility of 0.5 and this applies to 98 per cent of scans conducted, resulting in $0.5 \times 0.98 = 0.49$, which is added to the utilities of the other branches (i.e. $0.5 \times 0.01 + 1 \times 0.01$) giving an overall utility of 0.51, shown in Fig. 6.1.

The decision not to do a CT scan gives a utility of 0.50. The figures are very close, so the overall picture is neither for nor against doing a CT scan on every stroke patient, if the main purpose is to diagnose and treat non-vascular pathology. Indeed, if a branch is included for the later diagnosis of some non-vascular pathology which becomes clinically obvious, then the utility of not doing a CT scan will rise. If value is given to the 'usefulness' of a positive

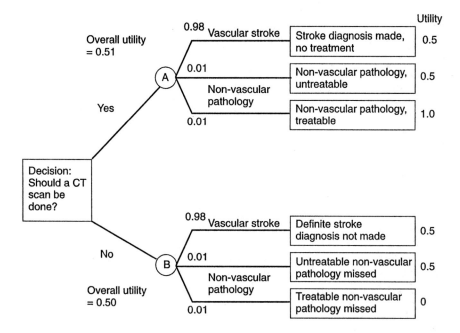

Fig. 6.1 Decision analysis examining the utility of performing a CT scan for the purpose of detecting non-vascular pathology.

diagnosis even when there is no treatment, the overall utility of doing a CT scan will rise.

Alternatively, life expectation after CT scanning could be used as the measure of outcome. In this case the detection of treatable non-vascular pathology (i.e. subdural haematoma, meningioma) would be awarded the full life expectation (assuming negligible surgical mortality) at the average age of onset of the stroke. Life expectations can be obtained from life tables; the expectation for a 70-year-old is around 15 years. The life expectation for a patient suffering a stroke is about 5 years. If these life expectations are used instead of the arbitrary measures of utility, and it is assumed that half non-vascular pathology is treatable, doing a CT scan for a patient will 'buy' 5.05 years of life, and not doing a CT scan will produce 4.9 years.

The value of a year of handicapped life compared with a year of normal life could be weighted to give a more refined comparison of the decision to do or not do a CT scan. The principles would be the same.

Aspirin for every stroke patient?

The beneficial effects of aspirin in secondary stroke prevention must be taken into account (Antiplatelet Triallists Collaboration 1994*b*), and it has been suggested that every patient considered for antiplatelet treatment after stroke should have a CT scan to exclude a cerebral haemorrhage (Consensus Conference 1988). It is argued that without CT scanning it would not be safe to give aspirin because patients with haemorrhagic lesions might get worse. Decision trees can be used to quantify the utility (or increased value) of the information that thrombo-embolic strokes are potentially treatable. A second decision tree is shown in Fig. 6.2. The utilities used are again arbitrary, but it is unlikely that there would be great disagreement on their rank ordering. The decision to do a CT scan is rewarded with a far higher overall utility (0.87) than not doing a CT scan (0.50), largely because the 80 per cent of diagnoses of thrombo-embolic stroke are of greater value now that a treatment is available (assuming that it would be unsafe to give aspirin without scanning first).

The whole process can be made much more sophisticated by introducing estimates of recurrence rates, strokes, and deaths avoided by aspirin treatment, and patients harmed by being given aspirin after a haemorrhage. In the UK, with 100 000 first strokes per year, a policy of universal scanning might be expected to prevent 285 non-fatal recurrent strokes and 142 deaths per year, along with 540 successfully treated cerebellar haematomas and other non-vascular pathology. An alternative policy of treating all 1-month survivors with aspirin would marginally increase the number of ischaemic strokes and stroke deaths prevented, but as well as the patients who suffered missed surgically treatable pathology, would result in 3300 patients who had had haemorrhages being treated with aspirin. If 2 per cent (66) of these are harmed per year by aspirin treatment, the small benefit is reversed, but the difference is still fairly small. A policy of universal CT scanning is therefore supported in terms of patient outcomes, but scanning is much more useful in terms of diagnostic, diagnostic thinking, and therapeutic efficacy.

Magnetic resonance imaging (MRI)

This modality has excellent technical efficacy for imaging the brain. In general MRI is more expensive, slower, and more prone to failure because of movement or claustrophobia than CT, but the technology is changing rapidly, and fast scan times are now possible. Moreover, in acute stroke, CT is more sensitive in the detection of haemorrhage, diagnosis of which is the prime objective of an early scan. MRI has the advantage of optional add-ons, such as diffusion- and perfusion-weighted images, and magnetic resonance angiography, which are emerging as useful research tools in acute stroke evaluation, with outstanding sensitivity, and the ability to age an ischaemic lesion and suggest where viable tissue remains (Koroshetz and Gonzalez 1997; Lutsep et al. 1997; Warach et al. 1997).

In many ways the evaluation of MRI has been more thorough than that of CT. Sensitivity for stroke diagnosis within 24 hours is excellent, and clearly

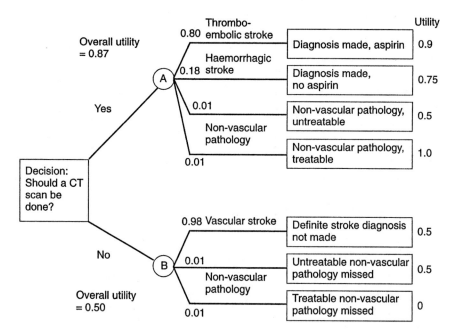

Fig. 6.2 Decision analysis examining the utility of performing a CT scan for the purpose of deciding on treatment with aspirin.

superior to CT (sensitivity, 0.82–0.92 (Kertesz *et al.* 1987; Bryan *et al.* 1991; Kenton *et al.* 1997); specificity, 0.92 (Bryan *et al.* 1991)), even for lacunar strokes where the sensitivity of CT is poor (sensitivity, 0.74–0.78 (Rothrock *et al.* 1987; Arboix *et al.* 1990)). Moreover, the subtlety of early CT scan changes makes inter-observer reliability less good (Bryan *et al.* 1991). After 48 hours the two techniques are about as sensitive as each other.

Some studies have examined the impact of MRI on clinical decision making. A Canadian group studied 116 patients who had both CT and MRI within 10 days of stroke onset (Shuaib *et al.* 1992). Localization of the stroke was superior on MRI in 9 of 39 patients with cerebral cortex lesions, and 23 of 25 with brainstem or cerebellar lesions. MRI demonstrated multiple infarcts in different territories, suggesting embolism, in 22 cases. Diagnosis was changed in 16 per cent of cases after MRI, and management was changed in 19 per cent. This was mostly to commence anticoagulation, but in one case, anticoagulation was discontinued (when an aneurysm was identified). In 10 per cent a precise vascular aetiology was clear after MRI (carotid or vertebral occlusion, one case of carotid dissection). In 14 per cent the diagnosis of ischaemic stroke was clinically unsuspected. A diagnosis of infarction was refuted by MRI in 2 per cent, as was a CT diagnosis of venous thrombosis (thereby avoiding angiography). The scale of these benefits is a little surprising, and the work needs to be replicated. It remains unclear whether any benefit in outcome resulted from the additional scanning and anticoagulation. A British study of the usefulness of MRI requests (for all diagnoses) reported a change of diagnosis in 20 per cent of cases, increased confidence in the diagnosis in 30 per cent, and change of management in 27 per cent. Consultants' reasons for requesting scans were to increase accuracy in the identification (47 per cent), location (5 per cent), and quantification (14 per cent) of disease. Diagnostic, work up, and therapeutic efficacy were confirmed, but at a moderately high financial cost. The investigators measured quality of life before and after the scan, and found that it fell slightly, but this is impossible to interpret in the absence of a control group who did not have an MRI scan, so we are unable to comment on outcomes efficacy (Szczepura et al. 1991).

A more ambitious study sought to quantify changes in doctors' diagnostic thinking resulting from an MRI result in a range of neurological diseases (Hirsch et al. 1996). The investigators estimated the likelihood ratio directly, by asking doctors to guess the probability of each of their differential diagnoses before and after the MRI. This is no easy task, and will have entailed considerable measurement error. In 76 per cent of cases the probability of the presumed diagnosis changed. MRI shifted the doctors' estimates towards more certainty, either confirming a diagnosis or ruling it out. The likelihood ratio was greater than 100 in 26 per cent of cases, and was greater than 10 in a further 5 per cent. Twenty-four per cent thought that the MRI changed diagnostic thinking, mostly preventing the need for further tests. As expected, the test was most useful where there was greatest diagnostic uncertainty (probabilities of 0.25–0.75). Change of therapy resulted in 34 per cent, and 47 per cent claimed that prognosis had changed. This study is interesting for having attempted to quantify several higher levels of investigational efficacy, but is open to the criticism that doctors ordering tests are likely to try to justify themselves when questioned.

Other investigations

Investigation of stroke patients should be aimed at detecting those patients with non-vascular pathology, those with unusual causes of stroke, possibilities for secondary prevention, and assessing co-morbidity. The Oxfordshire Community Stroke Project reported that only 4 per cent of 244 patients with an apparent first stroke turned out to have non-atheromatous, non-embolic causes for their symptoms and signs (Sandercock et al. 1989). A further 105 had no discernible cause for their stroke, but the majority of patients had risk factors: hypertension (52 per cent), co-existing ischaemic heart disease (38 per cent), diabetes (10 per cent), and a past history of transient ischaemic attack

(14 per cent). The authors considered that a full blood count, erythrocyte sedimentation rate (ESR), blood glucose, urea and electrolytes, syphilis serology, chest radiography, and ECG should be sufficient to identify most patients with non-vascular pathology.

The routine ordering of chest radiographs after stroke has been questioned. In a hospital with a policy of universal CT head scanning of stroke patients, CT scan records were used to identify 435 consecutive cases. Eighty-six per cent of these patients had an admission chest radiograph, but 78 per cent of these were technically unsatisfactory (rotated or poor inspiration). Technical efficacy was therefore poor. Abnormalities were detected in 16 per cent, implying reasonable diagnostic efficacy. Review of clinical records revealed that isolated cardiomegaly and old TB changes (33 plus 6 cases) had no impact on management. Six cases had metastases on CT scan. One was already know to have a mass on chest radiographs, and one had a previous lobectomy. One hilar mass was only appreciated after the head scan result was available. One case of multiple metastases was newly diagnosed, a clinical diagnosis of pulmonary oedema was confirmed in seven cases, and aspiration pneumonia was confirmed in six cases. Therefore in 14 cases (3 per cent) management was supported or altered, only five of which (1.3 per cent) were not suspected clinically (therapeutic efficacy). The value to clinicians of a normal test was not quantified, but the authors suggested that in the absence of specific clinical indications, chest radiography is not warranted in acute stroke (Sagar et al. 1996).

Echocardiography is often used to identify potentially cardioembolic sources for stroke, including left atrial and left ventricular thrombus, mitral stenosis, vegetations in endocarditis, atrial myxoma, patent foramen ovale, and aortic arch atheroma. Trans-oesphageal echocardiography has exceptional sensitivity for most of these diagnoses, approaching 100 per cent and about twice that of trans-thoracic echocardiography (good diagnostic efficacy) (Manning 1997). The problem is low specificity for identifying lesions that have caused (or will cause) emboli rather than cardiac lesions per se. For example, the 'diagnostic yield' of trans-oesophageal echocardiography after stroke is around 50 per cent. However, a study of people who had no history of stroke, found 46 per cent to have abnormalities, rising to 75 per cent in people aged over 75 (Lindgren et al. 1994b). Although these cardiac lesions might explain some of the increased stroke risk at this age, it is quite possible that they are merely 'passengers' and of no pathological significance. Current work is using trans-cranial Doppler to identify which cardiac lesions are associated with evidence of embolization into the carotid circulation (Markus et al. 1995; Molloy and Markus 1996; Ringelstein et al. 1998). As yet, there are no therapeutic trials of aspirin or warfarin based on echocardiographic or trans-cranial Doppler findings, which would provide evidence of therapeutic efficacy.

Investigation of the carotid arteries

The indications for, and effectiveness of, carotid endarterectomy are now well established (North American Symptomatic Carotid Endarterectomy Trial Collaborators 1991; European Carotid Surgery Triallists 1998). There is a need to define which patients to investigate further and how. The objective is to identify symptomatic, severely stenosed carotid arteries. Clearly, any investigation strategy is unwarranted if the patient does not want surgery, is not fit for major surgery, if the stroke aetiology is a bleed, or if available technical skill is limited, with surgical mortality and morbidity above about 5 per cent.

Non-invasive assessments

The OCSP clinical classification (together with CT scan or MRI) gives a reasonable guide to pathology and risk of recurrence, which should aid investigation strategy (see Chapters 4 and 13). Posterior circulation strokes are unlikely to represent symptomatic carotid disease, and these patients' carotid arteries need not be investigated. Lacunar strokes are generally due to small-vessel disease, but some are considered to be embolic or due to middle cerebral artery occlusion, and as the accuracy (sensitivity and specificity) of this diagnosis is the poorest of all the four clinical subtypes (Lindgren et al. 1994a; Wardlaw et al. 1996), a case can be made for further investigation. The prognosis in total anterior circulation strokes is so poor that carotid endarterectomy is unlikely to be considered unless a reasonable recovery is made.

The main clinical groups in whom arterial imaging should be considered are those with ipsilateral carotid territory transient ischaemic attack (or transient monocular blindness), and those with partial anterior circulation strokes, in whom recovery is good and recurrence frequent.

Stenosed carotid arteries might be expected to give rise to a bruit. The between-observer agreement on the presence of a significant cervical bruit is low, and might easily occur by chance (Chikos et al. 1983). The accuracy of a cervical bruit in detecting significant (> 75 per cent) stenosis is also very low, with both false positives and negatives, and a likelihood ratio of about 3 (Hankey and Warlow 1990). Clinical examination is unreliable and remains part of the ritual but should not be used to decide on the need for further investigation.

Use of duplex Doppler ultrasound is very widespread (Beech et al. 1996), but the test has limited sensitivity and specificity compared with angiography. For detecting 70–99 per cent stenoses, sensitivity is 0.71–0.93 and specificity 0.78–0.82. The likelihood ratio for a positive test is between 4 and 8, and between 0.09 and 0.32 for a negative test (Mittl et al. 1994; Kent et al. 1995; Srinivasan et al. 1995). Sensitivity for detecting a (non-operable) complete occlusion is good, but not perfect (about 0.92). The probability of a treatable carotid lesion in patients with carotid TIAs is around 20 per cent (Hankey and Warlow 1990). A positive ultrasound study will therefore lead to an increase in the probability of the patient having a treatable lesion to 50–67 per cent (i.e. odds × likelihood ratio; see Chapter 4), or a probability of having operable disease of 25–53 per cent if the ultrasound shows stenosis of less than 70 per cent. One study reported a negative predictive value of 0.90, implying that only 10 per cent of operable lesions were missed, but this figure will have been dependent on the prevalence of disease in the study population (Mittl *et al.* 1994). The accuracy of duplex scanning is very operator dependent, and the published data are likely to represent better than average performance.

A policy of evaluation by duplex alone will help to avoid carotid angiography in patients with negative results if it is accepted that over a quarter of these patients may have treatable lesions that will be missed. The proportion of false negatives can be reduced by considering angiography for patients with a lower degree of duplex-defined stenosis, say 50 per cent. Those with a positive result will then require carotid angiography to decide whether a potentially operable lesion is really present. The cost is more angiograms and more angiogram-related morbidity.

Carotid angiography

Carotid angiography has probably become more accurate with digital subtraction techniques, but reported estimates (compared with operative findings) of sensitivity and specificity in detection of ulceration are only 73 per cent and 63 per cent, a likelihood ratio of 1.97 (Chikos *et al.* 1983). Detection of stenosis is probably more accurate, although patients considered to have no ulceration or less than 50 per cent stenosis on angiography were (even prior to 1983) very unlikely to be operated on, and consequently the correlation with operative findings in these patients cannot be made. Certainly a positive carotid angiogram (i.e. 50 per cent or greater stenosis and/or ulceration) will increase the probability that an operable lesion is truly present to at least 90 per cent.

Carotid angiograms are subject to disagreement in their interpretation even when broad groups (such as 0–29 per cent, 30–69 per cent, 70–99 per cent, and 100 per cent stenosis) are used. Matters are not improved by the use of three different methods for calculating severity of stenosis, which, fortunately, are reasonably readily interconverted (Rothwell *et al.* 1994a). Kappa for inter-rater reliability (categorized mild, moderate, or severe) was 0.66–0.76, depending on the method. The standard deviation of differences in estimates of severity between observers varied from about 15 per cent for mild stenoses, to about 5 per cent for severe (70–99 per cent) stenoses. By definition 95 per cent of disagreements can be expected to be within two standard deviations either way, so the range of uncertainty is considerable (Rothwell *et al.* 1994*b*; Gagne *et al.* 1996). Consequently, a stenosis said to be 50 per cent by one radiologist could be assessed the next day by another radiologist as 70 per cent (and therefore requiring surgery) but be within the limits of disagreement between observers. Such wide between-observer variation is worrying and suggests that greater efforts in standardization of procedures are required (Young *et al.* 1996).

A further problem with conventional angiography is procedure-related morbidity. Some 4 per cent of subjects will experience neurological symptoms, and in 1 per cent these will be permanent. Risks are greater in those with tighter stenoses (Hankey *et al.* 1990*a*, *b*). Having been used as the basis for definitive treatment trials, however, it will remain the gold standard investigation until non-invasive methods are sufficiently developed to supersede it.

Magnetic resonance (MRA) and computed tomography angiography (CTA)

These newer techniques are of interest because they raise the hope that conventional angiography can be avoided (Ruggieri *et al.* 1992). MRA has the advantage of not requiring contrast injection, imaging the intracranial vessels, and can be performed as a short extension to MRI. However, up to 10 per cent of patients cannot tolerate MRA because of restlessness (Kenton *et al.* 1997). With current methods MRA is at least as good as duplex ultrasonography (sensitivity, 0.92; specificity, 0.75; compared with conventional angiography). Inter-observer reliability is excellent (k = 0.91; Bowen *et al.* 1994; Mittl *et al.* 1994; Kent *et al.* 1995; Vanninen *et al.* 1996). Technical and diagnostic efficacy are generally considered to be not yet sufficient to enable MRA to supersede conventional angiography, and access to MRA is still limited. CT angiography requires the use of contrast injection, and is less well evaluated (Knauth *et al.* 1997; Shrier *et al.* 1997).

A comparison of different investigation strategies (ultrasound alone, MRA alone, carotid angiography alone, or ultrasound and MRA with angiography in doubtful cases) for deciding on the need for carotid endarterectomy, using a decision analysis, has been reported (Kent *et al.* 1995). This showed that the combination strategy was the most cost-effective in terms of quality adjusted life years gained, although the differences between the different options were quite small. This work suggests that it may be reasonable to limit the use of angiography where MRI is available and duplex accuracy is known to be good.

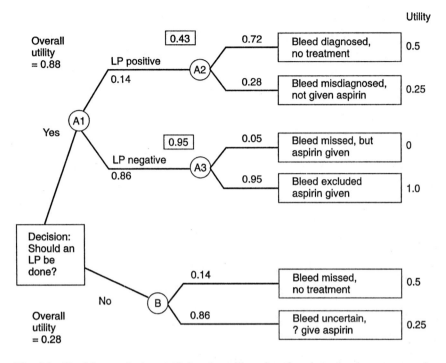

Fig. 6.3 Decision analysis examining the utility of performing a lumbar puncture for the purpose of deciding on treatment with aspirin.

Lumbar puncture

Lumbar puncture has two main uses: first to diagnose infection (meningitis, syphilis) in patients who may present with signs suggestive of a stroke; secondly, to distinguish subarachnoid haemorrhage and primary intracerebral haemorrhage from a cerebral infarction. With the advent of CT scanning, and because of the danger of tentorial herniation following lumbar puncture in patients with unsuspected mass lesions, this latter indication has fallen into disuse.

With increased interest in the use of antiplatelet agents after minor thrombotic strokes, the use of lumbar puncture to exclude cerebral haemorrhage might be thought helpful in centres without access to CT scanning, since it has a high specificity and variable sensitivity, ranging from 72 to 90 per cent (Harrison 1980; Britton *et al.* 1983). It is possible to construct a decision tree for the use of lumbar puncture in deciding which patients to treat with aspirin, as shown in Fig. 6.3. At circle A1, the probability of a positive result (i.e. haemorrhagic or xanthochromic tap) is 14 per cent, and of a negative result, 86 per cent. The circle A2 shows the true positive probability (i.e. the sensitivity, which is 72 per cent), and the false positive probability (i.e. 1 − sensitivity). At circle A3, the true negative probability (i.e. the specificity, which is 95 per cent) and false negative probability are used. Once again arbitrary utilities are used to calculate the overall utility of either decision. The balance is clearly in favour of doing a lumbar puncture. The tree could be made more complicated by including the small risk of coning, which is probably less than 1 in 1000 and may actually be balanced by the small benefit of diagnosing unsuspected meningitis or neurosyphilis.

The decision tree favours doing a lumbar puncture largely because of the high probability that a clear CSF will be found which will lead to the possibility of treatment with aspirin, but a very small chance of treating a haemorrhagic stroke with aspirin inadvertently. The practical problems with such a policy would need to be examined before it could be recommended. For example, if prophylactic subcutaneous heparin is given to stroke patients, there is a risk of developing a haematoma around the lumbar puncture site which may lead to cord compression and paraplegia (Ruff and Dougherty 1981).

Summary

1. The efficacy of investigations can be thought of at several different levels, including technical efficacy, diagnostic efficacy, therapeutic efficacy, and patients' health status outcomes.
2. The currently recommended criteria for performing a CT scan are for patients with an atypical clinical course, young patients, where there is diagnostic doubt, and when antiplatelet or anticoagulant therapy is to be started. This includes most stroke patients who are not moribund.
3. Clinical decision trees may be a useful adjunct to weighing the risks and benefits of particular courses of action. CT scanning for all patients is supported by its greater overall utility. Interestingly, lumbar puncture is also supported by decision analysis.
4. Newer imaging modalities such as MRI offer outstanding technical efficacy (nice pictures), and have also been shown to be useful in clinical diagnosis and management, but not in altering outcomes.

7 Severity

Is it a bad stroke?

The severity of disease can be described in many different ways, ranging from the patient's perception, the amount of physiological disturbance, and the consequent disability and handicap caused, to the burden for society (Stein *et al.* 1987). The severity of a stroke may be assessed in terms of the amount of brain damaged (e.g. size of the lesion found on CT), the extent of any arterial lesion(s) demonstrated on angiography, or the function of the brain (by positron emission tomography (PET) scanning, or presence of symptoms and signs of decompensation). Alternatively, the severity of a stroke may be measured by the distance walked in a fixed time, the ability to climb stairs, or the ability for self-care. From a social perspective, severity may be measured by impact on work, enjoyment of usual sex life, and social engagement. The pathological differences between types of stroke and the alternative ways of assessing severity make a simple answer to the question 'Is it a bad stroke?' difficult.

Impairment, disability, and handicap

A useful model that has gained wide support is the World Health Organization's *Classification of Impairments, Disabilities and Handicaps* (World Health Organization 1980). Although it is tempting to consider that a linear relationship exists between each level of markers of severity (e.g. motor impairment leads to difficulty walking outdoors, which in turn leads to the handicap of not being able to meet friends), in practice it is much more likely that many factors, such as personality, intelligence, and wealth will operate to either reduce or increase the impact of disease.

Figure 7.1 shows that impairments due to stroke may lead to disability and handicap, but it is possible for impairments to lead to handicap without disability intervening. For example, a stroke may resolve leaving no disability but leads to the loss of livelihood—a severe handicap—because the patient's

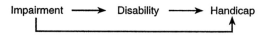
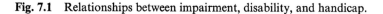

Fig. 7.1 Relationships between impairment, disability, and handicap.

driving licence is taken away. Similarly, some impairments may cause disability but no apparent handicap. In this case, a stroke may lead to poor balance, causing difficulty climbing stairs—a disability, but the provision of a stair lift permits the patient to continue leading the same sort of life as before the stroke occurred. Not all impairments lead to disability or handicap. An upper quadrantic visual field loss would lead to no disability or handicap for most patients, but in a keen squash player is a disastrous handicap. Finally, patients may suffer with disabilities and handicaps that are due to other pathological processes, unrelated to the stroke.

The impairments, disability, handicap model is not a complete description of the effects of a disease. It ignores the burden of disease on the family and society and requires the concept of impairment to be widened to accommodate the concept of biological (i.e. anatomical, physiological, and psychological) severity. The biological severity and degree of impairment caused by a stroke are not terribly useful indicators of severity because no one single marker (e.g. analogous to staging for cancer) exists that covers the spectrum of conditions that can result from a stroke. Furthermore, multiple problems which are common amongst older stroke patients cannot be accommodated.

Reasons for measuring severity

Prediction

The heart of the question 'Is it a bad stroke?' is to do with prognosis of individual patients. The question can be re-phrased as 'Which biological features, impairments, disabilities, and handicaps lead to good and bad outcomes?' The relationship between indicators of severity and outcome is confused because often the outcome of interest (e.g. ability to walk or use an affected arm, return home, time spent in hospital, survival) may also be used as a measure of severity. A useful approach to this question is to consider severity at different points in the natural history of the stroke. At onset, prediction of early survival (say, to 1 month) is of importance, together with the likely length of time in hospital. The best indicators of survival at onset are the level of consciousness over the first 24 hours, urinary incontinence persisting for a week, gaze paresis, and impairment of swallowing (see Part 4). Predictors of discharge by 1 month at the onset of stroke include the degree of arm and leg weakness, conscious level, continence of urine, and age (Barer and Mitchell 1989).

Later on, different clinical features of severity are likely to be more important because of the deaths of the most severely affected patients. In a series of patients included in a trial (and therefore not truly representative of all stroke patients admitted to hospital), mobility, age, dressing ability, continence of urine, and power in the affected limbs assessed at 1 month all contributed to prediction of discharge at 3 months (Barer and Mitchell 1989). In a more representative series, it is probable that pre-stroke ability and cognitive impairments would also have an impact on early discharge.

A point that deserves emphasis, is that no matter how many severity indicators are measured, prediction is not sufficiently accurate to determine management of an individual patient. Measurements made at onset of the stroke will correctly predict 1-month survival or discharge from hospital in two-thirds to three-quarters of cases. The rest will be wrongly assumed to have a poor prognosis. As time passes, the accuracy of prediction improves, so that by 1 month measures of severity will correctly predict discharge from hospital by 3 and 6 months in four-fifths of cases (Barer and Mitchell 1989). None the less, it is not possible with present severity indicators to give clinical guidance about which patients should receive rehabilitation and which patients should be resettled in institutions. The best that can be done is to continue with rehabilitation efforts in all survivors until it is self-evident that a good outcome will not be achieved.

An important goal is to measure the extent to which rehabilitation does or does not improve disability and reduce complications of stroke among patients who turn out to require institutional care. It may be argued that resources are wasted on patients who stand no chance of achieving discharge from hospital, and without such evidence it will be difficult to support present customs of continued rehabilitation until the need for institutional care is obvious in the face of ever tighter financial constraints and limited rehabilitation resources.

The target for the future should be the development of severity measures that are reliable, easy to use, and predict important outcomes with much higher accuracy. It is vital that representative series of patients are used for this purpose, and that predictions are assessed in at least two independent series of patients to improve the validity of severity measurement. It would also be helpful if more clinically relevant groups (such as, alive at 3 months but severe weakness of limbs) of patients were analysed, rather than pooled analyses of consecutive series of patients.

Comparison

Indicators of severity are of use when making comparisons between groups. It is of great public interest to compare outcomes, such as mortality, between different hospitals, and is now part of British health services policy. The extent to which outcomes vary is determined to a large extent by the type of patients seen, and in particular by the severity of strokes suffered by patients. A severity measure can therefore be used as a control for any differences in the case mix treated in a particular place. The simplest way to apply this in practice is to make comparisons of outcome only between stroke patients suffering similar types of stroke. For example, if two hospitals had different 1-month death rates for stroke patients, the explanation might be that one hospital had developed a superior acute treatment strategy for stroke. An alternative explanation is that the treatments are identical, but that the severity of strokes seen at each place is different. To control for differences in severity, simple indicators are likely to be the only measures routinely available. In this case, comparisons of patients grouped by their conscious level on admission to hospital could be made. Any differences in 1-month death rates are then more likely to be due to differences in clinical practices in the two locations.

Targeting

A further use for simple measures of severity is in targeting of treatments. The concept of triage has been used successfully in a trial of a stroke unit to select patients likely to survive the acute stroke and require rehabilitation (Garraway *et al.* 1981). Triage requires a measure that can be applied rapidly and with reasonable accuracy so that decisions about treatment can be made quickly. In such cases level of consciousness is likely to be the best indicator to use. But even this apparently simple measure can be difficult to apply in practice. A patient who is drowsy on admission has impaired consciousness but may survive the acute phase. A patient who is deeply unconscious and unresponsive to painful stimuli is highly unlikely to survive the acute phase, and the decision to give supportive treatment, such as intravenous fluids and antibiotics, must be made with this knowledge. Whether supportive treatments given to unconscious patients result in longer survival in a disabled state is not known. However, because most early deaths are due to primary brain damage it is unlikely that supportive treatments have much impact on the natural history of the disease process.

Despite much information about prognosis and predictors of good and poor recovery (see Chapter 15), it is remarkably difficult to decide which patients should be given high levels of rehabilitation (or be treated on a stroke unit) early in the course of a stroke.

Selection of patients who will benefit most from rehabilitation is a desirable reason for targeting scarce resources. Such thinking clearly prejudges whether rehabilitation makes any difference to recovery, but given that these services exist (and evidence to support their use can be found, see Chapter 10), methods of selection are required because in many hospitals there are insufficient rehabilitation resources. There is an understandable tendency to put patients who stand a good chance of getting better onto stroke units because of the need to ensure a steady throughput of patients. This a self-fulfilling prophesy; patients selected for their chances of spontaneous recovery will tend to do well. Those not selected because of adverse prognostic signs will tend to do badly. Logically, rehabilitation resources should be directed at those patients who without further treatment will probably have a poor and limited recovery. Further research is needed to define who those patients are and their ability to benefit from rehabilitation.

Outcome

Severity may be an appropriate index of outcome for some interventions, particularly acute drug treatments which aim to reduce the consequences of the initial vascular process. In such cases, it is feasible that treatment will result in a reduction of patients categorized as suffering a severe stroke. However, this approach is likely to obscure treatment effects, as most severity indicators are too broad and therefore insensitive to change. Combining various variables that are good indicators of prognosis into an overall score and then measuring the difference in the score at entry into treatment trial and at a specified time after entry has been used successfully to assess the effects of acute treatment in stroke (Barer *et al.* 1988*b*). This has the effect of allowing for the disparate impairments caused by strokes but has the potential disadvantage of weighting improvements in limb power equally with improvements in speech, for example.

Impairments

A wide range of stroke severity scales has been developed for assessing patients entered into clinical trials (Tables 7.1, 7.2). In some cases, these scales are used explicitly to provide measures of outcome (Lyden and Lau 1991), whereas in other cases a more vague objective of 'evaluation of stroke patients at the acute stage' is given (Treves *et al.* 1994). These scales all share a common grounding in the clinical examination.

   In a useful review of these (and other) scales, substantial variation in inter-rater agreement for similar items was noted, suggesting that further work on standardizing methods of assessment is needed and that comparability between scales is limited (D'Olhaberriague *et al.* 1996). The selection of items for such severity scales is variable and there does not appear to be consensus among neurologists on what to include or exclude. For example, it is remark-able how little attention is given to identifying higher cortical impairments that may have major implications for communication and rehabilitation.

   A logical approach to selecting items for a severity scale is to examine the ability of items to predict outcomes such as mortality, disability, or depend-ency on others. Several investigators have examined the relationship between severity scales and outcomes (Weingarten *et al.* 1990; Gladman *et al.* 1992; De Haan *et al.* 1993). Single impairments (i.e. conscious level, urinary incon-tinence) performed as well as more complex multivariate scales in prediction

Table 7.1 Examples of stroke severity scales based on impairments

Full title	Abbreviation	Reference
Edinburgh Clinical Neurology Examination	Edinburgh exam	Lindley *et al.* (1993)
Stroke Data Bank	SDB	Shinar *et al.* (1985)
National Institutes of Health Stroke Scale (a)	NIHSS (a)	Brott *et al.* (1989a)
National Institutes of Health Stroke Scale (b)	NIHSS (b)	Goldstein *et al.* (1989)
Mathew Scale	Mathew scale	Gelmers *et al.* (1988b)
Canadian Neurological Scale	CNS	Cote *et al.* (1989)
Italian Stroke Scale	Italian scale	Tomasello *et al.* (1982)
Unified Neurological Scale	UNSS	Treves *et al.* (1994)
European Stroke Scale	ESS	Hantson *et al.* (1994)
Scandinavian Stroke Scale	SSS	Roden-Jullig *et al.* (1994)

Table 7.2 Stroke severity scales: items included (see Table 7.1 for abbreviations and references)

Sign	Edinburgh exam	SDB	NIHSS (a)	NIHSS (b)	Mathew scale	CNS	Italian scale	UNSS	ESS	SSS
Higher cortical impairments										
Language/dysphasia	+	+	+	+	+	−	−	−	−	+
Consciousness	+	+	+	+	+	+	−	+	+	+
Confusion	+	−	−	−	−	−	−	−	−	+
Orientation	−	−	−	−	+	+	−	+	−	+
Visuo-spatial function	+	−	−	−	−	−	−	−	−	−
Neglect	−	−	+	+	−	−	−	−	−	−
Power										
Weak arm, R/L	+	−	+	+	+	+	+	+	+	+
Weak hand	+	+	−	−	−	−	−	+	−	+
Weak leg, R/L	+	+	+	+	+	+	−	+	+	+
Weak face	+	+	+	+	+	+	−	+	+	+
Gait	−	−	−	−	−	−	−	−	−	+
Other signs										
Cerebellum	+	+	+	+	−	−	+	+	+	−
Speech/dysarthria	+	+	+	+	−	+	−	+	+	+
Cranial nerves	+		−	−	−	−	+	−	+	−
Pupillary responses	−	−	+	−	−	+	−	−	−	−
Hemianopia	+	+	+	+	+	−	+	−	+	−
Extraocular movements	+	+	+	+	+	−	−	+	+	+
Sensory loss (hand)	+	+	+	+	+	−	−	−	−	−
Reflexes	−	−	−	−	+	+	+	−	−	−
Babinski's sign	−	−	+	−	−	−	+	−	−	−
Tone	−	−	−	−	−	−	−	+	−	−
Neck bruit	−	+	−	−	−	−	+	−	−	−

+, Included; −, not included.

of outcomes, and these scales had only limited power to explain variation in disability outcomes.

Inevitably, the utility of a specific measurement must be related to its purpose. If the purpose is to measure outcomes following an acute treatment, the various severity scales that have been developed are of doubtful value. The scores are neither comprehensive in coverage, nor has sensitivity to change following stroke (or treatment of known efficacy) been documented. Interestingly, the relationship between stroke impairment scales and Barthel ADL Index, Oxford Handicap Scale, and a quality of life indicator (Sickness Impact Profile) showed that less than half (Barthel, 48 per cent, Oxford Handicap, 37 per cent; and SIP, 33 per cent) of the variation was explained by impairment scores (De Haan et al. 1993). Patients and health service commissioners are unlikely to be impressed by data on efficacy based on changes in a summed list of impairments, some of which are critical to successful independent life, some of which are irrelevant, and some of which may improve independently of any treatment.

If the main purpose is to make case-mix adjustments to outcomes found in trials (where randomization has not resulted in adequate balance between groups) or where observational data from routine sources are compared, the much simpler method of assessing conscious level appears to work just as well and is more likely to be recorded accurately.

Disability

Measures of disability, particularly activities of daily living scales, have gained in popularity as indicators of severity because of a notion that they form a common pathway through which the effects of several, diverse impairments, together with coexisting diseases, may express their combined effects. Disability measures can be seen as moving the focus from the level of cell or organ to the person, and are relevant to the aims of rehabilitation and of patients themselves. Moreover, organ- or system-specific disability scales, as well as general activities of daily living scales, can be used.

Disability measures have been thought suitable for a wide variety of purposes, including improving confidence in assessing disability, improving communication between professionals, improving identification of problems, and as a means of standardization of clinical methods (Wade and Collin 1988). In addition, disability measures of severity may be helpful when making comparisons between different diagnostic groups, for epidemiological and health care delivery studies, and to monitor progress clinically. However, even measures that are used widely suffer with problems that need to be overcome. Most scales suffer from 'ceiling' and 'floor' effects that lead to patients with more extreme severities of stroke to either score at the top or bottom of the scale, thus reducing sensitivity to change. Allied to this problem, most scales are not complete descriptors of activities of daily living and are made up of very low order activities.

In an attempt to increase the range of activities considered, the Nottingham extended activities of daily living scale was developed (Nouri and Lincoln 1987). However, none of the disability measures commonly used in stroke research and clinical practice cover the wide domains of disability conceptualized in the WHO Impairments, Disabilities, and Handicaps taxonomy. This classification identified 13 disability domains: locomotion, reaching and stretching, dexterity, seeing, hearing, personal care, continence, communication, behaviour, intellectual functioning, consciousness, eating–drinking–digesting, disfigurement. Many, if not all, of these are highly relevant to stroke patients and it is an interesting reflection on the research conducted over the past few decades, that so little attention has been given to domains other than mobility and self-care. The Office of Population, Censuses, and Surveys (now the Office for National Statistics) carried out important work producing a disability scale based on the WHO taxonomy, which was used in a national prevalence survey of disability in Britain (Martin *et al.* 1988). This disability scale has been compared with the Barthel ADL Index and shown to describe the full range of disability better (Wellwood *et al.* 1995). It deserves to be much more widely used in stroke research as it provides a more complete description of disability, is well validated, and has in-built utilities based on general population valuations which would be useful in cost-effectiveness analyses.

It is common for disability to be confused with dependency and for both to be mixed up with autonomy (Wilkin 1987). All three are useful concepts when thinking about stroke severity. Dependency, in contrast to disability, relates to the social context within which abilities are used. For example, many older men are dependent on others to wash their clothes and cook for them as these were (but no longer are) socially sanctioned gender-specific dependencies. These older men do not lack the ability to perform these tasks of washing, ironing, and cooking but they habitually do not do them. Autonomy refers to the control individuals have on their own lives: a very disabled person who cannot walk may be dependent on others to get around, but has complete autonomy in deciding where to go. These related concepts are vital to the proper assessment and management of stroke patients, who are often assumed to have no autonomy because of disability and dependency.

Handicap

Handicap is defined by the WHO as follows: 'In the context of health experience, a handicap is a disadvantage for a given individual, resulting from an impairment or disability, that limits or prevents the fulfilment of a role that is normal (depending on age, sex, social and cultural factors) for that individual'. Measuring handicap is concerned with estimating the *disadvan-*

tage associated with impairments and disabilities, whereas disability is concerned with the *performance of tasks*. It is possible for people to be very badly disabled (for example, paraplegic) but to suffer very little disadvantage because of the facilities, help, and other resources available to them, and the attitudes of those around them. Measures of handicap are potentially of greater value to patients, who need to minimize the effects of illness on their lives. Unfortunately, comparatively little effort has gone into this area, in part because of the diverse meanings of the term 'handicap', and the need to view handicap in terms of individuals and their immediate environment. In practice, much rehabilitation is properly concerned with reducing handicap, but because the tools of measurement are not well developed, it is remarkably difficult to demonstrate that much rehabilitation effort is worthwhile. Severity of handicap also suffers from the disadvantage of appearing rather a 'soft' measurement, and therefore even if improvements occur, it might be thought that they are due to subjective biases rather than real benefits.

The Oxford Handicap Scale was derived from the Rankin Scale (see Chapter 15), substituting the words 'interferes with life style' or 'restriction of life style' for 'disability' (UK-TIA Study group 1988; Bamford *et al.* 1989). It is unlikely that this scale represents a real advance over the original Rankin Scale, it only covers aspects of physical independence, but it does have the merit of simplicity.

An alternative, widely used approach to measuring handicap is the Frenchay Activities Index (Wade *et al.* 1985c). This is not based on the WHO definition of handicap but comprises some disability items (cooking, washing, housework, shopping) and some social engagement items (going to clubs, participation in games, car trips) and does not assess disadvantage due to stroke in a systematic or comprehensive way.

More recently, a new strand of research has focused on measurement of handicap using the WHO definition and dimensions of handicap (i.e. mobility, occupation, independence, social integration, orientation, and economic self-sufficiency). To develop a quantitative approach to measuring handicap, the London Handicap Scale (Harwood *et al.* 1994b,c) used the concept of utilities to assess the severity of descriptions of handicapped states (see Chapter 6). Utilities reflect preferences and values, and hence, disadvantage. While stroke patients' utilities could be used, in practice interviewing patients to obtain utilities is difficult. Of greater relevance to state-funded health care are utilities obtained from panels of 'judges' who are representative of the general population from whom stroke patients arise. The task is then simply to describe an individual's health status using the WHO dimensions and then apply a valuation of that health state obtained from the judges to derive a handicap score. An individual's true handicap determined in this way is similar to that obtained from a handicap score to the extent to which the individual's views and values coincide with those of the judges. While this is a serious assumption to make, evidence suggests that patients' and general public utilities do not differ much (Ebrahim *et al.* 1991). Furthermore, as the general public pay for health care in the UK, it can be argued that it is their views that are most relevant in determining the value to be placed on specific health states.

The London Handicap Scale has been assessed for validity and reliability and performs reasonably well. Concurrent validity has been demonstrated against the Oxford Handicap Scale, Barthel ADL Index, Nottingham extended ADL index, and Nottingham Health Profile. Factor analysis shows only one major component, which explained 60 per cent of the variance in scores, suggesting that the scale is measuring a single construct, related to but different from other aspects of the health experience of stroke patients.

Burden of illness

The burden of illness concept is of value in measuring the effects of different types of illness, can accommodate multiple problems in the same patient, can cope with the diversity of stroke, and can be measured in a variety of more objective ways. Indicators range from the financial cost of an episode of illness, the number of days in hospital, and the days of work lost, but can also include the emotional and social effects on the family. However, burden of illness indicators do not correlate directly with other measures of severity, particularly biological or impairment measures. For example, a stroke causing minimal motor paresis with early recovery may lead to a major burden of illness in some patients who embrace the sick role so completely that their families and work suffer. At the other extreme, a stroke damaging most of the brainstem of an elderly patient with no relatives may lead to a very rapid death which will cause a very small burden of illness to society.

Each of these levels of severity (biological/impairment, disability, handicap, burden of illness) is affected by other factors, which explain in part why the relationship between each step in the hierarchy is not direct. Figure 7.2 shows some of these factors.

It might be thought that severity measures are complicated enough, but whatever level or type of severity is considered, indicators are not likely to be dichotomous (i.e. severe, not severe) nor are they unidimensional. For example, the duration, treatability, prognosis, and intrinsic 'nastiness' of indicators of severity may all need to be considered, depending on the reasons for measurement. Moreover, severity is not a static attribute of an illness but changes with time, and methods of aggregating severity measures over time are needed. Ageing also has an impact on severity measures, as the same biological or disability level of severity will have different consequence and implications at different ages. Finally, it is important to be clear whose value systems are used to decide on which measurements of severity of stroke are

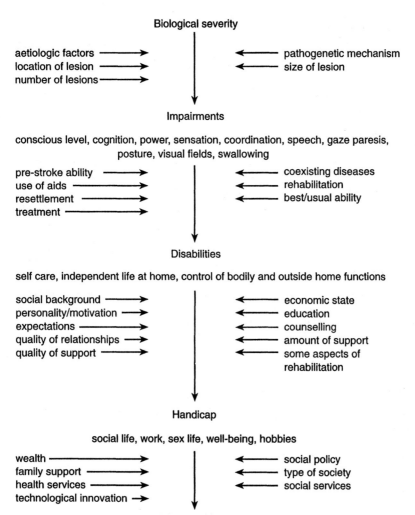

Fig. 7.2 The relationships between biological severity, impairment, disability, and handicap.

relevant. It should not be assumed that professional views of what is a severe or important illness are the same as the views of patients, relatives, or friends.

Summary

1. The severity of stroke may be measured in terms of its biological effects, the impairments, disabilities, handicaps, and burden on society that these produce.

2. Severity measurements may be used to predict outcome, the need for services, triage patients for management, and to permit better comparisons of the results of treatment.

3. Stroke severity scales are of limited value in assessing outcomes. Adjustment for differences in case-mix between groups is more simply done by use of conscious level alone.

4. Disability and handicap scales provide means of assessing stroke severity independent of underlying pathology. They can provide comprehensive and useful assessments of outcomes of stroke services, including acute treatments.

5. A severity measure is not a simple dichotomous variable (i.e. severe stroke versus not severe stroke). Several dimensions are involved (duration, treatability, associated symptoms, intrinsic 'nastiness'), and the relationship between them is not easily predictable.

6. Relationships between impairment, disability, and handicap are not linear or direct. Many factors have an influence on the severity of disease, and an understanding of these factors may provide new approaches to helping stroke patients.

PART 3 MANAGEMENT

- Prevention

- Acute treatments

- Rehabilitation

- Preventing recurrence

8 Prevention

Why prevent?

> It is better to be healthy than to be ill or dead. That is the beginning and the end of the only real argument for preventive medicine. It is sufficient.
> *(Rose 1992)*

The idea of prevention is attractive, but preventative interventions must still be judged by the same criteria as any others. They must be effective, affordable, acceptable, humane, accessible, and equitable. Indeed, the target population will be more or less healthy, so evaluation should be even more stringent than usual. The costs of prevention in terms of resources, time, inconvenience, and changes to life style must be carefully weighed against likely benefits. Failure to do this may lead to poor prioritization, and lack of understanding of important motivational factors will lead to poor compliance and reduced effectiveness.

The potential for prevention

Four strands of evidence suggest that much of the mortality and morbidity associated with stroke is preventable:

● variation in time and place, both between and within countries, implies that stroke risk is not immutable;
● observations that migrants adopt the risk of their host environment supports this;
● many personal characteristics, such as blood pressure, smoking, and physical activity, are associated with a gradient of stroke risk: the lower the risk factor, the lower the occurrence of stroke;
● experimental evidence from randomized controlled trials has demonstrated reductions in incidence of stroke following reduction of risk factors (e.g. blood pressure).

Evidence for prevention

Pathological evidence

One approach to prevention is to identify convincing mechanisms for the pathogenesis of stroke and intervene to reverse them. There is elegant anecdotal evidence that paradoxical embolism of venous thromboses, via a patent foramen ovale, to the cerebral arterial circulation, is a cause of strokes (Manning 1997; Cerebral Embolism Task Force 1989). Patent foramen ovale is relatively common, being found in approximately 20 per cent of post-mortem examinations. Should we seek to identify and close these defects surgically?

Similar arguments were, for many years, the main justification for performing carotid endarterectomies (Warlow 1984). The mechanism was convincing: carotid stenosis due to atheromatous plaques, plaque fissuring, and either occlusion due to thrombus on the plaque which could propagate into the middle cerebral artery, or embolization into the middle cerebral artery. Remove the plaque surgically and you remove the risk of stroke. Before a preventative treatment can be justified, however, further evidence is required. We need to know that a risk factor is important, and also that doing something about it alters the subsequent risk of stroke.

Aetiological evidence

Observational studies, such as case-control and cohort studies, provide evidence to support causal relationships between risk factors and disease. In some cases, this evidence seems very biologically plausible, is consistent with other studies, and results in a general view that intervention is justified without any need for randomized controlled trials, or because randomized controlled trials would be difficult or impossible to mount. Almost all the evidence for two important interventions, stopping smoking and increasing physical exercise, is based on observational studies, but is unlikely ever to be confirmed in large-scale randomized trials. Observational studies, however, should always carry an 'interpretation warning'—the findings may be due to bias or confounding.

For example, it would be very helpful to know whether oestrogen replacement therapy (HRT) prevented coronary heart disease and stroke in women. Until recently, there were no randomized controlled trials to provide evidence but the use of HRT can be considered as an 'exposure' in cohort or case-control studies. HRT was suggested to half the risk of stroke in one cohort study (Paganini-Hill *et al.* 1988). As medical therapies are not prescribed at random, it is entirely possible that any benefits observed in this study are due to selection bias or confounding. Women given HRT vary in many ways, apart from their medication. They tend to be of higher social class, may have been selected to exclude women with hypertension or other evidence of vascular disease, and are kept under closer medical supervision than other women. Unfortunately, other cohorts have failed to confirm the protective effect of HRT, and the first of a number of randomized controlled trials that are being carried out to examine this question suggested that HRT was actually associated with an excess of strokes over placebo treatment (Hulley *et al.* 1998).

Another problem in assessing efficacy of preventive interventions is 'confounding by indication'. People with high blood pressure are at greater risk of stroke, but are also those most likely to be treated with antihypertensive drugs. If such treatment does not completely reverse the excess risk, the treatment will appear to be associated with stroke. One cohort study found a relative risk of 1.5 for stroke amongst treated hypertensives, even after taking account of their blood pressure (Boysen *et al.* 1988). Treatment for hypertension appears to increase the risk of stroke! It is easy to dismiss results like this for an intervention where there is better evidence of effectiveness from randomized trials. In other cases, such as HRT, where the 'real' effect is more uncertain, we may be more easily misled.

A further example that highlights the dilemmas of over-reliance on observational, rather than experimental, data comes from the area of dietary interventions. Intake of β-carotene, an antioxidant, is associated with a much lower risk of cardiovascular disease in cohort studies (the relative risk comparison is for high versus low intake of β-carotene) (Jha *et al.* 1995). A biologically plausible protection mechanism exists to support high intakes of β-carotene. In four randomized controlled trials that have now been published examining the impact of dietary supplements of β-carotene on cardiovascular disease in people at high risk of cancers, quite the opposite picture emerges (Fig. 8.1; Egger *et al.* 1998). The consistency of observational epidemiology and randomized controlled trials seen in blood pressure and cardiovascular risk is not mirrored here, nor should we blindly assume that all epidemiologically supported observations are true.

Randomized trials

If two (or more) possible treatments are assigned randomly amongst a population of patients, the groups receiving each treatment will be similar in everything except the treatment they are receiving. This will be true if the randomization procedure is unbiased, and the groups are large enough for chance variation in other important factors to be small. Randomization can avoid the effects of both known and unknown factors which might otherwise distort the results. Maintaining this balance is the reasoning behind the slightly counter-intuitive practice of analysing trials according to 'intention to treat'. All patients are analysed according to the group to which they were randomized, rather than analysing only those patients who stayed on their assigned treatment. The size of the difference between active treatment and placebo groups will be underestimated, but at least the direction of the difference will not be biased.

An example is the Stroke Prevention in Atrial Fibrillation (SPAF) trial, which assigned 421 patients with non-valvular atrial fibrillation to anti-

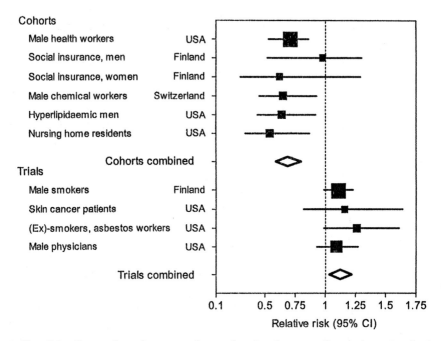

Fig. 8.1 Comparison between observational cohort studies and randomized controlled trials: β-carotene and cardiovascular disease risk (from Egger *et al.* 1998).

coagulation with warfarin or placebo. The two groups were well matched for a wide range of possible prognostic factors, although 55 per cent of the placebo group had a history of hypertension compared with only 49 per cent of the warfarin-treated group. Follow-up was for a mean of 1.3 years. There were 18 strokes or other systemic emboli (the predefined primary outcome events, 7.4 per cent/year) in the placebo group, compared with six in the anticoagulated group (2.3 per cent/year). Many of these strokes actually occurred in patients who had been withdrawn from active treatment or who were inadequately anticoagulated. The relative risk on treatment was 0.67 (95 per cent CI, 0.27–0.85). At this point in the trial, and in the light of the experiences in other similar trials, the investigators decided that the benefits of anticoagulation were clear, and stopped the trial as they felt it would be unethical to continue giving patients placebo (Stroke Prevention in Atrial Fibrillation Investigators 1990*a,b*, 1991). The 'real' benefit of anticoagulation over placebo will be somewhat greater than the estimate from the trial, because of the number of strokes that occurred off active treatment. Against this, trials that stop early tend to overestimate the size of effect, since they are more likely to be stopped when the difference between treatment arms is, by chance, larger than the 'real' difference (Pocock 1992).

We need to know two things about a treatment from a trial. First, whether the difference in stroke incidence between the different treatments could have occurred by chance and, secondly, how big the difference is between the treatments. To get reliable information on the magnitude of the benefit in prevention, where small effects applied to many people may be worthwhile, we need very large trials. The problem with randomized trials is that they require elaborate organization, clinicians must be comfortable with admitting uncertainty about the best treatment for their patients, and trials are expensive.

Systematic review and meta-analysis

Randomization in small or moderate-sized trials does not guarantee the avoidance of chance imbalances between treatment groups. Nor can such trials exclude the play of chance in making one treatment appear more or less beneficial than another. The magnitude of apparent benefits can be very different in different trials, and there will often be wide confidence intervals to the estimate of the size of benefit from any one individual trial.

Systematic review is a method of obtaining all the relevant data, and (when appropriate) pooling the results of trials (or other epidemiological studies) (Thompson and Pocock 1991). The extent to which different treatments or different populations can be considered similar enough to combine data is debated. The best systematic reviews search the literature carefully, make efforts to find unpublished data, retrieve data from the original investigators where possible, and apply quality criteria to determine which studies to include. The Cochrane Collaboration Stroke Group undertakes and disseminates comprehensive overviews which are regularly updated (Counsell et al 1995; Warlow et al 1998). Such 'cumulative' meta-analyses give the best current estimates of whether a treatment is effective, how effective it is, and where research data are lacking (Lau et al. 1993).

Blood pressure lowering

A good example of this approach examined the relationship between blood pressure and stroke, and the extent to which the 'epidemiologically expected' benefits of blood pressure reduction were achieved during trials of anti-hypertensive drugs (MacMahon et al. 1990). Data were assembled from seven cohort studies, involving 420 000 people who were observed for an average of 10 years and who experienced 843 fatal and non-fatal strokes. In addition, the results of 14 randomized, controlled trials of antihypertensive drugs, involving 37 000 participants, were combined.

Together, the observational studies showed an exponential increase in stroke risk with increasing blood pressure. Each 10 mmHg increase in diastolic pressure was associated with an 2.3-fold increased risk of stroke, across the range 76–105 mmHg (equivalent to a relative risk of 0.44 per 10 mmHg decrease in diastolic pressure). The combined analysis had enough precision to examine the shape of the curve at its extremes, whereas individual studies included too few strokes to do this. There was no evidence of a threshold or J-shaped curve, with an increased risk for lower levels of blood pressure. This is important, because it implies that reducing blood pressure reduces risk regardless of the actual level of blood pressure. What matters is the baseline risk of stroke, contributed to by age, blood pressure, smoking, previous stroke or heart disease, and so on. There is no such thing as categorically defined hypertension which needs treatment in isolation from other cardio-vascular risk factors (MacMahon *et al.* 1990).

The hypertension treatment trials lasted, on average, 5 years and reduced diastolic blood pressure by 5–6 mmHg. Strokes in the trials therefore occurred, on average, after only 2–3 years of blood pressure reduction. There were 484 strokes in placebo groups, and 289 in active treatment groups, a relative risk on treatment of 0.58 (95 per cent CI, 0.50–0.67). The relative risk expected from the observational studies for such a blood pressure decrease was very similar, suggesting that virtually all the expected benefit of reducing blood pressure therefore seems to be gained within 2–3 years of treatment (Collins *et al.* 1990).

Cost-effectiveness, cost-utility, and decision analyses

All treatments are associated with costs. Drugs and operations cost money, taking tablets and monitoring their safety and effectiveness is time consuming and inconvenient, operations are debilitating in the short term and may leave long-lasting complications, drugs have side-effects and life-style modifica-tions may be resented or mean that enjoyable activities are avoided. In some cases the adverse effects can all but eliminate the gains of treatment. For example, in a comparison of warfarin and aspirin for atrial fibrillation, the superiority of warfarin in preventing ischaemic strokes was greatly offset by the extra intracerebral haemorrhages caused by anticoagulation (Stroke Prevention in Atrial Fibrillation Investigators 1994, 1996).

When is the cost of taking treatment worthwhile? Clearly this depends on how big a problem we are attempting to avoid, and the potential benefits of taking the treatment. We can evaluate this formally in a cost-effectiveness analysis. The costs in monetary terms are compared with the desirable effects of treatment offset by any adverse effects. Using the example of atrial fibrillation, it has been estimated that a comprehensive treatment programme for Swedes with atrial fibrillation would reduce both costs and stroke morbidity, if haemorrhagic complications were low, with 34 individuals being treated to avoid one stroke each year, and net savings of £9000 per stroke avoided; whereas if risk of haemorrhage was high, 83 patients would need

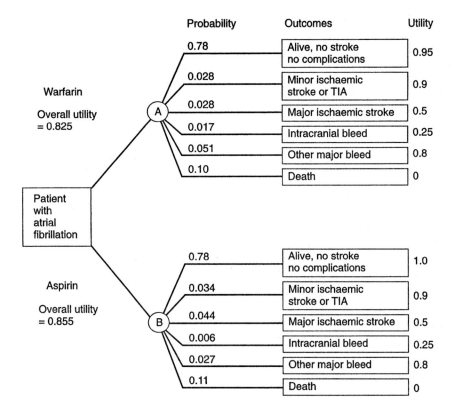

Fig. 8.2 Decision tree analysis of treatment with warfarin or aspirin for the prevention of stroke among people with non-rheumatic atrial fibrillation.

treating to avoid one stroke, at a net cost of £14 000 per stroke (Gustafsson *et al.* 1992) (discussed more fully in Chapter 1).

This approach requires us to compare the benefits of avoiding ischaemic strokes with the detriment of haemorrhage, taking tablets, attending for anticoagulation control, and so on. Cost-utility analysis attempts to measure effectiveness on a single scale of value, worth, or desirability (called 'utility'). Each outcome is valued on a scale of 0 (equivalent to death) to 1 (equivalent to full health). Utilities are measured on a ratio scale, and can be used to adjust figures for survival differences between treatments for quality ('quality adjusted life years' or QALYs).

Decision analysis is a modelling technique for combining the desirability of various outcomes with their probability (see Chapter 6 for some simple examples). Both aspirin and warfarin are associated with lower stroke incidence in atrial fibrillation compared with placebo. Which is preferable overall? Or do the side-effects and inconvenience of either make it worth taking a chance on having a stroke? Figure 8.2 illustrates a decision analysis for warfarin versus aspirin (with probability figures taken for someone aged under 75 over 3 years in the SPAF-2 trial (Stroke Prevention in Atrial Fibrillation Investigators 1994), and utilities estimated by the authors).

This example emphasizes that the great majority of patients are alive and stroke- and complication-free after 3 years. Taking warfarin is certainly inconvenient (reflected by the slightly reduced utility of 0.95 compared with taking aspirin, which, for the sake of argument, we have considered to be of trivial inconvenience). In spite of there being fewer ischaemic and total strokes in the group taking warfarin, overall, taking aspirin appears to be at least as desirable an option.

A simple decision analysis such as this makes a number of assumptions, which may be challenged. The number of outcomes considered could be expanded, especially to refine the type and severity of strokes and haemorrhages. The probability of each outcome will depend on the age and clinical characteristics of the individual, and the period of time over which observation is made. Some features may be uncertain, such as the acceptability of the anticoagulation monitoring service (determining how may people default from treatment) and the closeness of control (determining the number of haemorrhages). The utilities of the various outcomes could be estimated in a more sophisticated way, and may indeed vary from one individual to another. Finally, some account might be taken of the human tendency to want (and therefore value) benefits sooner and costs later, a process known as 'discounting'.

A simple decision analysis may be reasonable for a one-off choice, such as whether to undergo a carotid endarterectomy, but is clearly inadequate for an ongoing treatment as is required in atrial fibrillation. More appropriate is a model where individuals can be assigned to one of a number of states (such as alive and well, major stroke, minor bleed, dead) after a short period of time (for example, 6 months) under different treatments. These states become the starting point for the next 6 month period, and the whole process is continued until a predetermined time period has elapsed or until the whole population has died. This sort of model is called a Markov model, and can be performed readily on a computer. Assumptions about initial risk and rates of complications can be varied in what is called a sensitivity analysis (to see how 'sensitive' the final outcome is to each assumption).

Such a decision analysis has been published for the choice between warfarin, aspirin, and no therapy, over 10 years, for a 65-year-old man with no contraindications to therapy (Gage et al. 1995). As we might assume would happen in clinical practice, warfarin was swapped for aspirin if a haemorrhage occurred, and aspirin or no initial therapy changed to warfarin if a stroke or TIA occurred. Non-cerebral haemorrhages were presumed to alter quality of life for 1 month only, and third strokes were assumed to be fatal. Ten states of health were described, including various severities of stroke and haemorrhage and death. Probabilities of entering these states were obtained from the trials already described. High-, medium-, and low-baseline stroke risk cases were considered based on co-morbid risk factors (Atrial Fibrillation Investigators 1994).

The utilities applied to each of the health states were determined empirically in a separate study (Gage *et al.* 1996). Eighty-three people with atrial fibrillation, 84 per cent of whom were treated with warfarin or aspirin, and 20 per cent of whom had had a previous stroke, were presented scenarios describing life with a mild, moderate, or severe stroke, and describing taking warfarin or aspirin. The 'time trade-off' method was used, and the results validated by also using the 'standard gamble' (Torrance 1976). The time trade-off asks respondents how much time in a given state of health they would be willing to 'trade' for a shorter period of perfect health. The ratio of the two time periods gives the utility for the state of health. This assumes that 2 years in a state of health with a utility of 0.5 are valued the same as 1 year in a state of perfect health (utility 1.0). The standard gamble proposes a treatment which could restore a given state of health to a perfect one, but at the risk of instant death. The size of the risk is varied until the treatment and continuing in the state of health are equally desirable. The utility of the state of health is then 1 minus the risk which would be accepted. The worse the state of health, the greater the acceptable risk in avoiding it. A slight variation (involving time in a dreamless, unrefreshing sleep) was used to value the treatment options.

There was great variation between respondents in their valuations of all the states of health, from < 0 (worse than death) to 1 (equivalent to perfect health). The mean (median) utilities were 0.76 (0.94), 0.39 (0.03), and 0.11 (0) for mild, moderate, and severe stroke. The major stroke scenario was rated as equivalent to or worse than death by 82 per cent of respondents, while the equivalent figure for moderate stroke was 47 per cent. Almost all respondents had a utility of 1.0 for aspirin therapy. Mean utility for warfarin therapy was 0.987, although 10 per cent rated it worse than 0.95, suggesting that the majority of patients do not consider anticoagulation much of a disadvantage.

The decision analysis demonstrated the crucial importance of baseline risk in determining the cost-effectiveness of therapy (Table 8.1). For high-risk cases, warfarin therapy was cheaper than aspirin therapy (because the cost saving associated with avoiding strokes was greater than the cost of therapy and managing complications). For medium-risk patients warfarin therapy was more expensive than treatment with aspirin, and the extra cost per QALY was $8000. Both active treatments were more effective and cheaper than no initial therapy. For low-risk cases, the extra cost per QALY of warfarin over aspirin was $370 000, and the cost of warfarin over no therapy was $14 000 per QALY. Amongst low risk patients, aspirin therapy may be preferred as the tiny benefit in terms of QALYs can only be achieved at considerable cost. In

Table 8.1 Results of a decision analysis comparing warfarin, aspirin, and no treatment among people with non-rheumatic atrial fibrillation

Risk level	Annual stroke risk (%)	Quality adjusted life years gained by treatment			Extra cost per QALY warfarin versus aspirin
		Warfarin treatment	Aspirin treatment	No treatment	
High	5+	6.51	6.27	6.01	Cheaper
Medium	2.6–4.5	6.60	6.46	6.23	$8000
Low	<1.6	6.70	6.69	6.51	$370 000

the sensitivity analyses, annual stroke rate was the most important determinant of cost-effectiveness. Also important were the assumptions about the effectiveness of aspirin, the rate of major haemorrhage (which, if twice that seen in the trials, would be enough to abolish any advantage of warfarin over aspirin for medium-risk patients), the utility of warfarin treatment (if reduced to 0.92, the fifth percentile, warfarin was no longer preferred to aspirin for low- or medium-risk patients), and age (warfarin therapy is more cost-effective in 75-year-olds, despite higher bleeding risk, but less so in 55-year-olds).

The results of the utility determination study emphasize a fundamental problem with this sort of analysis. Not only are there assumptions made about being able to predict how a health state will be valued when it has never been experienced, but individuals varied greatly between each other. Some of this variation will have been measurement error, but some of it is real. The published decision analysis is useful for public health purposes, and as a general guide to clinical practice. However, it is no alternative to finding out how each individual perceives the inconvenience of prophylactic therapy and fears the occurrence of a disabling stroke. This is not easy, especially in busy practices, as the ideas are difficult and take much explanation. Computer-assisted, individualized, decision-aid programmes are increasingly available as research tools and will undoubtedly be introduced to clinical practice in the future.

The measurement of utilities is still very crude, and this is unfortunate as the actual numbers can be very important in making decisions. It has been pointed out that changing the utility of antihypertensive therapy from 0.99 to 0.98 (taking account of inconvenience, side-effects, and so on) abolishes all the apparent gain from treating mild hypertension (Fletcher 1992).

Discounting

If I am owed £100 I would rather have it now than in a year's time. If you offer £110 in a year instead of the £100 now, I would accept, implying that I discount money at a little under 10 per cent/year. Similarly, I would prefer to repay a debt later rather than now, and would prefer a health benefit now than in the future. The problem with all preventative treatments is that their monetary cost occurs early, as do many unwanted effects (such as peri-operative debility or stroke after a carotid endarterectomy, or side-effects of an antihypertensive drug). The benefits, if they occur at all, occur in the future. Most people see preventative measures as a sort of insurance premium, and are happy to bear the cost so long as the likelihood of benefit is large enough. For many preventive treatments the individual is unlikely to benefit, even where the treatment is of proven efficacy. When a middle-aged smoker chooses to stop, he affects his chances of being alive 20 years later by less than 10 per cent (Rose 1992). Eighty-two middle-aged mild hypertensives get no benefit from 10 years of antihypertensive treatment, while one of them avoids a stroke, and over a quarter of them develop side-effects (Medical Research Council Working Party 1985). Most people and their doctors greatly overestimate the risks of disease and the potential for risk reduction through medical treatment.

There is little empirical evidence about how health effects are discounted. Most studies assume that the financial discount rates used in accountancy apply. The decision analysis described above used a 5 per cent rate, and tested rates between 0 and 10 per cent. In some respects, patients who adopt an 'it will never happen to me' attitude and are non-compliant with medication or other advice are identifying the problem of discounting. They would rather not sacrifice their freedom from medication or their undesirable pleasures (smoking and over-eating) now, for an uncertain benefit in the future.

Who to treat?

Individual risk

Ultimately it is up to the individual patient to decide whether they wish to receive or take treatment. It is a doctor's, or other health professional's, responsibility to know what treatments are effective, and to help counsel and educate patients in a way that is understandable to them. There is a tendency amongst both doctors and patients to think in terms of absolutes. Treatments work or they do not. In reality, most treatments reduce risks rather than abolishing them completely. Sometimes the change in risk is very small. For example, in a randomized controlled trial of carotid endarterectomy for carotid stenosis not associated with symptoms in the ipsilateral cerebral hemisphere, 5.1 per cent of the operated group suffered ipsilateral stroke or died over 5 years of follow-up, compared with 11 per cent in the medically managed, control group. This gives a small absolute difference of 5.9 per cent (just over 1 per cent/year), but a large relative risk of 0.47 (Asymptomatic Carotid Atherosclerosis Study 1995). The difference was unlikely to have occurred by chance ($p = 0.004$). In this setting carotid endarterectomy does not alter the risk of stroke very much, but it is easy to interpret these results as saying that endarterectomy for asymptomatic carotid stenosis 'works' and therefore should be performed. In fact 100 such operations must be performed to prevent just one stroke in the next year.

Variables with high relative risk are likely to be of direct aetiological importance. The crucial factor in determining whether intervention is worthwhile for an individual is the absolute risk difference between exposed (i.e. treated) and unexposed (untreated) states (the 'attributable risk'). An intervention that reduces the chances of a stroke from 50 to 25 per cent is clearly more likely to benefit an individual than one reducing risk from 2 to 1 per cent, even though the relative risks are 0.5 on treatment in each case.

What determines the absolute risk difference is largely the individual (baseline) risk, which depends on age, sex, blood pressure, smoking status, cardiac history, and so on. A preventative treatment reducing risk by half will therefore be of more significance to a 70-year-old male hypertensive smoker (annual risk of stroke 6 per cent, risk difference on treatment 3 per cent), than a 30-year-old woman without other risk factors (annual risk of stroke 0.012 per cent, risk difference on the same treatment 0.006 per cent).

Numbers needed to treat

These risk differences are more difficult to understand and communicate than the relative effects of treatment. Use of numbers needed to treat (NNT) is an alternative way of communicating risk differences and is gaining in popularity (Cook and Sackett 1995). For example, the MRC Mild Hypertension Trial studied 17 354 men and women aged 35–64 years with diastolic blood pressure 90–109 mmHg for an average of 5 years. Half were assigned to propranolol or bendrofluazide, and half to placebo. Sixty strokes occurred in the treated group and 109 in the placebo group, giving rates of 14 and 26 per 10 000 patient years. The rate ratio (or relative risk on treatment) is 0.54, implying that risk is almost halved, which sounds impressive. The annual risk difference is $26-14 = 12/10\,000$, which means that 12 people will have avoided strokes by taking treatment per 10 000 patients treated for 1 year. In other words, $10\,000/12 = 833$ patients have to be treated for 1 year to avoid one stroke. This is the number needed to treat and is the reciprocal of the risk difference.

Of course, over longer periods risk accumulates. One stroke is avoided if 83 people are treated for 10 years. Still, 82 people are treated 'unnecessarily'. Moreover, of the 83, four would develop diabetes, 10 gout, and nine impotence severe enough to warrant stopping the drug (if given bendrofluazide). Treatment of mild hypertension in middle-aged people certainly 'works', but when the risks and benefits are presented in this way, many people would choose to forgo the benefits. Raised blood pressure will need monitoring, and if it becomes more severe, or as the individual ages, or acquires other risk factors, the benefits of treatment will increase. Stroke is relatively rare in middle-aged men, regardless of their blood pressures. As baseline risk increases, the NNT falls.

A further example illustrates the very small NNTs that arise when baseline risks are very high. A 76-year-old man with atrial fibrillation, a history of hypertension, and heart failure has an 8.1 per cent annual risk of stroke (compared with 0.26 per cent for the men in the placebo arm of the MRC hypertension trial) (Atrial Fibrillation Investigators 1994). Anticoagulation reduces the risk by 68 per cent to $(1 - 0.68) \times 0.081 = 0.026$ or 2.6 per cent/year, a risk difference of 5.5 per cent. The number needed to treat, for a year, to avoid one stroke is therefore $1/0.055 = 18$.

Modifiable risk factors

Data on the effectiveness of interventions vary in their quality. For some interventions there are good meta-analyses of results from randomized controlled trials which give the best estimates of the size of the effect. The stroke module of the Cochrane Library maintains regularly updated meta-analyses of the effectiveness of many interventions (Warlow et al. 1998). Others are unlikely to be tested in randomized trials in the foreseeable future, but are thought important enough to promote in their absence. Included in this category are physical activity, stopping smoking, weight reduction, and close glycaemic control in diabetes.

The best estimate of the magnitude of effect of the most important interventions is given in Table 8.2. This estimate is given as a relative risk (RR) on treatment compared with none, or in some cases an alternative (specified) treatment. The numbers needed to treat (NNT) statistic can be calculated from these by estimating the absolute (baseline) risk for the particular population involved, using the methods described in Chapter 2:

$$NNT = 1/[(\text{individual (baseline) risk} \times (1 - RR)].$$

The relative risk has only been imprecisely estimated for some treatments, which means a range of NNTs is generated. It must also be accepted that there is further uncertainty in estimating baseline risk, so the NNT is only a broad guide to treatment efficacy.

Primary and secondary prevention

It is conventional to split prevention into those activities intended to reduce the incidence of disease in those who have yet to suffer any clinical event

Table 8.2 Interventions to prevent stroke

Risk factor	Intervention	Evidence	Relative risk (95% CI) on treatment	Source
Life-style factors				
Salt intake	Reduction	Systematic review of RCTs, blood pressure end point	About 0.75 per 50 mmol Na/day	Law et al. (1991b)
Smoking	Stopping	Cohort studies	0.5 after 2 years	Kawachi et al. (1993), Wannamethee et al. (1995b)
Inactivity	Moderate exercise	Cohort studies	0.55 (0.4–0.8)	Wannamethee et al. 1998
Obesity	Weight loss	Cohort studies	0.5 per 6 kg/m²	Shinton et al. (1991), Abbott et al. (1994a)
Drug interventions				
Blood pressure	Drugs	Systematic reviews of RCTs	0.58 (0.5 (0.67) per 5–6 mmHg diastolic	Collins et al. (1990)
Isolated systolic hypertension	Drugs	RCT	0.64 (0.50–0.82) for 12 mmHg systolic fall	SHEP Co-operative Research Group (1991), Staessen et al. (1997)
Cholesterol	HMG CoA reductase inhibitors ('statins')	Systematic reviews of RCTs (secondary end point)	0.69 (0.57–0.83)	Blauw et al. (1997), Crouse et al. (1997)
Atrial fibrillation	Warfarin (INR 2–4)	Systematic reviews of RCTs	0.32 (0.21–0.5)	Atrial Fibrillation Investigators (1994), Barnett et al. (1995)
Atrial fibrillation	Aspirin	Systematic reviews of RCTs	0.79 (0.62–1.0)	Barnett et al. (1995), Atrial Fibrillation Investigators (1997)
TIA/minor stroke	Aspirin	Systematic reviews of RCTs	0.75 (0.67–0.83)	Antiplatelet Triallists Collaboration (1994b)
Post myocardial infarction	Warfarin	Systematic reviews of RCTs	0.45 (0.23–0.70)	P. Smith et al. (1990)
Diabetes	Close glycaemic control	None for stroke outcomes	0.58 for IHD/PVD outcomes	Diabetes Control and Complications Trial (1995)

Surgical interventions			
Symptomatic carotid stenosis (70–99%)	Surgery (versus medical)	RCT	0.55 (after 3 years including surgical mortality/ morbidity)*	North American Symptomatic Carotid Endarterectomy Trial Collaborators (1991), European Carotid Surgery Triallists (1998)
Asymptomatic carotid stenosis (60–99%)	Surgery (versus medical)	RCT	0.47 (after 5 years including surgical mortality/ morbidity)*	Hobson et al. (1993), Asymptomatic Carotid Atherosclerosis Study (1995)

RCT, randomized controlled trial; IHD, ischaemic heart disease; PVD, peripheral vascular disease.
* The effect of these interventions cannot be described by a single relative risk. Surgical morbidity produces an immediate hazard after which strokes accumulate more slowly in surgical patients. Relative risks are given for 3–5 years.

(primary prevention) and those interventions for people who have established disease, which are intended to reduce recurrence (secondary prevention). In practice, these distinctions are fairly artificial as many people have asymptomatic evidence of cardiovascular disease, and this trend increases with age. What really matters is the baseline level of risk at which an intervention is used. For example, older cholesterol-lowering drugs were shown to be beneficial only among people at high risk of cardiovascular disease (so-called secondary prevention) but were actually harmful among those at low risk of disease (Davey Smith *et al.* 1993). By contrast, the newer and safer HMG CoA (3-hydroxy-3-methylglutaryl coenzyme A) reductase inhibitors (statins) are effective across a broad range of cardiovascular disease risk, covering both primary prevention and secondary prevention baseline risks of disease (*Effective Health Care Bulletin* 1998). Consequently, in Table 8.2 both primary and secondary prevention areas are included, although a further discussion of the issues of preventing recurrence is given in Chapter 13.

Which antihypertensive agent?

The majority of the data on blood pressure reduction which have used mortality and stroke incidence end points have used thiazide diuretics and β-blockers (Amery *et al.* 1985; Medical Research Council Working Party, 1985, 1992; Coope and Warrender, 1986; Wilhelmsen *et al.* 1987; Wikstrand *et al.* 1988; Dahlof *et al.* 1991; SHEP Co-operative Research Group, 1991). In addition there are data on the calcium-channel blockers nitrendipine (Staessen *et al.* 1997), and in a weaker trial, nifedipine (Gong *et al.* 1996).

The association between blood pressure and stroke is almost certainly causal. Any method or agent that reduces blood pressure will probably therefore be effective. Although most have only been evaluated in terms of their ability to reduce blood pressure, some agents will be useful because of dual indications (ACE inhibitors in heart failure or diabetes, β-blockers or calcium-channel blockers in angina, α-blockers in benign prostatic hyperplasia). The effectiveness and overall tolerability of all the currently available classes of drugs is similar and reasonable (Lewis *et al.* 1996; Philipp *et al.* 1997), although there is good evidence that methyldopa is not well tolerated (Croog *et al.* 1986).

Side-effects

The presence of a risk factor, such as hypertension, is not a disease *per se*, and any benefit accrued in terms of quality adjusted life years from avoidance of stroke, ischaemic heart disease, and death will be easily lost if large numbers of patients suffer treatment side-effects in the early years of treatment. The same goes for non-pharmacological methods (Stamler *et al.* 1989; Law *et al.* 1991*b*; Alderman 1994; Appel *et al.* 1997). If these are perceived as an unwanted imposition which diminishes quality of life, they cannot be considered 'side-effect free'. Indeed, promoting physical activity in older age may be associated with an increased risk of injury (Ebrahim *et al.* 1997). Determining whether a symptom is due to a drug is not always easy. A common side-effect reported soon after starting is suggestive, but is essentially an uncontrolled observation. We will never know what would have happened if a placebo had been prescribed. Many patients in placebo groups report 'side-effects', and patient information sheets distributed with drugs list many side-effects which are often then experienced by the suggestible. Sometimes an '*n* of 1 trial' will be required, where a placebo is given in sequence with the active drug, the order unbeknown to the patient (and, if possible, the doctor). The effects, or side-effects, can then be judged against a control (Guyatt *et al.* 1986; Mahon *et al.* 1996). As therapy will generally have to continue for many years, side-effects are generally not to be tolerated, and drugs should be changed until a suitable one (or combination) is identified.

Hypertension is generally undertreated, in the UK at least (W. C. S. Smith *et al.* 1990; Coppola *et al.* 1997). Current guidelines emphasize that some groups, such as diabetics, need vigorous control of blood pressure, on the basis of their increased risk of vascular events (Sever *et al.* 1993; UKPDS 1998). There is reluctance to reduce blood pressure, however, which is not above an arbitrarily defined limit (often 160/90). Current thinking suggests that for patients at high risk, especially in 'secondary prevention' populations, the lower the (tolerated) blood pressure, the better (Hansson 1998).

How long should preventive treatments be given?

Evidence is strongest in the area of blood pressure control with antihypertensives. Here, drug trials have been conducted for 5 years on average. As the relationships between blood pressure and cardiovascular disease risk are seen both at younger and older ages, and treatment effects are still apparent up to the age of 80 years, there is a rationale for maintaining drug treatment for longer than the 5 years for which good evidence is available. A recent case-control study reported an increase in risk of intracerebral haemorrhage in people who had stopped taking antihypertensive medication and was sufficiently newsworthy to be cited in the *Lancet* (Bonn 1998). Since the patients in the study were not randomly allocated to stopping or continuing medication, it is possible that other confounding factors, determining both increased likelihood of stopping medication and increased risk of cerebral haemorrhage (e.g. heavy alcohol intake), explain the observed association rather than the speculative ('thinning of the arterial wall caused by many antihypertensive agents ... render the wall more vulnerable to injury when exposed to high blood pressures after drug withdrawal'), but biologically plausible, mechanism given for the finding.

In other areas, it is clear that stopping smoking is likely to be beneficial only if a person remains a non-smoker. Similar arguments probably apply to physical activity, where it has been shown that taking up light or moderate activity is associated with a reduced risk of cardiovascular disease, even in people with pre-existing disease (Wannamethee *et al.* 1998).

High-risk and population approaches

Individuals whose personal risk of stroke is high, by virtue of their age, medical characteristics, and behaviours, have most to gain from prevention. In Chapter 2, we saw how only 40 per cent of strokes occur in individuals with hypertension (defined as systolic blood pressure > 160 mmHg). A treatment that reduced their risk by 50 per cent would only prevent 20 per cent of cases of stroke, since hypertension is uncommon (12 per cent of the middle-aged population described). The majority of strokes occur in people who are 'normotensive' with blood pressures between 120 and 160 mmHg (since there are many more of them than there are hypertensives). We also saw that reduction in blood pressure has the same effect on relative risk of stroke regardless of the starting blood pressure. Rose pointed out that small downward shifts in the distribution of blood pressures would have a disproportionate effect on overall cardiovascular mortality and morbidity (Rose 1992; Cook *et al.* 1995). Really big changes in the burden of disease will involve changes in the whole population, not just those at high risk.

This observation will hold wherever a risk factor has a graded, continuous association with risk, and where the distribution of the risk factor is approximately normal (with the bulk of the population falling towards the centre of the distribution). In stroke epidemiology, blood pressure, homocysteine, body mass index, and glucose tolerance fulfil these criteria, and so, to an extent, does physical activity.

Can we use a population approach as part of a prevention strategy? For each risk factor, it means every individual in the population reducing his or her risk, even those who are at low risk. The high-risk approach is easy to translate into clinical terms. Anyone who is at high risk should have all possible risk factors reduced as much as possible. Someone at low absolute risk may not benefit from intervention, especially where potent therapies with potential adverse effects are involved. For these treatments a high-risk approach is the most cost-effective. A population approach must involve interventions which are relatively risk free, and will broadly involve life-style alterations. A paradox is that although everyone in a population must reduce risk to reduce the overall burden of disease, the majority of individuals will not benefit from the change. Indeed, the time spent shopping for a healthy diet and taking exercise is probably greater than the extra life expectancy achieved by making such healthy life-style changes (Grover *et al.* 1994)! Such changes will therefore have to be perceived as cost free, or desirable in their own right. This will usually mean societal or cultural changes. Interventions are therefore required at the policy and governmental level. The means of intervention will be legislation, the press, advertising, commercial and peer-group pressure. The main targets are diet, exercise, and smoking.

Salt reduction

The great majority of salt in the diet is in processed foods, including bread, breakfast cereals, cooked meats, and tinned food (James *et al.* 1987). Salt is a flavour enhancer, and is valued by the food industry for making otherwise bland food taste interesting. Unfortunately, we habituate rapidly to the taste of salt, so a low-salt diet is perceived as tasteless (Beauchamp *et al.* 1983). It is unlikely that food manufacturers will reduce salt content in food voluntarily, therefore the only mechanisms for promoting this are government regulation, or consumer pressure, which might be promoted via the press, and regulation on food labelling (Godlee 1996). But what is the evidence for this public health approach to prevention?

The relationship between a population's urinary excretion of sodium (a proxy for dietary intake of salt) and the mean level of blood pressure and proportion of the population labelled hypertensive was confirmed by the Intersalt Study, conducted in 52 population samples around the world (Intersalt Cooperative Research Group 1988). The relationship within populations, at the level of individuals, has proved much harder to define. Part of the problem may be that measurement of habitual dietary sodium intake is notoriously unreliable, as there is great day-to-day variation. Mischaracterization of the exposure variable in this way will have weakened the observed association. A series of meta-analyses suggested, however, that the association between salt intake and blood pressure was stronger than previously assumed, the ecological, cross-sectional, and intervention studies were consistent with each other, and that moderate reductions in dietary salt have the potential to make very large reductions in stroke incidence (Frost *et al.* 1991; Law *et al.* 1991*a,b*).

A more recent updated analysis of the Intersalt data attempted to correct for regression dilution bias (that is the extent to which estimation of true urinary sodium excretion was unreliable owing to only a single measurement being taken) (Elliott *et al.* 1996). The new analyses made dramatic differences to the conclusions reported in the earlier paper, as the predicted reduction in systolic blood pressure associated with a 100 mmol reduction in urinary sodium excretion went from 1.6 mmHg to 4.3 mmHg. Such large differences would translate to a change from a 4 per cent reduction in cardiovascular disease mortality to a 21 per cent reduction associated with a 100 mmol fall in urinary sodium excretion (Davey Smith and Phillips 1996). The method of adjusting for regression dilution bias in a univariate way is relatively straight-forward and was carried out in the original report. A subsample of the participants had a duplicate urinary sodium excretion measurement taken and the correlation coefficient between the original and duplicate measures was 0.46. To make adjustments for this innate variation within individuals, sodium–blood pressure regression coefficients were divided by 0.46. Alter-native, more complex multivariate methods of adjustment attempt to allow for the additional covariation with body mass, age, sex, and potassium, and produced smaller estimates of within-individual variation which therefore produced larger regression coefficients and a much larger predicted impact on reducing the risk of disease (Dyer *et al.* 1996). Certainly, if these estimates are reliable, then as the meta-analysts who have compiled both observational and experimental data have commented: 'few measures in preventive medicine are as simple and economical and yet can achieve so much' (Law *et al.* 1991*b*). However, other meta-analyses have not concurred on the extent of likely blood pressure reduction with salt restriction, probably due to different criteria for selection of studies included (Ebrahim and Davey Smith 1996, 1998; Midgley *et al.* 1996; Cutler *et al.* 1997).

Scientific evidence can be assembled and analysed to make different points, and this is true in the case of salt, blood pressure, and mortality, which has now become a major area of conflict between the salt industry, academics, and public health (Swales 1989; Stamler *et al.* 1993; Hanneman 1996; Law 1996; Alderman 1997a,b; Elliott 1997). Most salt restriction trials are of very short duration; very extreme reduction in intake is feasible but many people rarely tolerate this for long. If the evidence from trials of salt restriction in humans that were longer than 6 months' duration is included (i.e. an attempt to collate evidence relevant to the public health question of habitual dietary change and its effectiveness over a reasonable period of time), much smaller estimates of blood pressure change result (about −1 mmHg and −2.8 mmHg systolic blood pressure in normotensives and hypertensives, respectively) (Ebrahim and Davey Smith 1998).

Only two studies have examined the relationship between dietary sodium intake and mortality directly, one in hypertensives (Alderman *et al.* 1995) and the other in a general population (Alderman *et al.* 1998). These two large observational cohort studies found that the higher the dietary intake of sodium (and total calories), the lower the all-cause and cardiovascular disease mortality rate. The studies with apparently the most relevant outcomes appear to give the wrong answers. As always, considerable caution is required in interpreting observational studies. Dietary recall is notoriously inaccurate for classifying intake, and the range of salt intakes reported in this study was quite low. Bias and confounding are impossible to exclude, no matter how carefully a study is performed. Furthermore, it is unlikely that the effects of individual dietary constituents is simple and direct. It is more likely that diets comprise interacting components (Davey Smith and Ebrahim 1998) and that 'diets as a whole may be more important determinants of health outcome than an individual component' (Alderman *et al.* 1998).

There would seem to be no alternative to large-scale randomized controlled trials to settle the uncertainty, although with the practical problems inherent in undertaking trials of life-style changes there would still be the risk of inconclusive results. One large, long-term, randomized trial of sodium restriction has already reported equivocal findings. Sodium intake in the intervention group was reduced by 48 mmol/day after 6 months compared with the control groups, although this was less than intended, and the difference reduced progressively over the following 3 years. As often happens, the control group also reduced its sodium intake. The trial design also involved some subjects reducing weight, which complicated interpretation as there was a strong negative interaction between the effects of weight loss and sodium reduction on blood pressure (both interventions together had less effect on blood pressure than the sum of the effects of the two interventions separately). However, the effect of salt intake reduction was to reduce blood pressure after 6 months by 1.6/0.8 mmHg compared with the control level, and this was only slightly attenuated after 3 years. Weight reduction was rather more effective in reducing blood pressure, but the changes were small compared with those achievable by drug therapy (Trials of Hypertension Prevention Collaborative Research Group 1997).

The scientific question about the true strength of the relationship between salt intake and blood pressure remains open. This raises an important (and unanswered) question about what strength of evidence is required to justify changes in health and social policy, especially when commercial interests and consumer preferences are at stake, and they seek to influence the discussion (Taubes 1998). If the most optimistic estimates are true, reduction in salt intake offers a powerful means to influence future cardiovascular morbidity and morbidity. If these results are explained by confounding and bias, then the considerable effort require to effect changes in salt consumption would be futile.

This discussion of salt restriction and prevention of cardiovascular disease highlights the difficulty in moving to public health policy from ecological studies between populations, observational studies of individuals within populations, experimental data testing interventions unlikely to be of relevance to public health interventions, and using intermediate end-points (in this case blood pressure) rather than clinical events. Similar problems apply in the areas of promoting physical activity, smoking cessation, and multiple risk-factor interventions. Perhaps the most important point to draw from all of this was made by Sir Austin Bradford Hill many years ago: 'All scientific work is incomplete—whether it be observational or experimental. All scientific work is liable to be upset or modified by advancing knowledge.

That does not confer upon us the freedom to ignore the knowledge we already have, or to postpone the action that it appears to demand at a given time.'

Summary

1. The possibility of preventing stroke is supported by secular and geographic variation in occurrence, falling risk among migrants from countries of high stroke risk to those of low risk; graded relationship between risk factors and stroke; and the effects of altering risk factors reported in experiments.

2. Observational epidemiological data on high blood pressure are supported by evidence from trials. By contrast, observational relationships between β-carotene and cardiovascular disease are not supported by randomized controlled trials.

3. Systematic reviews are useful for obtaining estimates of effects of intervention. This information should be supplemented by cost-effectiveness, cost-utility, and decision analyses, which have the ability to take other factors, besides efficacy, into account and may result in different policies and practices.

4. Primary and secondary prevention strategies depend on the baseline level of cardiovascular risk among the population. In primary prevention, numbers needed to treat to avoid an event are large, as baseline risks are low. Small harms from intervention may offset any benefits. In secondary prevention the numbers needed to treat are more manageable as baseline risks are higher, and riskier treatments may produce overall benefits.

5. Population approaches to reducing risk of stroke can be contrasted with high-risk approaches. High-risk approaches are feasible for control of high blood pressure and use of aspirin in people with atrial fibrillation and established cardiovascular disease. Population approaches have a theoretical justification but little is known about their practical implementation.

9 Acute management

Admission to hospital

The first decision at the onset of a stroke is whether the patient requires hospital admission. The main reasons for admission are diagnostic (is it really a stroke?), to avoid or treat complications, to start rehabilitation early, to give treatment to prevent further strokes, and because of needs for nursing care that cannot be given at home. At present there is no established acute treatment for the neurological damage resulting from a stroke, but this is an area of intense research activity. If convincing and consistent benefits are shown for thrombolytic or neuroprotective drugs, not only will there be an additional reason for seeking hospital admission, but administering therapy will likely require very rapid access.

It is reckoned that between 25 and 50 per cent of all strokes in the UK are not admitted to hospital, but are managed at home by primary health care teams (Wade and Hewer 1985a; Bamford et al. 1986). In practice it is remarkably difficult to know how many people are not admitted to hospital, because unless a special project is set up to count them, they are not routinely noted. From estimates of incidence of stroke and numbers of patients admitted to hospital, it is possible to make a guess at the proportion of patients kept at home. In Nottingham this estimate was around 30 per cent (Barer et al. 1984). Incidence may vary greatly from place to place even within a single region (Wolfe et al. 1993), making such estimates unreliable. Admission rates are often higher (80–95 per cent) elsewhere in the world (Terent 1989; Jorgensen et al. 1992; Anderson et al. 1994a; Asplund et al. 1995; Fogelholm et al. 1996), and it is likely that they have increased in the UK over the past decade.

Data from the Oxfordshire Community Stroke Project have been used to examine the question of why patients are admitted to hospital (Bamford et al. 1986). The main reasons for admission in Oxford were severity of the stroke (assessed by degree of motor impairment and level of consciousness at 24-hours after onset) and living alone. These findings were confirmed in a similar study from Bristol (Wade and Hewer 1983, 1985a; Wade et al. 1985a). Family doctors gave their major reasons for admission as the need for nursing care (87 per cent), uncertainty about the diagnosis (42 per cent), and to start medical treatment for intercurrent illness (30 per cent). The rapid out-patient and domiciliary service provided by the neurology team was only helpful in 5 per cent of cases in keeping them at home.

It is perhaps surprising that neither the neurologists involved in the study, nor the family doctors viewed early access to rehabilitation services as a relevant reason for admission. It is worth noting that this series of cases had already been 'screened' by the study neurologists, and comprised only patients who really had suffered a stroke. Diagnostic uncertainty may be a significant reason for admission if all patients with a possible stroke are considered.

There is no doubt that some patients with severe strokes can be looked after at home, although it is doubtful whether those living on their own can be managed successfully without admission. Nor is it certain whether the rehabilitation, education of the patient and family, and medical treatment aimed at preventing a recurrence of the stroke will be adequately managed by a family doctor, who, in the UK, will only see around four or five new strokes each year. Whether managed in hospital or at home, provision must be made for supply of pressure-relieving mattresses, ensuring safe swallowing and proper continence management, and management of the frequent medical complications that occur after a stroke (Kalra *et al.* 1995; Davenport *et al.* 1996*b*; Johnston *et al.* 1998). A specialist diagnostic service, as used in the Oxford project, would apparently only reduce the demand for hospital admission by around 5 per cent. A well-organized, rapidly responding nursing team might be able to keep a much higher proportion at home, since in 42 per cent of those admitted this was the sole reason for admission. However, the rehabilitation needs of patients are unlikely to be well served unless coordinated multidisciplinary teams are available to assess patients at home, initiate, and monitor management.

The expectations of patients and their relatives are also important factors in determining hospital admission. Patients are afraid, and value the reassurance of hospital admission, and the implication that they are being 'cared about'. Hospitals and health care have important cultural, as well as medical, significance and these aspects should not be ignored (Pound *et al.* 1995).

Management at home

The Bristol Home Care Study was set up to decide whether providing a multidisciplinary team would reduce the use of hospital resources (to a point where the team would be self-funding) and improve the social and emotional adjustment of patients and their families, with no detriment to the functional recovery of patients (Wade *et al.* 1985*a*). Patients allocated to the trial were defined geographically to avoid problems of individual randomization of patients. This caused problems later on because the trial area appeared to have a higher stroke incidence, which was probably the result of increased ascertainment of milder strokes. The extra strokes in the trial area may have used hospital beds, leading to a similar number of bed-days used between control and trial areas. Patients and their relatives did not appear to adjust to the impact of a stroke any better in the trial area, nor was there any difference in patterns of disability.

The multidisciplinary team was mostly comprised of part-time staff, but followed the practices of hospital teams, with weekly team meetings, and division of work between nurses, occupational and physiotherapists, and a social worker. The type of staff and style of management needed to treat patients in their own homes compared with hospital is probably different. The team provided around 100 person-hours a week to about five new patients per week, and probably 20–30 patients were current cases requiring attention. This is a substantial workload and if each profession carried out its assessments, its treatment, and monitored progress, there would be considerable time pressure. A generic worker, skilled in nursing, rehabilitation, and social work, who would provide most of the care and treatment required (but linked to a hospital team for advice and support) might be a better model of management to assess in the community.

Among the reasons discussed for the failure of the scheme to produce the hoped-for outcomes was the sense of competition felt between hospital teams and the new service. The home care team lacked a direct responsibility for the acute management of stroke patients, and therefore was unable to actively encourage use of the service. One of the problems of health service evaluation, highlighted by this study, is that the intervention must be working well (i.e. known, respected, and used) before it can be tested fairly. Controlled trials of health services are difficult to do, or as in this case, difficult to interpret, because the recording of strokes was more efficiently done in the trial area, leading to a potentially biased assessment of the effects of the intervention. The authors considered that an individual randomized study design was not feasible, and under these circumstances either a multi-centre trial with randomization of several districts, or even a 'before-and-after' assessment of the changes produced by the home care team might have been preferable to the comparison of trial and control areas. A new single-centre trial, randomizing patients to hospital admission or home care, has been set up in Bromley, UK, which overcomes some of the problems of the Bristol trial and will report in the next few years (L. Kalra, personal communication). Because of the costs of such studies, it would be worth evaluating new services using observational designs, such as cohort studies and before-and-after comparisons, initially. Services that look promising could then be selected for more reliable evaluation using large, randomized controlled trials.

Relying on observational studies alone, however, can be misleading. In one study, the chances of short- and long-term survival, independence, and living at home a year later were twice as great after the introduction of an organized stroke service as they were before. Correction for multiple indicators of case-mix all but abolished the apparent advantages of the new service (odds ratio for adverse outcomes 0.9; 95 per cent CI, 0.7–1.5). The patients admitted seem to have changed more than the service did. It is worth noting that this study could not exclude moderate-sized, but still worthwhile, benefits from organized care (Davenport *et al.* 1996*a*).

Centralization of a health district's care for stroke patients has been recommended by an expert panel (Consensus Conference 1988). Responsibility for the care of stroke patients who never come into hospital will remain with the family doctor but a rapid response of stroke services to these patients could be achieved by use of the existing domiciliary visiting arrangements for consultant medical staff, and through domiciliary physiotherapy services with suitably trained, generic workers.

Reduction in the hospital costs attributable to stroke patients might be achieved by use of early discharge schemes (Rodgers *et al.* 1997; Rudd *et al.* 1997; Townsend *et al.* 1988). These schemes have the advantage of being available to all patients admitted to hospital, but it is still unclear whether they can match the outcomes achieved by the best in-patient care, or if they are cost-effective (see Chapter 10).

Acute treatment trials

Stroke is not homogeneous in either its pathogenic mechanism or in the impairments, disabilities, and handicaps it produces. The desired effects of treatment are ambiguous. Survival is desirable, but not if it means survival in an obtunded state. Measurement of changes in the underlying pathophysiology of acute stroke is only recently becoming feasible with magnetic resonance imaging and positron emission tomography. The potential treatments to be used may be useful in thrombo-embolic disease but positively harmful in haemorrhagic stroke. Consequently, attempts to determine the effects of treatments for acute stroke have been difficult.

Power

The most common problem of stroke trials is that they have been too small. This leads to difficulties in interpretation of trial results for two reasons. First, since stroke is such a heterogeneous condition, the findings of a small positive trial may be difficult to apply to individual stroke patients. Secondly, the study, if negative, may be too small to exclude an important treatment effect, that is, it has a low power. This second point often causes confusion, and may be clarified by Table 9.1.

A treatment that appears to be effective in a trial may be a rogue result, but the chances of thinking that the treatment is effective when in reality it is not effective (i.e. a false-positive result) is given by the *p*-value associated with the treatment effect. The conventional statistical approach is to define effects that

Table 9.1 Comparison of the results of a clinical trial with the true effects of a treatment

	True treatment effect	
Treatment effect in trial	Not effective	Effective
Not effective	Agreement, not effective	False-negative trial result, 'power' (type II error)
Effective	False-positive trial result (type I error) (p < 0.05)	Agreement, effective

might have occurred by chance only once in 20 similar trials as significant, and therefore likely to be 'true'.

Trials that do not produce significant differences between treatment groups are commonly referred to as 'negative' trials and are often misinterpreted. No evidence of effect is popularly confused with evidence of no effect. A trial that does not produce a statistically significant effect may be true (i.e. the treatment really is ineffective). Alternatively, it may be that the trial is hiding a real effect because it is too small and cannot exclude a true treatment effect. The best clue that a negative study has low power is to examine the 95 per cent confidence intervals (CI) of the differences in outcome between treated and control groups, and then to ask whether the upper limit includes an effect that would be clinically useful. If it does, then the trial should not be interpreted as indicating that the treatment is ineffective.

Since stroke is such a common disease, even small acute treatment effects (of the order of 5–10 per cent improvements in outcomes) may be useful if considered in the context of the whole population. For example, a treatment that produced a 10 per cent reduction in mortality (e.g. from 30 per cent 1-month mortality to 27 per cent 1-month mortality) amongst the 100 000 first strokes in England and Wales, would lead to a saving of 3000 lives. The catch is that to detect such small differences very large trials—'mega-trials'—are needed. Mega-trials were pioneered in evaluating treatments for heart attack, and have some features which distinguish them from smaller trials. To make such large trials work requires the co-operation of a large number of investigators in different centres. It also means that registration, randomization, and data collection must be kept as simple as possible. Outcome measures, in particular, must be simple enough to apply easily and must be valid, but because of the very large numbers involved in these trials, relaxation of usual standards of reliability is acceptable. If there is a true difference between two treatment groups, a mega-trial will have adequate power and, therefore, a good chance of detecting it, even though some patients are recruited for

Table 9.2 Sample size requirements for each group in randomized controlled trials with a power of 80 per cent and significance level of $p < 0.05$

Event rate in control group	Clinically important difference (i.e. control – treatment) to be detected					
	0.5%	1%	5%	10%	20%	30%
1%	8150	2500	250	106	47	29
5%	31 600	8400	470	160	58	33
10%	58 160	14 950	725	219	71	38
20%	101 800	25 700	1130	313	91	45
40%	151 000	38 000	1570	407	107	48

whom the treatment is ineffective, and despite the use of rather crude outcomes (such as 'dead or dependent versus not') (van Gijn and Warlow 1992).

Various charts and tables are available to determine how many subjects are needed to ensure that a trial has adequate power to detect specified differences, or they can be calculated from simple formulae (Kirkwood 1988). These calculations do not decide what is a clinically 'important' difference; this requires clinical judgement, together with an appreciation of the numbers of patients who will have to be treated to obtain a beneficial outcome (e.g. life saved, recurrent stroke prevented). In general, trials of treatment require many hundreds or thousands of subjects in each group if the outcome of interest is survival (or a dichotomous improvement versus not improved). Table 9.2 illustrates how the clinically important difference to be detected affects sample size.

Which measure of outcome?

Disability, handicap, and quality of life matter most to patients, but devising simple, robust, valid, reliable, and responsive measures of these for use in large-scale trials has proved difficult (Harwood et al. 1994b; Ebrahim 1995). Consequently, different outcomes have been used inconsistently (Roberts and Counsell 1998). They are prone to measurement error and their relationship to neurological impairment is complex (Harwood et al. 1997). Many things besides limb weakness contribute to poor quality of life, but the physical and social environment, and personal relationships, are hardly likely to be influenced by thrombolytic or neuroprotective drugs. Demonstrating and quantifying changes in measures of disability, handicap, and quality of life therefore requires big trials, and false-negative trials are a potential problem. None the less, these outcomes are important, and are required in informing health policy decisions.

Big trials are expensive, and one way around this is to measure an intermediate outcome that can be measured more precisely, but is related to the outcome of chief interest (Barer *et al.* 1988*b*). For example, a small trial designed to measure the rate at which cerebral oxygen metabolism recovers in patients given a new drug will have sufficient power to detect an important difference because the number of subjects required is determined by the variance of the outcome measured. As a general principle, it is essential to use outcomes that are closely related to the type of treatment given, and also to measure more global indicators such as handicap or quality of life, which may, or may not, show associated changes if treatment is beneficial. Acute drug treatments that do not have an impact on simple outcomes such as impairment, mortality, and hospital bed-days, but appear to have an impact on quality of life or activities of daily living, will be unusual. Trial power can also be increased by using repeated measures before and after the intervention to reduce measurement errors and therefore variance, but often this is not logistically possible.

Unless deaths are counted along with neurological and functional outcomes, imbalance between treated and control groups can occur (Barer *et al.* 1988*b*). If more patients in one group die, and these are the most severely affected, the survivors in this group will spuriously appear to be less disabled (because the more disabled ones have died). With days spent in hospital, patients who have died may be counted as contributing the maximum number of days of follow-up. For discharge from hospital, those discharged to institutions and those who have died should be counted together as having a 'bad' outcome. The tactic of counting death as equivalent to the worst outcome amongst survivors ensures that the balance achieved by randomization is not upset, and therefore that comparisons remain valid. Of course, this does not 'quantify' death, and careful choice of statistical analysis is needed.

Generalizability

Do the patients included in a trial bear any relationship to patients looked after by the majority of clinicians? If trial patients are highly selected, which they often are, then it is highly unlikely that they will be similar to the typical stroke patient. This is a particular problem in acute treatment trials because generally the patients should have neuroradiology to define the type and location of the stroke; should not have other pathological processes that might interfere with measured outcomes; should have treatment started very early in the course of the event so that potentially reversible pathogenetic mechanisms can be influenced; and should be in hospital to ensure uniform assessment, randomization, and other supportive treatment.

The typical stroke patient is old, with numerous other medical and social problems, is often kept at home, never goes near a CT scanner, and if admitted to hospital, is seldom there within the first few hours of the event. Consequently trials that try to ensure that the patients randomized are as homogeneous as possible may end up by producing a trial result that is of limited relevance to the practising clinician—the problem of generalizability. Moreover, unduly restrictive entry criteria severely limit recruitment to trials, and this may outweigh the advantages of a homogeneous group for statistical analysis and biological interpretation (LaRue *et al.* 1988; Dorman and Sandercock 1996).

There is no quantitative way to decide the extent to which a trial can or cannot be generalized to the patients seen in different settings. A judgment must be made by the individual clinician. Trials must strive to comply with an epidemiological maxim: 'validity first, generalizability second' (Hennekens and Buring 1987). If a trial result is not valid, because of bias, there is no point in trying to generalize it. It is better to define the groups to whom a valid result apply, and it will often be reasonable to assume generalizability unless there is a good reason to think otherwise. Trialists can help by their descriptions of the patients they actually studied. In particular, the age range of patients studied, the proportion with other medical problems, early case fatality, the setting from which patients were obtained (e.g. community, specialist neurology centre), and details of the patients not suitable for randomization. These non-randomized patients are the key to interpretation of a trial. If their death rate, for example, is markedly different from those included in the trial, it implies that substantial selection has occurred, making it less likely that the trial results will apply to all cases.

Another technique that helps decide the relevance of a trial to other patients is subgroup analyses, but these should be specified in advance, rather than produced following inspection of the trial results (data dredging). Subgroup analysis after data inspection, while tempting, runs a major risk of generating false-positive findings (so-called type I errors). The subgroup analyses that should usually be specified, which are of importance, are: male/female differences in outcome, age effects, and stroke severity and pathological type effects. However, even in mega-trials, it is extremely unlikely that sufficient numbers of participants will be recruited to have adequate power to reject subgroup null hypotheses.

Randomization

Balancing out the factors that have an influence on outcome after stroke is important if a valid comparison is to be made between treated and placebo groups. If we possessed complete knowledge about the prognosis of stroke, then a case could be made for allocating patients to treatment groups according to such knowledge. Randomization is simply a method for balancing out both known and unknown factors that may have a bearing on the outcome of interest. The effect of chance dictates that two groups allocated at random should only differ to an extent determined by chance variation.

It is possible, however, for simple randomization to go wrong and for the play of chance to lead to large imbalances between groups. An example of this effect was an early trial of the use of steroids to reduce cerebral oedema (Mulley et al. 1978). Nearly twice as many patients unconscious to the point of being insensitive to pain were randomized to the placebo group. This imbalance is surprising and is statistically unlikely, but not impossible. In this case, although the treatment groups were poorly balanced the bias was weighted in favour of the treatment group having a good outcome, but an insignificant result was obtained. Unless a trial is very large, it is worth stratifying the randomization process (i.e. randomizing severe and milder strokes separately), so that major imbalances in the most important prognostic factors do not occur. Computer programs are available that reduce imbalance amongst important, prespecified, prognostic factors, while retaining the random allocation principal ('minimization' methods) and should be used more widely in small trials (Treasure and MacRae 1998).

Consistency

A single positive trial result will not alter clinical practice, nor should it. It might be a fluke result, it might only apply to a highly selected group of patients, or other deficiencies in the trial design (e.g. short follow-up, losses and withdrawals, side-effects of treatment, unrecognized imbalances between groups, etc.), all of which make most clinicians naturally conservative about trying new treatments on their patients.

A trial of haemodilution in acute stroke highlights the need for a cautious approach to a single trial. An initial report of haemodilution by venesection and infusion of dextran 40 applied to 102 patients admitted to a stroke unit showed clear benefits in the proportion returning home, and in the functional and neurological recovery rate (Strand et al. 1984). Surprisingly, these investigators, having obtained a positive result, decided to set up a much larger multi-centre trial to test the effects of treatment in a more typical setting than the specialist stroke unit (Scandinavian Stroke Study Group 1987). In all 373 patients were randomized, but this time no benefits of treatment were found in the whole group, or in any subgroup (Scandinavian Stroke Study Group 1988).

The last word on haemodilution was from an Italian study (Italian Acute Stroke Study Group 1988), which randomized 1267 patients, carried out CT scans on nearly all of them, and disappointingly demonstrated no benefits in survival or disability. Subgroup analyses did not pick out any benefits for those treated very early, for infarcts compared with haemorrhages, or for those patients with high haematocrits at the outset.

The message is quite clear—treatments that look like winners must be subject to further evaluation. With increased demand for research funds and a natural human tendency for novelty, it is difficult to ensure that replicate trials are done.

Reporting of trials

A major advance in the conduct of trials has been agreement among investigators, and adoption by journal editors, for standard approaches to trial reporting. The Consolidated Standards of Reporting Trials (CONSORT) guidelines provide an explicit checklist which includes issues such as the number of eligible patients, the methods of random allocation and blinding, and data presentation (Altman 1996; Begg *et al.* 1996). In the past, investigators have reported trial findings in idiosyncratic ways that often hide what happened to every participant. While such reporting was not often deliberate, major problems of trial interpretation ensue if intention-to-treat analyses cannot be carried out.

Aspirin and heparin in acute stroke

Until recently the role of aspirin and anticoagulation in acute stroke and 'stroke in evolution' was unclear. Practice was very variable, with 10 per cent of UK physicians treating acute stroke at least sometimes using low-dose subcutaneous heparin (Lindley *et al.* 1995). A meta-analysis of available data was consistent with a moderate benefit, but was also consistent with no benefit at all (Sandercock *et al.* 1993).

The situation is now very much clearer thanks to two mega-trials, the International Stroke Trial (IST) and the Chinese Acute Stroke Trial (CAST). In the IST 20 000 patients with acute stroke (within 48 hours) were randomized between receiving heparin (25 000 IU/day or 10 000 IU/day) or placebo. The design also randomized patients to receive 300 mg/day of aspirin or no aspirin, in a 2 × 2 factorial design (i.e. patients were randomized to one of four possible groups: aspirin alone, heparin alone, heparin and aspirin, no treatment). Treatment was for 14 days or until discharge if sooner. Almost all had a CT scan, 87 per cent prior to randomization (International Stroke Trial Collaborative Group 1997). CAST randomized 21 000 patients to 160 mg/day of aspirin or placebo for 4 weeks or until discharge (Chinese Acute Stroke Trial Study Group 1997).

Heparin

At 14 days, there was no difference in the number of deaths between patients treated with heparin (9.0 per cent) and no heparin (9.3 per cent) (risk ratio 0.97). After 6 months, 62.9 per cent of patients in each group were dead or dependent. Fewer recurrent ischaemic strokes in the treated groups were offset by an identical increase in the number of recurrent haemorrhagic strokes. The higher dose of heparin was associated with more deaths and non-fatal strokes within 14 days than the lower dose, but there was no difference in the combined end point of death or dependence at 6 months with the lower dose. No subgroup, including patients with atrial fibrillation or different stroke subtypes, benefited significantly more or less than the average.

Despite these findings, in a *Lancet* commentary on the IST study, Bousser suggested that in patients with atrial fibrillation, it would be 'more appropriate to start secondary prevention straight away with anticoagulants rather than with aspirin. And, the negative global results for heparin obtained should not deter the clinician from prescribing it, to prevent deep vein thrombosis ...' (Bousser 1997). It is remarkable that in the face of clear evidence of lack of benefit in thousands of patients, and clear potential harms, a clinician is swayed by indirect evidence (anticoagulants are more beneficial than aspirin in atrial fibrillation), small trials (e.g. prevention of deep-vein thrombosis) with inadequate ability to detect serious harms, and subgroup analyses. In part this reflects ignorance of epidemiological reasoning, and in part a heritage mentality based on clinical science grounded in pathophysiology. Indeed, Bousser, supporting Caplan (1991a), suggests that 'the clinician should identify mechanisms and causes of ischaemic stroke in order to individualise treatment'. The best treatment for the individual comes from an appraisal of their individual risk obtained through an understanding of the factors which determine recurrence (see Chapter 13) followed by application of the best estimates of risk reduction which are obtained either from meta-analyses or from mega-trials. Clinicians who believe that they can tease out a subgroup (from trial reports, pathophysiological reasoning, or their imaginations) that will do better or worse than the pooled average estimates derived from trials and meta-analyses are deluding themselves and not helping their patients.

Aspirin

This had a small but definite effect in reducing death or dependency, but only when the results of the two trials were combined. In IST, aspirin treatment resulted in a small, statistically uncertain, reduction in deaths within 14 days (9.0 compared with 9.4 per cent, risk ratio 0.96), and a small, statistically significant, reduction in death or recurrent stroke (11.3 compared with 12.4 per cent, risk ratio 0.91). After 6 months, there was a small reduction in the combined end point of death and dependency with active treatment (62.2 compared with 63.5 per cent, risk ratio 0.98). Again, no subgroup benefited significantly more or less than any other. In the Chinese trial, patients were, on average, younger than in the IST, and had lower absolute risks of death,

Table 9.3 The pooled effects of aspirin in acute stroke

	Number of participants	Recurrent stroke (%)	Haemorrhagic stroke (%)	Deaths all causes (%)	Deaths/non-fatal strokes (%)
Aspirin	20 207	496 (2.45)	205 (1.01)	1231 (6.09)	1662 (8.22)
Control	20 190	636 (3.15)	168 (0.83)	1327 (6.57)	1843 (9.13)
Number need to treat		145	555 (harm)	208	110

recurrent stroke, and dependency after 4 weeks. Aspirin reduced deaths from 3.9 to 3.3 per cent (risk ratio 0.85), reduced death or non-fatal stroke from 5.9 to 5.3 per cent (risk ratio 0.89), and reduced death or dependency from 31.6 to 30.5 per cent (risk ratio 0.97). Taken together with IST and one much smaller previous trial, this gives pooled odds ratios for death or non-fatal stroke of 0.89 (95 per cent CI, 0.83–0.95), and 0.95 (95 per cent CI, 0.91–0.99) for death or dependency (Table 9.3).

The actual numbers of events avoided by using aspirin in the acute phase are small. The difference in death rates between aspirin and control groups is only 0.5 per cent and the combined end point of deaths and non-fatal stroke is less than 1 per cent. Thus for every 1000 patients treated, nine deaths or non-fatal strokes will be avoided, but this could be as few as 3 and as many as 15 events avoided. Detecting treatment effects as small as 0.5–1 per cent requires trials of this size, and it might be thought that such effects are simply too small to be worth having. Despite these small effects, these two acute aspirin trials provide evidence for early prescribing, since aspirin should be prescribed for long-term secondary prevention, so long as haemorrhage has been excluded with reasonable certainty. This strengthens the case for routine CT head scanning soon after stroke. The two trials do not tell us one way or the other whether it is safe to give aspirin early without CT scanning to exclude a haemorrhage. The intracranial haemorrhages caused by aspirin mean that such action would probably be risky.

A mega-trial has the potential to answer a question once and for all, but is still prone to the effects of chance, bias, and confounding, even if much less so than smaller trials. Strictly, of course it only answers the question that it was designed to answer. Problems may arise if many randomized patients receive trial medication outside the trial protocol, where it appears to be 'clinically indicated', as possibly happened in the case of nitrates in the ISIS-4 trial after myocardial infarction, producing a so-called 'null bias' (ISIS-4 Collaborative Group 1995; Woods 1995). In CAST more than half the participants received another (non-trial) treatment, including thrombolytics, calcium antagonists, glycerol, and herbal medication. Fortunately the results do not seem to have been affected as these treatments are largely ineffective.

Thrombolysis

Great excitement, particularly in the USA, has followed the publication of a randomized, placebo-controlled trial demonstrating reduced death or dependency in patients given intravenous tissue plasminogen activator (tPA, alteplase) within 3 hours of the onset of acute ischaemic stroke (NINDS rt-PA Stroke Study Group 1995). This has led to considerable efforts to re-educate the public about the urgency of seeking medical attention in the face of a possible stroke ('brain attack'), and expediting admission to hospital, evaluation in hospital emergency departments, CT scanning, and treatment delivery. Is this effort justified?

The National Institute of Neurological Disorders and Stroke (NINDS) study involved 624 patients in a two-stage experiment. All had CT head scans to exclude haemorrhage, and no contraindications to thrombolytic therapy. Follow-up CTs were performed to detect treatment-related haemorrhages. Half the patients were treated within 90 minutes of stroke onset, the rest within 180 minutes. The first stage examined changes in a 42-point neurological impairment score in 291 patients, 24 hours after stroke onset. The median score on entry was 14, with a range of 1 to 37. The majority of these patients were, therefore, no more than moderately severely affected. After 24 hours there was a small difference in the neurological score between the tPA and placebo groups, and in the proportion who had made a complete neurological recovery (median scores 8 versus 12; relative risk for improvement 1.2; 95 per cent CI, 1.0–1.4; $p = 0.06$; both in favour of tPA treatment). Outcomes at 3 months were also determined (see Table 9.4).

The second stage included a further 333 patients and was designed to test the effect of treatment on death and disability measured by global health and activities of daily living rating scales (the Barthel, Rankin, and Glasgow scales) 3 months after the stroke. High thresholds were used to denote favourable outcomes, which essentially implied complete recovery (e.g. 19/20 on the Barthel scale, and a Rankin score of 0 or 1).

There were no differences between the results of the two stages of the study, nor in any subgroup defined by stroke subtype, severity, or time to treatment, so the results have been combined (Table 9.4). There was a small reduction in mortality in the tPA group (17 compared with 21 per cent, $p = 0.30$). More patients treated with tPA had complete or almost complete recovery on each of the four outcome scales, ranging from 43 per cent versus 27 per cent on the Rankin scale, to 34 per cent versus 21 per cent on the neurological score. Active treatment gave a 35–67 per cent (relative) increased chance of a favourable outcome, and the number needed to treat per favourable outcome was 6–9 patients. Eleven per cent of tPA-treated patients had an intracranial haemorrhage, of which 60 per cent were symptomatic and 26 per cent fatal. Thus, about 3 per cent of treated patients had fatal intracranial bleeds, but 13–16 per

Table 9.4 Three-month results from the NINDS tPA trial, results from two parts of the trial combined and recalculated from data in the paper

	Number (%) with favourable outcome		Risk ratio (95% confidence interval)	p-value
	tPA (n = 312)	Placebo (n = 312)		
Survival	259 (83%)	246 (79%)	1.31 (0.9–2.0)	0.30
Barthel index	162 (52%)	120 (38%)	1.35 (1.1–1.6)	0.0007
Rankin score	133 (43%)	83 (27%)	1.60 (1.3–2.0)	0.00003
Glasgow score	142 (46%)	98 (31%)	1.45 (1.2–1.8)	0.0003
NIH stroke scale	107 (34%)	64 (21%)	1.67 (1.3–2.2)	0.0001

cent experienced a more favourable 3-month outcome. In comparison, 4 per cent of placebo group patients had bleeds, one of which was fatal.

Four questions must be answered before accepting the results of this trial:

1. Is there any alternative explanation for the results, other than a beneficial effect of tPA?
2. How does this trial compare with other similar trials?
3. Is treatment cost-effective, especially as implementation will require a substantial investment in reorganizing systems, including providing 24-hour rapid-access CT scanning?
4. Could routine practice replicate the results achieved under the strict protocols of a trial?

Alternative explanations

An imbalance in the proportions of the two groups who had been taking aspirin before their strokes (tPA 26 per cent and placebo 18 per cent) did not seem to affect the results. There was also an imbalance in the proportion of lacunar strokes between groups (in favour of the tPA group). Statistical adjustment for this and other differences slightly increased the benefit in favour of tPA. There may also have been differences in other unknown prognostic factors, as the trial size would have been inadequate to eliminate them entirely (Friedman 1996). Despite the monumental effort involved in running a trial such as this, the numbers enrolled were quite small, and a chance result is possible, despite the highly statistically significant p-values. The estimates of the size of the benefits are imprecise, and although the results are consistent with a quite large benefit (a relative risk of favourable outcome up to 2.2), it may also have been trivial (relative risk 1.1).

Concordance with other studies

There have been a number of other thrombolytic trials, using streptokinase (Multicentre Acute Stroke Trial—Italy 1995; Donnan *et al.* 1996; Multicentre

Acute Stroke Trial—Europe 1996), tPA (Hacke *et al.* 1998), and smaller trials using a variety of agents (Wardlaw and Warlow 1992).

The two European Co-operative Acute Stroke Studies were the most similar to the NINDS trial. ECASS-I (Hacke *et al*, 1995) used a slightly higher dose of tPA, entered patients up to 6 hours after stroke onset, and excluded mild or very severe cases. Between 5 and 15 per cent of stroke admissions at participating centres were randomized. This study showed a small benefit for tPA in terms of neurological and functional outcomes, at the cost of an increased mortality rate. On intention-to-treat analyses, 30-day mortality was 18 per cent in the tPA group, and 13 per cent in the placebo group, but 36 per cent of the tPA group were independent on the Rankin Score, compared with only 29 per cent for placebo (odds ratio 1.15; 95 per cent CI, 0.98–1.35). Seventeen per cent of the trial population were declared 'protocol violators' after randomization (albeit blind to treatment allocation), with more of the tPA group being excluded. Protocol violators, particularly those whose initial CT scans already showed signs of infarction, had a high mortality, especially from intracranial bleeding. The investigators made much of the significant advantages for active treatment after exclusion of this group. Unfortunately post-randomization exclusions are prone to introduce major biases, and conclusions based on them must be considered unsafe. There was also a failure to take adequate account of the different death rates in comparisons of some of the functional outcomes, introducing a bias in favour of tPA.

ECASS-II randomised 800 patients within six hours of a stroke, using the same dose of tPA as the NINDS trial. CT criteria excluding signs of major infarction were more restrictive than in ECASS-I. After 90 days 40 per cent of tPA treated patients had a favourable outcome on the Rankin Scale (0-1) compared with 37 per cent on placebo treatment (relative risk 0.91), a difference which could have arisen by chance. There was no difference in deaths between the groups (10 per cent), nor any advantage for the subgroup randomised within three hours. A 'post hoc secondary analysis' re-defining success to include patients with only minor disability (Rankin 0-2) showed a slightly larger, and statistically significant benefit (54 per cent vs. 46 per cent), but conclusions based on such 'data-dredging' are risky. The original end-point (with Rankin grades 0 or 1 being 'favourable') was presumably chosen to maximise the chances of demonstrating the efficacy of tPA on the grounds that it aims to 'cure' strokes. Six other pre-defined end-points were all essentially the same in the two groups (Hacke *et al* 1998).

Unfortunately to make thrombolysis safe it appears that it is necessary to exclude the most severely affected patients (reflected in the much lower mortality rate in ECASS-II compared with ECASS-I, and the high spontaneous improvement rate in the placebo group). This is the group that stands to gain most from intervention. More sophisticated selection of patients for thrombolysis is required, and newer magnetic resonance methods may provide this.

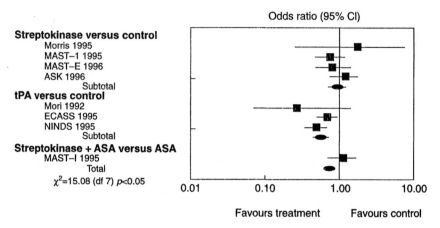

Fig. 9.1 Meta-analysis of trials of thrombolysis in acute stroke: effect on death or dependency at the end of trial follow-up. (From Wardlaw *et al.* 1997, redrawn with permission of the author and *Lancet*).

A meta-analysis has been performed of 12 trials of thrombolysis, including 3435 patients of whom 694 died and 1001 were functionally dependent at the end of follow-up. In actively treated patients fewer were dead or dependent compared with control-group patients (61.5 per cent versus 68.0 per cent; odds ratio 0.75; 95 per cent CI, 0.63–0.88) (Fig. 9.1). However, early case fatality was higher in treated patients compared with controls (21 per cent versus 12 per cent; odds ratio 1.99; 95 per cent CI, 1.6–2.5), and thrombolysis was associated with more symptomatic haemorrhages, some of which were fatal. Patients treated within 3 hours of stroke onset did not suffer an excess of deaths and were substantially less likely to be dead or dependent (odds ratio 0.55; 95 per cent CI, 0.42–0.71). There was marked variation in early case-fatality between trials (but not death or dependence as a combined outcome) which makes conclusions based on pooled results uncertain (Wardlaw *et al.* 1997).

The evidence on the use of thrombolytics in acute stroke is consistent with a worthwhile reduction in death and severe disability, but probably at the cost of increased early case-fatality. The current best estimate from meta-analysis is a 25 per cent odds reduction for death or severe disability but with a 36 per cent increase in the odds of death. This implies that the extra deaths due to thrombolysis were among patients who would have survived with moderate to severe disability without treatment. If, as some work has suggested (Solomon *et al.* 1994; Gage *et al.* 1996), survival in disabled states is valued very poorly, this is a reasonable trade-off. However, there is considerable variation between people on their valuations of health states, making the gaining of individual informed consent to a treatment which may improve the chances of a good recovery, but at the expense of increased risk of death, very difficult for an ill patient in a rushed environment. For many stroke patients, the very fact of surviving a potentially fatal event is cause for celebration (Pound *et al.* 1995).

Cost-effectiveness

No formal analysis has been done, and in any case this would not be able to take account of the capital investment in CT scanning, acute stroke units, and the recurrent staff costs required. Given the high costs of long-term instit-utional care, a moderately effective treatment could be worthwhile, despite high implementation costs.

Translation of trial results into routine practice

The results achieved in trials probably represent the best that could be achieved in terms of efficacy and safety, and for the time being, any attempt to introduce thrombolysis into routine practice would probably not yield com-parable results. The high proportion of 'protocol violators' in ECASS, who fared badly, illustrate some of the potential problems even within the confines of a randomized trial.

The NINDS study only randomized about 3 per cent of over 17 000 potential subjects screened for inclusion (NINDS t-PA Stroke Study Group 1997). Some did not have stroke, but many who did were too late for inclu-sion. Currently very few patients reach hospital within 2 hours of stroke onset (which is what is required given about an hour for evaluation and investi-gation once in hospital). For example, in Copenhagen, 7 per cent of patients were admitted within 1 hour, and less than a quarter were admitted within 3 hours (Jorgensen *et al.* 1996). In Leicester, an accurate time of onset was only determined in 70 per cent of cases, but 25 per cent of patients were admitted within 2 ½ hours (Harper *et al.* 1992). Reasons for delay include awaking with stroke, living alone, failure to call medical help, progressive symptoms, and ambulance delays. In the NINDS trial, every aspect of the admission process was scrutinized to reduce time to treatment, including public and ambulance personnel education, advance warning of arrival by ambulance crews to emergency departments, expedited 24-hour CT scanning (even using the CT scanner to get a chest radiograph), dedicated stroke emergency teams without conflicting clinical duties, and protocols for supply and preparation of tPA infusions (NINDS t-PA Stroke Study Group 1997). All this implies the need for considerable overcapacity in the hospital emergency medical system to cater for very few patients.

Use of thrombolytic therapy outside of randomized trials is premature. A recent national UK survey of consultants managing stroke patients (Ebrahim and Redfern, 1999) has shown that they remain sceptical of the efficacy of thrombolytics, and that their use of these drugs is still as low as it was in 1992

(Lindley *et al.* 1995). In the near future, patients may expect that fast-track procedures are available for those who do get to hospital in time, and accept possible treatment risks of thrombolytic drugs.

Other treatments

The search for new treatments for acute stroke has been built on an understanding of the pathogenesis of stroke. The main mechanisms that seem important in determining the extent of damage are cerebral oedema, blood flow in the area around the lesion, neuronal metabolism, neural protection and growth, and neurochemical abnormalities in ischaemia (Table 9.5).

The drugs listed in Table 9.5 are of some interest as they show that even with a pathophysiological understanding of the ways in which stroke affects the brain, apparently logical treatments are without effect. This lack of success in so many early drug trials almost certainly resulted in the nihilism which still surrounds stroke care. However, many treatments, including corticosteroids, naftidrofuryl, glycerol, and calcium antagonists, have not been evaluated in trials with sufficient numbers of participants to exclude moderate benefit (or harm). Many newer neuroprotective and other agents are being evaluated, and there is a danger that these, too, will be abandoned for want of adequately sized trials (Dorman and Sandercock 1996; Del Zoppo *et al.* 1997; Dyker and Lees 1998; Lees 1998).

Several of these areas have been systematically reviewed by the Cochrane Stroke Group and detailed reviews are available on websites or CD-ROM. Further reviews of use of mannitol, fibrinolytic agents, calcium antagonists, antioxidants, and piracetam are planned for completion in the next 2 years (Cochrane Library, 1998 issue 3). There are still several areas which have not yet been examined systematically and it is hoped that investigators with interests in the acute treatment of stroke will collaborate with the Cochrane Stroke Group to complete and maintain reviews of some of the older treatments (e.g. barbiturates, naloxone, and hypothermia) which may have been inadequately evaluated in underpowered, small trials.

Summary

1. Patients admitted to hospital tend to have more severe strokes and to live alone. The need to investigate patients to exclude diseases that may mimic stroke is not well recognized amongst primary health care doctors.

2. The proportion of stroke patients admitted to UK hospitals varies from 50 to 75 per cent. The chief perceived reason for admission is for nursing care.

3. Admission to hospital may ensure rehabilitation is started early and

Table 9.5 Mechanism of action of various drugs used in the treatment of acute stroke

Mechanism	Drug	Reference
Reducing oedema		
	Steroids	Qizilbash et al. (1998)
	Barbiturates	Sila and Furlan (1988)
	Glycerol	Rogvi-Hansen and Boysen (1998)
Improving blood flow		
	Haemodilution	Asplund et al. (1998)
	Vasodilators	
	Nimodipine	Gelmers et al. (1988a), TRUST Study Group (1990)
	Naloxone	Baskin and Hosobuchi (1981), Frederico et al. (1991)
	Prostacyclin	Bath and Bath (1998)
	Naftidrofuryl	Steiner and Rose (1986)
	Vasoconstrictors	
	Theophylline	Mohiuddin et al. (1998)
Reducing neuronal metabolism		
	β-Blockers	Barer et al. (1988a)
	Naftidrofuryl	Steiner and Rose (1986)
	Barbiturates	Safar (1980)
	Hypothermia	Thomas (1984)
Thrombus directed therapy		
	Antiplatelet agents	
	Aspirin	Chinese Acute Stroke Trial (1997), International Stroke Trial (1997)
	Oxypentifyline	Bath et al. (1998)
	Anticoagulants	Counsell and Sandercock (1998a)
	LMW heparins	Counsell and Sandercock (1998b)
	Thrombolytic agents	Wardlaw et al. (1998)
	Streptokinase	Sloan (1987)
	Tissue plasminogen activator	Hacke et al. (1995), NINDS rt-PA Stroke Study Group (1995)
	Fibrinogen depletion	Liu et al. (1998)
Neuroprotective agents		
	NMDA antagonists	
	Magnesium	Muir and Lees (1995)
	Selfotel	Grotta et al. (1995), Davis et al. (1997)
	Gangliosides	Candelise and Cicconi (1998)
	Vinpocetine	Bereczki and Fekete (1998)
	Lubeluzole	Grotta (1997)
	Piracetam	de-Deyn et al. (1997)
	Lifarizine	Squire et al. (1996)
Antioxidants		
	Ebselen	Yamaguchi et al. (1998)
	Ginkgo biloba	Garg et al. (1995)
	Tirilazad mesylate	STIPAS Study Group (1994), Haley et al. (1996)
Cell membrane effects		
	Citicoline	Clark et al. (1997)
	Calcium-channel blockers	
	Flunarazine	Franke et al. (1996)

complications avoided. A single trial of a domiciliary management team did not succeed in reducing the use of hospital beds, and consequently was not considered a viable alternative to hospital admission.

4. No current acute treatment is successful in substantially reducing the mortality or limiting the brain damage caused by strokes. Aspirin started in the acute phase is associated with small benefits, and thrombolytics in highly selected patients may produce modest benefits, but with moderate risk and probably increased early mortality.

5. Clinical trials have suffered with problems of low power to detect important treatment effects because of small sample sizes, have excluded patients not completing treatment, and have often studied highly selected patients who are atypical of many stroke patients.

6. Future studies must be large, should include patients broadly representative of all stroke patients, should be pragmatic in design, and should measure simple outcomes appropriate to the intervention. These outcomes are usually death, days in hospital, or a functional end point such as independent living.

10 Rehabilitation

The nature of rehabilitation

Rehabilitation is 'about the tertiary response to insult or disease' (Goodwill and Chamberlain 1988), so is concerned with the prevention of complications of disease. The effects and complications of stroke are discussed in Chapter 14, but rehabilitation is about more than prevention of complications. It is concerned with reablement (the restoration to former abilities and rights) and resettlement (the use of new or prosthetic environments). The World Health Organization defines rehabilitation as 'the combined and coordinated use of medical, social, educational and vocational measures for training or retraining the individual to the highest possible level of functional ability'. Using this definition, a case could be made for everyone, sick or well, receiving their share of 'rehabilitation'!

The rehabilitation approach involves a multidisciplinary team, comprising the patient, the family, therapists, nurses, social workers, and doctors. Team members assess the patient's disease in terms of impairments, disabilities, and handicaps, together with the burden on the family and local services. Priorities for treatment and goals are then defined with the patient and family, and specific therapy may then be started. Non-specific therapy begins with the assessments, priority and goal setting, which encourage the patient and family to begin to understand the nature of the disease and its effects. Regular team meetings are held to monitor progress towards goals, redefining them if necessary, and starting or stopping specific therapies.

Specific therapies may include the Bobath approach (Bobath 1970) which emphasizes the developmental approach to recovery (e.g. the patient must achieve sitting balance before proceeding to standing), together with a normal bilateral, rather than hemiplegic, pattern of movement and posture. Some therapists prefer the Brunnstrom methods, which make use of the pathological tonic reflexes to maintain posture and carry out activities. The former method aims to avoid inhibitory pathological reflexes, whereas the latter tries to enhance them. Both methods have their proponents, but neither has been evaluated in placebo-controlled trials, or compared with each other.

Occupational therapists in the UK usually adopt a 'practice makes perfect' eclectic approach, giving the patient plenty of opportunity to relearn skills such as dressing and washing. Some daily living skills may require the temporary or permanent use of aids or appliances, which the occupational therapist is trained to provide. Social workers will often be concerned with advice on coping with the burden of care, as well as practical advice about financial matters, arranging domiciliary services or resettlement into more appropriate environments. This may mean institutional care, but can also be provided in a range of supported non-institutional options. Rehabilitation may take place in various settings, the acute hospital ward, a stroke unit, a day hospital, an out-patient clinic, or at home.

Evaluation of rehabilitation

The favoured method for deciding whether any treatment, drug or health service, is effective is to conduct a randomized, controlled trial. If the treatment received can be made 'blind' to either recipient or provider, and preferably both, the trial removes a powerful source of potential bias. Given the complexity of the rehabilitation process, it is not surprising that the development of suitable summary outcomes to evaluate the effects of rehabilitation has been slow. The tailor-made, therapist-dependent packages of treatment are also very difficult to standardize. An hour spent with a physiotherapist who has the ability to develop a good rapport may be worth days of therapy with another therapist with poor social skills.

Evaluation of rehabilitation has many problems that may be categorized into the following groups: the patients, the interventions, and the outcomes.

The patients

Spontaneous recovery
Stroke patients will either die or recover to some extent. This basic information about natural history is fundamental, but explains why many therapies appear to be effective when studied without a concurrent control group. The before-and-after comparison is a fallacious way of assessing whether a treatment has made a difference because allowance is not made for spontaneous recovery. Since before-and-after comparisons mimic the usual clinical approach to treatment, they can be quite persuasive evidence to the scientifically naive. Spontaneous recovery can be best allowed for by making comparisons between groups randomly allocated to one or other form of therapy (or indeed, no therapy if this is ethical).

Heterogeneity
Stroke patients may look fairly similar to an untutored eye, but to a therapist the challenge is the uniqueness of each patient. This uniqueness applies not just to the type and location of the lesion causing the stroke, but also to the patient's previous abilities, coexisting diseases, social circumstances, personality, emotional response to the stroke, and aspirations.

Evaluations of effectiveness can cope with this problem in two ways. One is to reduce the sources of variation between patients by selecting only those with a particular type of lesion, affecting a particular part of the brain, causing a particular impairment, and so on. For example, several trials have concentrated efforts on rehabilitation of the hemiplegic arm (Sunderland *et al.* 1992; Feys *et al.* 1998). This approach aims to get a valid answer to the research question posed, even if it will not be applicable to all patients. The second way is to study large numbers of patients so that the diversity of stroke and its consequences are well represented. The former approach may be self-defeating because of the limited availability of ideally matched groups of patients to compare. The Frenchay Arm Study, for example, took over 3 years to recruit 132 patients (Sunderland *et al.* 1992).

Numbers
The number of subjects available to be evaluated in trials may be too few, although in clinical practice there always seem to be too many patients requiring attention! As with any attempt to evaluate therapy, it is essential that a prior effort is made to calculate the number of subjects that will need to be compared to establish whether the null hypothesis (i.e. no effect of treatment) can be safely accepted if the study produces a negative result (see Chapter 9, Acute management).

Selection bias
A successful rehabilitation team chooses patients that it knows it can help. To a greater or lesser extent rehabilitation leads to selection biases. Selection of patients who are motivated enough to put up with continued attendance at the rehabilitation department will tend to produce better results than trying to treat every patient. Selection of therapists who are particularly 'good' with stroke patients to work on a unit may achieve better results than selecting therapists working in other settings or places.

The best way to overcome the problem of selection of patients is to set up explicit criteria for inclusion in a study of the effectiveness of rehabilitation, and to measure what happens to all those patients who are allocated to the programme, and not just those who finish it. Selection of individual patients for therapy is therefore removed from the therapists' control, and thus removes this potential source of bias.

The intervention

Therapy and therapists
Rehabilitation practice is built on experience with largely untested treatments, depends on interaction between patient and therapist, and between members of the rehabilitation team, and aims to treat the patient in an

individualized way. Although randomized controlled trials are generally agreed to be the best way of deciding whether complex interventions 'work' (Meade 1977; Garraway and Akhtar 1978), it is difficult to conceive of how a satisfactory trial can be set up when the intervention can be so variable. Rehabilitation does not fit comfortably into the model of a placebo-controlled drug trial. One solution to this problem has been to treat the intervention as a 'black box'. If one type of rehabilitation is more successful than another, there should be some measurable difference, on average, between groups treated in the different ways, so long as large enough numbers are studied.

A further problem with non-standardized therapies is that they will tend to vary over a period of time, and between places. At present Bobath-orientated physiotherapy is very popular in the UK, but this will probably wane. Terms such as 'Bobath', 'Brunnstrom', or 'neuroproprioceptive facilitation' approaches indicate ideologies rather than types of approach that can be documented, standardized, and replicated. Evaluation studies should, if possible, specify by report or direct observation the activities carried out with patients and their duration. Without this information it is impossible to distinguish the effects of types and amounts of therapy from the more nonspecific effects of contact with rehabilitation teams.

Ethics of rehabilitation

Rehabilitation is now a major part of health services, and despite relatively little scientific evidence of its effectiveness, is assumed to work, in both lay and professional minds. Consequently the opportunity to test whether a rehabilitation treatment is better than spontaneous recovery is rapidly disappearing because many people believe that it is now unethical not to offer all stroke patients access to rehabilitation.

Stroke patients' views of the benefits of rehabilitation are highly relevant in determining what we mean when we say a therapy does or does not work. Patients appreciate physiotherapy; they believe it can bring about functional improvement. The exercise component is valued as it is associated with keeping busy and active, and programmes conducted at home give structure to the day. Patients also find therapists a source of advice and information and a source of faith and hope (Pound et al. 1994). Perhaps surprisingly, evaluations of rehabilitation have ignored virtually all of these aspects. Not only should these patients' views be taken into account in developing outcome measures for use in trials of specific therapies, patients' valuation of exercise in its own right deserves to be tested as a specific intervention.

At present it is not clear whether specific forms of rehabilitation have any merits over and above practice and encouragement. The time-consuming and elaborate assessment and teamwork rituals of rehabilitation teams may be a poor use of time for the majority of patients. Only by establishing effectiveness can resource levels for rehabilitation be maintained or increased, but this must be achieved without disadvantaging individual patients by depriving them of what is believed to be useful, a paradox which calls for considerable ingenuity in study design.

The main ethical dilemma faced by rehabilitation teams is whether they are being wasteful of resources in continuing to carry out untested, unstandardized methods of treatment. Brocklehurst et al. (1978) showed that patients who recovered least got the most therapy (simply because they stayed in hospital longest). If there is doubt about the value of a therapy, then it should be put to a scientific test. The other side of this problem is that so little is known about what are the important components of rehabilitation. Consequently it is all too easy to conduct trials prematurely in the development of a therapy.

Dosage and timing of rehabilitation
On average, a stroke patient receives 30 minutes of physiotherapy and 10 minutes of speech therapy a day (Hewer 1973). A trial of speech therapy after stroke (Lincoln et al. 1984) which demonstrated no advantage from therapy over the expected spontaneous improvement in language recovery was fiercely criticized because the amount of speech therapy received was too little, and yet it was exactly what was used in usual clinical practice. Little is known about the optimum amount of therapy, and it is unlikely that the relationship is linear or cumulative.

Of equal importance may be the timing of rehabilitation. Early access to a rehabilitation team may be more important than the actual amount of therapy given. In the Edinburgh stroke unit trial (Garraway et al. 1980b), although stroke unit patients received fewer hours of therapy contact, they achieved independence sooner than medical ward patients. Stroke unit patients were seen by an occupational therapist much sooner than were medical ward patients, although timing of physiotherapy input was similar. This may mean that early access to the team is important, but it may be that the occupational therapy intervention is crucial. By contrast, a meta-analysis of stroke unit trials showed no effect of timing on the relative effectiveness of stroke unit therapy (Stroke Unit Trialists Collaboration 1997). Considerable uncertainty persists about what components of rehabilitation are important.

The outcomes

Relevance of outcomes to the goals of therapy
Rehabilitation has very wide-ranging goals, and is certainly concerned with more than gaining a level of independence in activities of daily living. Yet major candidate summary measures (such as discharge to institutional care) have many other determinants besides quality of rehabilitation. Part of the

difficulty is that therapists may define their success (or failure) in terms of 'intermediate outcomes', features which are considered to be important stepping stones on the path to improved overall functioning, but which are not particularly important in their own right. For example, physiotherapy concentrates on balance, spasticity, symmetrical posture and movement, and muscle weakness, aiming to promote independence in simple tasks such as walking and dressing. Overall success, however, may be defined as a return home to a spouse who has at last come to terms with illness in the family after much counselling and support; or it may be a patient who looks and feels happy, or at least accepting, of chronic ill-health. Good sitting balance may well make this easier to attain, but not necessarily so.

A further confusion is the concept of autonomy, which need not necessarily be related to dependency at all. Very dependent people can be totally autonomous in the control they exert over what happens to them and those around them. Indeed, it might be argued that the role of rehabilitation is to achieve the maximum level of autonomy for a patient, regardless of the degree of impairment and disability suffered. A useful method of considering the options for outcome measures is to classify them as relating to impairments, disabilities, and handicaps. Given the multiple interventions used in rehabilitation, it will usually be necessary to measure more than one outcome. In a review of 50 articles concerned with stroke rehabilitation, it was noted that there is an overemphasis on physical self-care indicators, with virtually no attention given to indicators of well-being, quality of life, satisfaction with care, or return to work (Seale and Davies 1987).

Repeatability, validity, and sensitivity to change
Outcome measures must perform well to be of any use. Measurement of any biological or social variable will show some random variation, but provided this variation is small compared with the effects of therapy that are to be detected then this does not matter. It is important to know how repeatable a measurement is when used at different times on patients who have not changed clinically (within-observer variation), and when it is used by different people (between-observer variation). Unfortunately the repeatability of most disability and quality of life measures is poor compared with that expected of biological and physiological measures, which increases the need for large numbers of participants in trials (Gompertz et al. 1993).

The validity of an outcome measurement is the extent to which it measures what is intended. Usually this means comparison with a superior method of measuring the same outcome. Measurements of disability and handicap do not lend themselves to comparison with a superior method, since the outcome used is usually only one of several methods of assessment, none of which is clearly better than any of the others. In these circumstances, it is useful to examine the extent to which the outcome concurs with other indicators that have some bearing on success or failure. For example, relating a disability measure with lengths of stay in hospital gives an indication that the disability measure is valid (Ebrahim *et al.* 1985). Imperfect validity (i.e. the measurement is related to, but not exactly the same as, what is intended) will further depress power, so trials will need to be larger.

The sensitivity of a measurement to changes in patient abilities or handicaps is an obvious requirement. Broad patient groupings such as the Rankin classification (Rankin 1957) are useful for describing the severity of strokes seen in a unit, for example, but useless for assessing improvement in anything but a mega-trial. Patients may have improved substantially, but not move up to a higher category. The extremes of the scale pose a further trap; patients may improve beyond the limits of the scale, particularly with the widely used Barthel activities of daily living scale (Mahoney and Barthel 1965). Equally, the lowest and highest limits of the scale do not correspond with the nadir and zenith of ability patients may experience.

Popular outcome measures

Widely used, popular measures have advantages (Wade and Collin 1988). It is claimed that use of a standard measure would improve the attention given to the subject of disability, would improve communication between staff, would improve problem identification, and would permit different research studies to be compared. These may be more apparent than real advantages. As noted by Seale and Davies (1987), rehabilitation is concerned with far more than ability in self-care. The Barthel ADL Index, advocated by Wade and colleagues, limits understanding of the scope of disability, the type of problems identified, suffers from marked ceiling effects, and when used routinely in clinical practice can reduce, rather than increase, communication between rehabilitation team members. The Barthel ADL Index may not be the best buy outcome indicator.

By far the most important criterion in choosing outcome measures is that they should be relevant to the stated goals of a rehabilitation programme, and should be scientifically tested to ensure repeatability, validity, and sensitivity to change. If the measure chosen is also a widely used, popular measure, so much the better, because this will aid others in interpretation of results.

Independent measurement of outcome

If a rehabilitation team has to decide whether its own endeavours are worthwhile or not, there will inevitably be a conscious or subconscious desire to see the best side of the service. This is a bias that is difficult to avoid without special safeguards. In routine clinical practice it is acceptable for patients and therapists to decide for themselves whether treatment is improving things.

When conducting more formal evaluation, this is likely to lead to the expected affirmative answer.

The best way to avoid this bias is for outcome measures to be made by people other than the therapists conducting treatment. This should give more objective results, but cannot be done blind to the patient's treatment status, since the patient knows whether treatment has been given and may tell the assessor. Self-assessments by patients themselves may also be prone to this sort of 'self-deception' bias and consequently are not an alternative to independent assessors. A further refinement of this method is to ensure that therapists are not informed of the trend that results are taking during the course of an evaluation study. The object of this is to prevent therapists from prejudging the overall outcome and either becoming more or less enthusiastic in their approach.

Studies of effectiveness

Randomized controlled trials of rehabilitation present major problems for the investigator. For many practical reasons, it is not generally feasible for a single centre to randomize more than a few hundred patients in a trial of a service innovation or reorganization, nor is it easy to organize multi-centre trials. For a variable intervention, applied to a heterogeneous condition, with no consensus on appraisal of benefits, a trial of this size is small, making type II statistical error likely. In such circumstances, systematic review and meta-analysis may provide a means of improving power.

Stroke units

Studies of stroke units were among the first trials of the impact of health services on stroke patients (e.g. Garraway et al. 1980a; Stevens et al. 1984; Sivenius et al. 1985; Indredavik et al. 1991; Kalra et al. 1993a; Kalra and Eade 1995; Kaste et al. 1995). In the UK plans to develop stroke units in each health district were put forward in 1974 (Royal College of Physicians of London 1974). The benefits that stroke units would bring were thought to be:

- concentration and coordination of scarce resources;
- education of staff;
- planning of progressive patient care;
- initiate research projects.

The main emphasis in this early report was on the research potential of stroke units and, in particular, the evaluation of whether patients in a stroke unit did better than those having usual care.

Do stroke units really save lives?

It is now widely accepted that stroke unit care saves lives and this view is largely the result of an important systematic review of 10 trials published in the *Lancet* (Langhorne *et al.* 1993) which demonstrated an odds ratio for mortality of 0.72 (95 per cent CI, 0.56–0.92) within the first 4 months of onset which persisted to 1 year. Does this result fall into the 'too good to be true' category? It is almost heretical to ask such questions, since the evidence flows in the direction that patients, investigators, clinicians, and policy makers approve. But could publication bias or faulty trial design (e.g. inadequate randomization), for example, have led to this finding? Random allocation was not performed in two of the trials, and in the others it was possible for investigators to 'fix' the process (e.g. sealed envelopes can be held up to the light and shuffled to suit the patient and investigator). The inclusion criteria used were very broad and led to great clinical heterogeneity in the interventions compared; stroke units and rehabilitation teams were included in the same meta-analysis despite their inherent differences. The patients included in the trials were also very heterogeneous and in some trials there were imbalances between intervention and comparison groups, which is not surprising given the small size of most of the trials. Furthermore, the biological mechanism whereby stroke units may alter risk of mortality is not apparent.

Whenever a series of small, sometimes poorly performed trials are pooled, there is a great danger that spurious positive effects will be found as many of the biases in inadequate trials tend to push the results in favour of stroke unit care. Whenever systematic reviews throw up findings of this nature, there are two options: the first is to believe that the findings represent the truth and act on them; the second is to conduct a large mega-trial which will clinch the answer to the question by using a single protocol, standardized intervention, unbiased randomization methods, and blind assessment of outcomes. In other areas of health care where comparisons have been made between the results of meta-analysis and mega-trials it is apparent that caution should be taken in following the first option (Egger *et al.* 1997). By analogy with stroke units, the meta-analysis of in-patient geriatric consultation services (cited in Egger *et al.* 1997) found reductions in mortality and in institutionalization at 6 months (Stuck *et al.* 1993), but a large trial of comprehensive geriatric assessment failed to find the same benefits (Reuben *et al.* 1995).

Since the original *Lancet* publication, a further nine trials have been included in an updated review (Stroke Unit Trialists Collaboration 1997). Interestingly, with accumulation of more data, the mortality reduction associated with stroke units versus general medical ward care has attenuated (odds ratio, 0.80; 95 per cent CI, 0.60–1.00) and is of only borderline statistical significance (Table 10.1). Inclusion of institutionalization and dependency outcomes demonstrates benefits for stroke units compared with

Table 10.1 Meta-analysis of randomized trials of organized stroke care (from Stroke Unit Trialists Collaboration 1997)

Comparison	Stroke unit versus general medical ward	Mixed rehabilitation versus general medical ward	Stroke unit versus mixed rehabilitation
Number randomized	2060	647	542
Pooled odds ratio for death (95% CI)	0.80 (0.60–1.0)	0.92 (0.52–1.32)	0.82 (0.40–1.24)
Pooled odds ratio for death or institutionalization (95% CI)	0.72 (0.58–0.86)	0.74 (0.44–1.04)	0.90 (0.52–1.28)
Pooled odds ratio for death or dependency (95% CI)	0.68 (0.52–0.84)	0.64 (0.40–0.88)	1.01 (0.51–1.51)

general medical ward care; this result is more plausible, since the outcome does relate to one of the major goals of stroke unit care. Comparisons of stroke units versus mixed rehabilitation wards do not show convincing benefits, although confidence intervals are wide.

The greatest relative effects were found for death and dependency, with almost a 30 per cent reduction (overall pooled odds ratio 0.71; 95 per cent CI, 0.57–0.85). Absolute outcome rates were variable from trial to trial, but averaged (in the control group) 25 per cent dead, 47 per cent at home, and 34 per cent independent, giving numbers needed to treat for each of these outcomes of 22, 14, and 16. There were no substantial differences in benefits according to age, sex, stroke severity, type of medical department providing the service, timing of admission, or maximum duration of stay. Mean length of stay on the stroke units varied from 13 to 162 days, which was in some cases shorter, and others longer, than for the control group. Overall there was a small reduction in length of stay on the stroke units (8 per cent) or no difference, depending on how it was calculated.

It is unlikely that the scientific community of stroke researchers would be willing to mount a multi-centre mega-trial of stroke unit care, although it is interesting that in the similar area of cardiac rehabilitation, where systematic reviews of upwards of 40 small and often badly executed randomized controlled trials have shown 20 per cent reductions in mortality (Ebrahim and Davey Smith 1996), the English NHS Executive has commissioned a large, multi-centre trial because of doubts about the evidence of benefit (NHS Research and Development Programme 1997).

Checking for publication bias

One question that does arise is whether publication bias has occurred, such that small negative trials have not been published, whereas small positive trials are more likely to be published. The original stroke unit review

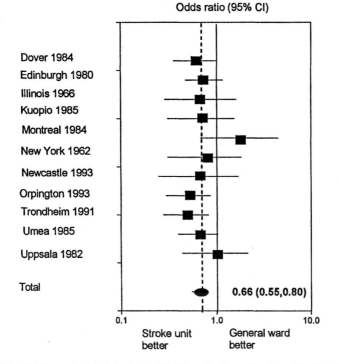

Odds ratio (95% CI)

Dover 1984
Edinburgh 1980
Illinois 1966
Kuopio 1985
Montreal 1984
New York 1962
Newcastle 1993
Orpington 1993
Trondheim 1991
Umea 1985
Uppsala 1982

Total   0.66 (0.55,0.80)

0.1   1.0   10.0

Stroke unit   General ward
better   better

Fig. 10.1 Meta-analysis of stroke unit trials: effects on death and institutionalization at final review.

certainly identified five further trials but data were not available at the time of analysis. The authors of the review examined the question of publication bias by determining how many patients would have to be studied to refute their findings on mortality and considered that if all the known, but as yet unreported, studies showed no effect on mortality, this would not make a difference to their conclusions. However, if these newer studies were methodologically better, it might be sensible to give them greater credence.

Another way of looking at publication bias is to construct a funnel plot (Vandenbroucke 1988). The odds ratios of treatment effects found in each study are plotted against its sample size (or some proxy measure, such as the standard error of the odds ratio). The scatter of odds ratios around the pooled estimate should be greatest where statistical power is weakest, that is small studies should be widely scattered around the bottom of the graph with the spread narrowing in larger studies—hence the shape of the graph should be that of a symmetrical inverted funnel. If publication bias has occurred, small studies which found no benefit of treatment should be missing from the base of the funnel. Figure 10.2 shows a funnel plot for the stroke unit trials which is

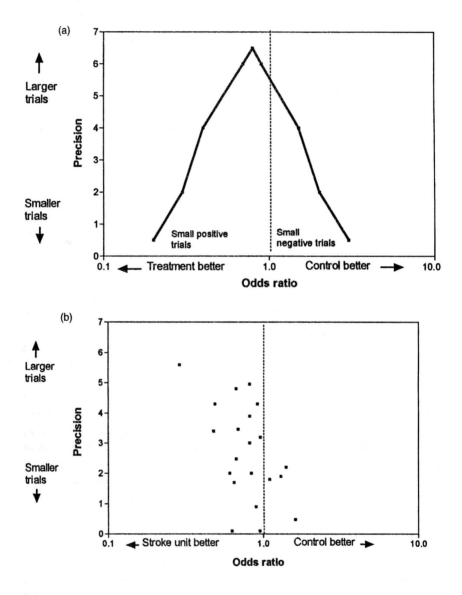

Fig. 10.2 Funnel plots. (a) A symmetrical funnel plot of trials. If small, negative trials are missing, this may be due to publication bias. (b) Stroke unit trials, funnel plot of mortality outcome. The plot is asymmetrical, but small, negative trials are not missing, so publication bias is not likely.

rather unusual. There is no evidence of publication bias (small negative trials are present) but there is clear asymmetry, suggesting that the meta-analysis may be suspect for reasons other than publication bias.

Visual inspection, particularly of a small number of data points, is unreliable and a further enhancement to assess symmetry of the effect versus precision (funnel plot) graph is to calculate a regression equation of the standard error of the odds ratio estimate on a standardized odds ratio (i.e. odds ratio divided by its standard error) (Egger *et al.* 1997). If the graph is symmetrical, the regression line will go through the origin and the intercept will (within sampling error) lie close to zero. In this case, the regression line for the original 10 trials does not go through zero but has an intercept of 1.14 (95 per cent CI, 0.52–1.76). A similar analysis for the 19 trials reported more recently (Stroke Unit Trialists Collaboration 1997) is even more asymmetrical, with an intercept of 1.82 (95 per cent CI, 0.84–2.82). The causes of funnel plot asymmetry are not only publication bias but include location bias (e.g. only English language trials), data irregularities (e.g. poor study design), and true heterogeneity where the size of the effect differs according to study size (Egger *et al.* 1997). It is possible that the smaller studies differed from the bigger trials in the type or intensity of intervention, or that the smaller studies had higher death and dependency rates, or that the smaller studies were more often badly designed. In this case, the most likely explanation for the asymmetry is that the smaller trials were all of rehabilitation whereas the bigger trials were of stroke units, and the investigators have, helpfully, provided separate estimates of efficacy for the different types of intervention. Asymmetry is worrying because it can generally be taken to indicate that the meta-analysis estimate of effect is substantially biased, that there is major heterogeneity of effect, or that it is a result of the play of chance. In this case, chance is a very unlikely explanation as even the 99 per cent confidence intervals of the intercept do not include zero. We must conclude that the evidence on the effectiveness of stroke units, although important and highly influential on health policy, is only of moderate strength.

Why might stroke units improve outcome?

These trials have been taken to demonstrate not only a means of reducing the mortality and disability associated with stroke, but also a model of service against which further innovations and development can be compared. Almost uniquely in rehabilitation, the demonstration that one form of care makes a difference compared with another makes both investigators and clinicians keen to believe the findings are true. The key question remains: what is it about a stroke unit that may make it more effective? Organization and enthusiasm *per se* are not biologically plausible explanations, but are merely

Table 10.2   Possible explanations for better outcomes on stroke units

---

- Amount of remedial therapy
- Therapy type or content
- Aids, appliances, orthoses, and seating
- Better identification of stroke-associated impairments and disabilities
- Assessment and management of co-morbidity
- Prevention, identification and management of complications (dysphagia, malnutrition, pneumonia, venous thrombosis, incontinence, pressure sores, depression)
- Continuity (nurses adopting therapy principles, routines, policies)
- Less competition for medical and nursing time
- Improved motivation and morale
- Communication, education, and involvement of relatives
- Increased self-directed therapy
- Realistic goal setting and prognostication
- Discharge planning
- Follow-up and outreach for late complications

---

facilitatory. Simply calling a ward a stroke unit in the face of resistance and resentment by staff, and in the absence of a change in 'process', is unlikely to be effective. A few possibilities are given in Table 10.2.

Several studies have tried to identify which of these features is important in practice. Coordinated multi-disciplinary team care, involvement of family and other carers in the rehabilitation process, specialization, and education of staff, patients, and carers were identified by trialists as the most important features differentiating their service from general medical care (Stroke Unit Trialists Collaboration 1997). Two authors stress the psychological component to stroke unit care (Indredavik *et al.* 1991; Kalra *et al.* 1993*a*). One study has demonstrated this explicitly, with better mood and adjustment among patients managed on a stroke unit than general wards, although psychological outcomes will be confounded by improvements in other aspects of health (Juby *et al.* 1996; Prince *et al.* 1997). Another trialist believed that therapy intensity was the key (P. Berman, personal communication). The surprising result of reduced mortality may have been mediated by prevention or swift treatment of complications of stroke or secondary prevention.

At least 60 per cent of admitted stroke patients suffer at least one medical complication. The appearance of a complication doubles the risk of death (Davenport *et al.* 1996*b*). In-patient stroke rehabilitation has been described as 'a medically active service' (Kalra *et al.* 1995). The reduction in disability and institutionalization might result in part from medical intervention (since debility resulting from acute illness limits the scope for remedial therapy), but also from rehabilitation or resettlement practices. Most of these features, however, should also be found on any rehabilitation or general geriatric ward, and this may be reflected in the subgroup analyses from the stroke unit meta-analyses (Table 10.1). The attractiveness of specialized units for staff, staff numbers, standardization of polices, education programmes, and a peer-group effect on, for example, morale or self-directed therapy ('home-work') between formal sessions are further possibilities which might be studied.

Amount and content of therapy

A number of studies have demonstrated, in small, randomized controlled trials, that aspects of physiotherapy or occupational therapy can improve various impairments, including arm weakness (Sunderland *et al.* 1992; Hanlon 1996; Aisen *et al.* 1997; Feys *et al.* 1998), trunk control (Dean and Shepherd 1997), unilateral neglect (Wiart *et al.* 1997), sensory loss (Yekutiel and Guttman 1993), and gait speed (Wade *et al.* 1992). These trials used novel techniques, or increased intensity of treatment compared with 'conventional therapy', to show their effects. In addition small trials have shown beneficial effects of acupuncture (Johansson *et al.* 1993), electromyographic (EMG) biofeedback (Glanz *et al.* 1997; Moreland *et al.* 1998), and functional electrical stimulation (Glanz *et al.* 1996). Effects have been quantitatively small, and tend to be greater on measures of impairment than disability. They do not tell us about the effectiveness of conventional therapy, and some of the more novel methods are not widely practised, but, as with the stroke unit trials, they show that impairments and disabilities are not immutable in the face of therapeutic endeavour.

The Frenchay Arm Study compared conventional with enhanced physio-therapy, the latter being an 'eclectic mixture' of Bobath exercises, EMG biofeedback, computer games, and behavioural management to encourage patient engagement, and to avoid overprotectiveness from relatives and learned disuse. The enhanced therapy group had a median of 129 minutes (range 8–399 minutes) per week of arm therapy, compared with the control group who had 53 minutes (range 0–265 minutes). Thus for most patients, although they received more therapy than usual, it is difficult to describe what they received as 'intensive'. Small gains were recorded in a measure of arm impairment, but there was no difference in an arm-directed disability scale or general disability. Besides low numbers, this study suffered from some initial imbalance between groups, and a differential death rate. Another arm study involved splinting the affected arm then asking the patient to rock in a rocking chair for 30 minutes a day for 6 weeks. The chair was arranged so arm function was required to prevent slipping out of it. At the end of therapy there were improvements on an arm impairment scale, but again not on disability scales (Feys *et al.* 1998).

Two meta-analyses have considered the question of rehabilitation intensity on outcomes (Langhorne *et al.* 1996; Kwakkel *et al.* 1997). These authors faced a fundamental problem in trying to find a common measure of 'exposure' and outcome, that is, how much therapy someone has had and how much good it has done. Duration of therapy is most often quoted, and 'high' intensity has generally meant about twice as much therapy. Many of the studies considered were of modest methodological quality, in part because of the paucity of 'blind' outcomes assessment. Effectiveness appeared to be considerably greater in studies without blind assessment, presumably because of bias. Increased intensity of physiotherapy resulted in lower rates in the combined outcome of death and deterioration, but only small differences in impairments and disabilities were found. The findings suggest that large trials examining intensity would be worth further investigation (Langhorne et al. 1996).

There is little direct evidence that patients treated on stroke units have more therapy, although therapy content may be different, as may other aspects of 'process' on stroke units. Kalra (1994a) found recovery to be greater and quicker, and discharge sooner, on his stroke unit. Patients on general medical wards received more physiotherapy and the same amount of occupational therapy in total, although this was spread over a longer hospital stay, so the therapy on the stroke unit was more intensive. Stroke unit therapy had less emphasis on transfers and personal ADL skills, and more on individualized care. Lincoln et al. (1996), using a non-participant observer technique, found relatively small but definite differences between activity on the stroke unit and the general wards. Time spent on formal therapeutic activities was low in both locations (about 35 minutes/day). However, stroke unit patients spent less time by their beds, more time interacting with nurses and therapists, slightly less time doing nothing, and had limbs positioned correctly more often. In a non-participant observational comparison of stroke unit, general ward, and geriatric rehabilitation ward care, similarities between stroke unit and geriatric rehabilitation ward were found, with patients in both settings being more often off the ward and engaged with relatives than those on the general ward (Pound et al. 1999). Inactivity on stroke units has been reported in other studies (Keith and Cowell 1987; Mackey et al. 1996; Newall et al. 1997) and the failure of patients to undertake therapeutic activity independently, or of staff to encourage them to do so, has been highlighted and is probably detrimental in any setting.

Kalra (1994b) also found that younger patients had a relatively greater benefit from stroke unit care than older patients, and he speculated that this might be because the comparators for older patients were the general geriatric wards, where multidisciplinary working was in place, and attention to avoiding or managing complications and co-morbidities was greater than on the general medical wards. The advantage of stroke unit care could simply be the avoidance of setbacks associated with suboptimal care elsewhere.

Table 10.3 Northwick Park out-patient rehabilitation study, main results (from Smith *et al.* 1981)

	Intensive, 4 days/week (n = 46)	Conventional, 3 half-days/week (n = 43)	No rehabilitation (n = 44)
Activities of daily living score at entry	22.0	21.5	21.1
Improvement in ADL from entry to 3 months	3.5	2.9	1.5
Improvement in ADL from entry to 1 year	3.5	2.9	0.6
% Deteriorating between entry and 3 months (95% CI)	2% (-2–6%)	10% (0.7–19%)	24% (11–37%)
% Deteriorating between entry and 1 year (95% CI)	6% (-2–14%)	11% (0.8–21%)	23% (9–37%)

Community and out-patient rehabilitation

Out-patient rehabilitation

Management after the hospital phase of stroke was studied in a trial set up to decide whether two different intensities—intensive (four whole days per week) and conventional (three half-days per week)—of out-patient rehabilitation were more effective than no rehabilitation (Smith *et al.* 1981). The control group received usual care but with the addition of visits by a health visitor. Although stroke is a common problem, finding sufficient patients to include in the trial was difficult, and recruitment of 121 patients took 6 years. This was largely because deaths and 'full' recovery excluded just over half of 1094 patients initially considered for the trial. Almost a third of the 1094 patients were excluded because they were considered 'too frail' to withstand the highest intensity of out-patient rehabilitation.

The patients were assessed at entry, 3 months, and 1 year, using a modified Barthel activities of daily living scale (Sheikh *et al.* 1979). This had been well tested for repeatability, with only small between-observer and within-patient variation. No other aspects of recovery were reported, although measures of motor power were made. The patients randomized were young (average age 63–65 years), two-thirds were men, and most had spent less than a month in hospital. Their average activities of daily living scores were very close to the bottom of the scale (i.e. almost 'independent'). The main findings are shown in the Table 10.3.

The timing of improvement is interesting. Little further improvement occurred in either therapy group after 3 months. If increased amounts of therapy are really associated with increased functional ability in a dose response fashion, it would be reasonable to assume that the cumulative effects of therapy over 1 year in the conventional group should have brought them up to at least the 3-month level of the intensively treated group. This did not occur. Rehabilitation, regardless of its intensity, appears to have benefits over no rehabilitation over a short time period. The first few months after a stroke are the period of most rapid spontaneous recovery. Early out-patient rehabilitation seems to build on this recovery, but to have no additional effects after this phase is over. More patients deteriorated in the group not receiving rehabilitation. The differences in deterioration rates at 3 months and 1 year were highly statistically significant. The mechanism of this effect is unclear.

Despite the criticisms levelled at this trial, it remains the best example of a well-executed trial of rehabilitation in this field. The patients were reasonably homogeneous, the intervention was practical although its components were not specified, a 'no treatment' control group was used, assessments were made independently of therapy, and an objective measure of outcome was used. The demonstration of a dose response relationship is a strong pointer towards a causal link between the better outcomes and the extra input. As well as providing positive evidence of benefit, it has paved the way for a much greater understanding of the difficulties in carrying out adequate evaluations of rehabilitation.

Early discharge and domiciliary rehabilitation

Rehabilitation does not necessarily have to take place in hospital. The time course of a 'stroke career' is long, and reducing handicap, and improving quality of life, can only take place in the context of a patient's home and social environment, and necessarily over a longer period of time than hospital care can provide. Different practical problems are faced at home, and the family may be more closely involved with treatment. At the same time, home therapy averts the need for lengthy and unpleasant ambulance journeys to hospital (Young 1994).

A trial from Bradford examined the effectiveness of domiciliary rehabilitation in comparison with day hospital attendance, for patients over the age of 60 who had residual disability after discharge from hospital for a stroke. Median time of discharge post-stroke was about 7 weeks, and median Barthel ADL Index was 15. Six months later, day hospital patients had received a median of 31 hours of physiotherapy and occupational therapy, compared with 17 hours for the home-treated patients. There were improvements in mobility and the Barthel ADL Index, more so in the home-treated group (odds ratio for maximum Barthel score 2.9, and for 'independent functional ambulation' odds ratio 2.7). Social activity was slightly, and statistically non-significantly, greater (odds ratio 1.9) and carer stress less (odds ratio 0.5) in the home-treated group. Walking outside and climbing stairs were areas where the greatest differences were seen (Young and Forster 1992).

A similar trial in Nottingham was more equivocal. There were no differences in an extended activities of daily living score, the Barthel ADL Index, or measures of social engagement and life satisfaction between hospital and home-treated groups, although home treatment was preferred for patients who had been rehabilitated on the stroke unit, whereas conventional care resulted in fewer deaths or transfers to institutional care amongst patients from the geriatric medical service. Total numbers of therapy sessions were comparable between the two groups, although they were concentrated differently, with half the hospital and three-quarters of the home-treatment group receiving some therapy (Gladman et al. 1993). A subsequent randomized trial demonstrated reduced disability in a group of patients given enhanced occupational therapy after discharge (Logan et al. 1997).

Other services have been developed to provide home-care packages to enable early discharge from hospital with ongoing rehabilitation. These, too, have been evaluated by randomized trials. In a London trial, 331 patients, about half the total stroke admissions during the study, who were able to transfer from bed to chair independently or with the help of a willing carer, were allocated to home rehabilitation for 3 months, or to further hospital care. About half of the hospital-care group were treated on a stroke unit. Home care was individualized, with up to one visit per day from each of physiotherapy and occupational therapy, along with up to 3 hours daily of Social Services generic personal care. There were no differences in outcomes (motor weakness, disability, cognition, anxiety and depression, carer strain, and satisfaction) 1 year later, although on average 6 days hospital stay per patient randomized were saved (Rudd et al. 1997). Small trials in Newcastle and Stockholm, operating similar schemes, confirmed these findings (Rodgers et al. 1997; Holmqvist et al. 1998).

Well-constructed home rehabilitation schemes appear to be at least as effective as hospital services (although the evidence is still incomplete) (Table 10.4). Caution must be exercised in interpreting studies in an area where services are changing and developing rapidly. Hospital stroke care has probably improved in recent years, and evaluation of early supported discharge schemes must ensure comparison with current best care, which means most patients with significant disabilities being admitted to a stroke unit or a generic rehabilitation ward. Rudd and colleagues' trial had a high proportion of stroke unit patients. One interpretation is that avoidance of complications, or the psychological effects of management by enthusiastic

Table 10.4 Randomized trials of early discharge and domiciliary rehabilitation schemes

Author	Intervention	Number randomized	Outcome measures	Result
Young and Forster (1992)	Home PT and OT versus day hospital	108	Barthel Index Frenchay activities index Motor Club assessment Functional ambulation Nottingham health profile GHQ-28 (carers)	Benefit on most measures
Gladman et al. (1992)	Home PT and OT versus conventional care	327	Extended ADL scale Barthel Index Nottingham health profile Social engagement (carer) Life satisfaction (carer)	No significant differences
Rudd et al. (1997)	Home PT and OT versus conventional care	331	Barthel Index Motricity Index MMSE, HAD, NHP 5 m timed walk Carer strain index (carer)	No differences in outcomes, mean 6 days less in hospital
Holmqvist et al. (1998)	Home PT and OT versus conventional care	81	Katz, Barthel ADL Motor score Social activities Aphasia, falls, 10 m walk Sickness Impact Profile	No differences in outcomes, mean 13 days less in hospital
Rodgers et al. (1997)	Home PT and OT versus conventional care	92	Placement Extended ADL Rankin Dartmouth Coop GHQ-30 (carers)	No differences in outcomes, mean 9 days less in hospital

ADL, activities of daily living; GHQ, General Health Questionnaire; HAD, Hospital Anxiety and Depression Scale; MMSE, Mini-Mental State Examination; NHP, Nottingham Health Profile; OT, occupational therapy; PT, physiotherapy.

and concerned therapists (Pound et al. 1994, 1995) is beneficial regardless of where rehabilitation takes place. Alternatively, in early discharge schemes there may be a trade-off between better remedial therapy (by virtue of its context and applicability in the patient's usual environment) on the one hand, and closer nursing and medical attention on the other (which might, for instance, lead to better recovery or containment of incontinence). A recent stroke unit trial used 'community rehabilitation' as its control group but still demonstrated substantial benefits for patients managed on the stroke unit (Ronning and Guldrog 1998). This, together with the other trials, suggests that stroke units and home rehabilitation schemes may offer different and complementary advantages to patients.

Social support after discharge

The long-term practical, emotional, and social problems for patients and their families after stroke have prompted attempts to provide, and evaluate, social support, advice, and counselling services. Services have included specialist outreach nurses, social worker visits, education sessions, cognitive behavioural therapy, and attempts to expand the patient's social network (Forster and Young 1996; Dennis et al. 1997; Evans et al. 1988; Friedland and McColl 1992). Randomized trials have been performed, which have failed to demonstrate any consistent benefit for these services (Table 10.5), but have raised interesting questions about how to assess them. Outcome measures such as the Barthel ADL Index, indices of social activity and perceived health status, adjustment to illness, mood, and carer stress may not be appropriate or sensitive enough. Measures of 'family functioning' have been somewhat more successful in recording the effects of counselling (Evans et al. 1988), but this outcome is beyond the repertoire of most health services researchers. Instead, a 'pot-pourri' of outcome measures has been used in these trials, perhaps in the hope that at least one of them will provide a result.

If the objective of social support is primarily humanitarian, to provide comfort in a time of crisis, frustration, and misery, crude rating scales may well be inadequate. Randomized trials are expensive and logistically difficult,

Table 10.5 Randomized trials of interventions to improve post-stroke psycho-social outcomes

Author	Intervention	Number randomized	Outcome measures	Result
Forster and Young (1996)	7–19 nurse visits over 12 months	240	Frenchay activities index Barthel Index Nottingham Health profile GHQ-28 (carers)	No significant differences, small improvement in activities score
Dennis et al. (1997)	0–17 social worker visits	417	Frenchay activities index Barthel Index, Rankin score GHQ-30 Hosp. Anxiety and Depression Social adjustment Carer hassles and satisfaction	No significant differences, some improvements in satisfaction and carer's mood
Evans et al. (1988)	Carer education, or counselling (CBT) by social worker	188	Carer knowledge Family function Use of social resources Patient adjustment	Improved with counselling
Friedland and McColl (1992)	6–12 sessions with social support therapist	88	Social support GHQ-28 Sickness Impact Profile Barthel Index	No differences

CBT, cognitive behaviour therapy GHQ, General Health Questionnaire so it would be sensible to use qualitative studies to characterize the research question closely before embarking on them. Qualitative (e.g. in-depth interview) methods should be used to explore the nature of benefits from patient and professional perspectives. From such work, more content-valid indicators, relevant to the concerns of patients and others, can be developed to aid quantitative assessment of possible benefits of such social support schemes.

Future developments

Refining the therapy

Previous evaluation studies have treated rehabilitation as a uniform therapy and equated the amount of therapy with its duration rather than considering its quality. The components of a rehabilitation programme are complex; some may be vital but other parts may be of less importance. It is necessary to define which components of rehabilitation are responsible for beneficial effects.

Single-case-study designs hold some promise for working out which techniques work and which do not. In general single-case studies mimic clinical practice. A patient's abilities are recorded to give baseline data, an intervention is tried and abilities are recorded again, and finally the intervention is withdrawn and further records of abilities made. This is called an A–B–A study design. In any disease with a spontaneous pattern of recovery this simple design will be inadequate since no control for spontaneous recovery is included. This can be overcome by recording a range of baseline abilities, some of which may be influenced by specific therapy and some of which will not. For example, in patients with dysphasia, recovery of naming ability may be improved by a practice regimen, whereas fluency of speech will not. If following a training programme, baseline measures of naming ability improve, but fluency does not, then it is more likely that the beneficial effects are due to therapy. This method is certainly not foolproof. If the natural history of recovery of different aspects of language differs, for example, (which it probably does) then a spurious conclusion of effective therapy may be made. Alternatively, single-case studies may be done when all spontaneous recovery has ceased. Demonstrating effects of therapy at, say, 1 year after a stroke makes it more likely that these are real. The single-case design has been used to evaluate perceptual retraining methods commonly used by occupational therapists (Edmans and Lincoln 1989). Therapy was shown to be of no use in a series of single-case studies. Single-case designs are an efficient way of testing potential therapies. Those that look promising should then be subjected to a randomized controlled trial to answer wider questions about the generalizability of the therapy and its cost-effectiveness.

A series of single-case studies showing benefits of similar magnitude in different patients adds further weight to concluding that a therapy is effective. Single-case studies should go a long way to disentangling the effects of rehabilitation. Interventions that require study are early mobilization versus a sequential sitting–standing–walking (Bobath) approach, physical strength and stamina training, biofeedback training methods, cognitive impairment practice regimes, and counselling.

Perhaps 'rehabilitation' is too nebulous a notion to evaluate in the same way as a drug or surgical procedure. Moreover, concentrating on effectiveness and efficiency as the sole arbiters of quality or value is less appropriate for rehabilitation than elsewhere. Issues of humanity, appropriateness, access, and equity are especially important for services directed towards vulnerable and neglected groups, such as stroke survivors. A number of studies have shown effectiveness for small elements of rehabilitation, not all of them well-established or widely available. Extending this work will require close definition of the objectives of an intervention or service, the identification of appropriate specific and generic outcome indicators, and standardization of the intervention itself. A prime candidate for further large-scale work must be intensity of therapy.

A final point to consider is the need for alternative models of care for some stroke patients. The emphasis on rehabilitation, either at home or in hospital, has resulted in neglect of the long-term care and palliative care needs of stroke patients. It is often forgotten that a very large number of strokes occur in very old people who have limited life expectancy. A rehabilitation model of care may deny them the options for palliation and a peaceful 'good' death. A study of quality of care in the last year of life of stroke patients showed serious problems of poor pain control, inadequate information, and doctors who were too 'rushed'(Addington-Hall *et al.* 1995). More research work on the long-term care needs and palliative care of stroke patients would be rewarding and likely to influence clinical practice and quality of life of a very neglected group of patients.

Summary

1. Rehabilitation aims to reduce the handicapping effects of disease by processes of reablement and resettlement. Its scientific study has been limited by the multiple levels at which therapy may have its effects, and the problems of defining suitable outcomes.

2. Evaluation of the effects of rehabilitation has to take into account the spontaneous recovery that occurs after a stroke, the heterogeneity of the impairments caused by strokes, the numbers of patients needed to make adequate measurements of treatment effects, and the effects of selecting patients for therapy.

3. The nature of therapy itself must be better defined so that the effects of standardized types and amounts of treatment can be compared.

4. Relevant outcomes that are repeatable, valid, and sensitive to change are needed. Rehabilitation has its effects at the handicap end of the spectrum of severity, but suitable handicap outcomes are not well developed.

5. Stroke units appear to reduce mortality over about a year by 18 per cent, death or institutionalization by 25 per cent, and death or dependency by 29 per cent. The precise elements of stroke unit care which lead to this outcome are unclear.

6. A number of small studies have demonstrated effectiveness for physiotherapy and occupational therapy, but the generalizability of these results is uncertain.

7. Out-patient rehabilitation improves performance in activities of daily living among younger patients suffering less severe strokes, and more intensive regimes appear to be more effective than less intensive regimes. Further studies are required to define the optimal duration of therapy, the necessary components of therapy, and its impact on a wider range of patients.

8. Early supported discharge and domiciliary rehabilitation schemes are logistically viable, are associated with outcomes which are probably no worse than those obtained in hospital, and may be better. Care must be taken to compare such schemes with the best current management, which is in-patient stroke unit care.

9. Attempts to design health service interventions which alleviate longer-term psychosocial distress have been made, but the results of evaluations have been disappointing. It is not entirely clear whether these studies have measured the most appropriate outcomes.

10. Single-case-study designs are an efficient method of testing potentially useful therapies. Treatments that produce benefits should then be evaluated using a conventional randomized controlled trial design.

11. Long-term care and palliative care for stroke patients are neglected areas of clinical practice and research.

11 Preventing recurrence

One in five strokes is a recurrent stroke (Jorgensen *et al.* 1997), and someone who has had a first stroke is at tenfold increased risk of another. Secondary prevention attempts to reduce the risk of recurrence, and it makes sense to target people who have already had a stroke or TIA as these individuals, with high baseline risk, stand to gain most. The distinction between primary and secondary prevention is not clear-cut (see Chapter 8). Many patients with apparent TIAs can be shown to have infarcts on neuroimaging, and prognostically TIAs and minor ischaemic cortical strokes behave similarly (Dennis *et al.* 1989a). All the risk factors for stroke described in Chapter 3 are likely to remain determinants of increased risk after a TIA or stroke. However, most evaluations of secondary prevention have not been concerned with reducing modifiable risk factors (e.g. alcohol use, smoking, physical inactivity) but have studied pharmacological interventions—anticoagulation, antiplatelet drugs, antihypertensives—and carotid surgery. A change in this emphasis might be of benefit, although trials of life-style modification are more challenging to conduct than drug trials.

Long-term anticoagulation

At least 17 randomized controlled trials of anticoagulation after either stroke in evolution or completed stroke had been reported by 1987 (Genton *et al.* 1977; Jonas 1988) and an up-dated Cochrane review of this evidence has been produced (Counsell and Sandercock 1998a). All the trials considered have been small and suffered from difficulties in precise diagnosis at entry to the trial. In general, subjects had evidence of a stroke but with a clear CSF on lumbar puncture which may not exclude a haemorrhagic stroke. Only one of the studies found any apparent benefit from treatment. This study (Carter 1961) found a reduction in mortality of 55 per cent in patients with progressing stroke, but because the numbers were small this apparently impressive difference was not statistically significant. Carter admitted to being uneasy about recommending anticoagulation because of its risks.

The risks of anticoagulation were apparent in another English trial (Hill *et al.* 1962). In an initial study it was found that death and bleeding were much more likely in those with a high (110 mmHg +) diastolic blood pressure. The trial protocol was immediately changed to exclude these subjects and then continued. Patients on active treatment had a higher death rate and 18 per cent of the subjects had an episode of bleeding. There was no difference in recurrent stroke rates.

Pooling of 11 comparable trials of 1136 subjects randomized to receive anticoagulation or no treatment gives an odds ratio of 0.86, a 14 per cent treatment benefit. However, the 95 per cent confidence limits are wide (0.62–1.19), indicating the benefit could be as great as 38 per cent or that those on treatment could do up to 19 per cent worse than those not treated. With the added problem of bleeding risks, post-stroke anticoagulation has never been popular.

It has been claimed that anticoagulation is of benefit in cerebral embolism. It is argued that because recurrence rates are so high, prophylaxis is necessary (Weksler and Lewin 1983). Emboli contain fibrin so anticoagulants, which inhibit formation of fibrin, might be expected to be effective. The evidence supporting this view is weak, including case series, which tend to give a biased view of treatment benefits, possibly because of publication bias (positive results get published, negative ones often do not). Of greater relevance is a trial of 1316 participants who had had TIA or mild stroke who were randomized to either aspirin or warfarin (INR 3.0–4.5) which was stopped early because of an excess of intracerebral bleeds in the warfarin group (Stroke Prevention in Reversible Ischaemia (SPIRIT) Study Group 1997). The trials show clear evidence of harm from long-term anticoagulation and no compensating evidence of dramatic benefits.

Anticoagulation in stroke and atrial fibrillation

In the eyes of most physicians, stroke in the presence of both atrial fibrillation and rheumatic heart disease is an indication to anticoagulate the patient (Bucknall *et al.* 1986). Starkey and Warlow (1986), in a critical review of the supporting evidence, demonstrated that only one randomized trial had been done and that this was small and showed no advantage of treatment (Baker *et al.* 1962). The evidence of benefit is derived entirely from selected case series, which are no substitute for properly controlled trials. It is now much too late to set up a trial of anticoagulation of patients with atrial fibrillation and rheumatic heart disease, not only because of established practice but also because of disappearing cases of rheumatic heart disease. However, such a trial would be of value and be feasible to conduct in poorer countries where rheumatic heart disease remains a common cause of stroke.

The role of anticoagulation in non-rheumatic atrial fibrillation (AF) is now clearer than it was when Starkey and Warlow (1986) stated that 'it is unsatisfactory and probably unethical as well to treat with anticoagulants patients with stroke and atrial fibrillation but without rheumatic heart disease until we know we are doing more good than harm'. At the time, an opposite Texan view (Sherman *et al.* 1986) concluded that the danger of treatment is worth the risk because of the seriousness of the condition. This is unusual reasoning, ignoring the need for treatment to actually work!

Since then, six randomized trials have provided evidence of the effectiveness of warfarin in the primary prevention of stroke in non-rheumatic AF—that is, before the occurrence of a TIA or stroke. Extrapolating these data to secondary prevention is tempting, and not wholly unreasonable, but patients with completed strokes or TIA are more likely to have advanced cerebral arterial disease and therefore could be at greater risk of harm from intra-cerebral bleeding. In any case, a third of strokes in patients with AF are not thought to be related to the AF, but to coexisting arterial disease. Fortunately, a good-sized randomized controlled trial has answered some of the questions. The European Atrial Fibrillation study group randomized 1007 patients to aspirin (300 mg), warfarin anticoagulation, or placebo, and in a further 2338 patients for whom anticoagulation was contraindicated, aspirin or placebo (European Atrial Fibrillation Trial Study Group 1993).

Forty-three (8 per cent/year) of the warfarin group suffered vascular death, stroke, myocardial infarction, or peripheral embolism, compared with 67 (17 per cent/year) for the placebo control group (relative risk (RR), 0.53; 95 per cent CI, 0.36–0.79: numbers needed to treat (NNT), 11 per year). Risk of stroke alone was reduced from 12 per cent to 4 per cent (RR, 0.34; 95 per cent CI, 0.20–0.57; NNT, 13). All-cause mortality was reduced by 18 per cent, but there were too few events to exclude this being a chance difference. 'On treatment' (explanatory) analyses showed even greater effects but these may be invalid because such analyses are no longer of all those randomized, and selection bias may explain the apparently better treatment effects. There was no waning of treatment efficacy with time.

Warfarin appeared to be more effective than aspirin (RR, 0.60; 95 per cent CI, 0.41–0.87; NNT, 19), and aspirin was slightly more effective than placebo (RR, 0.83; 95 per cent CI, 0.65–1.05; NNT, 25). Major bleeds occurred at the rate of 2.8 per cent/year for warfarin, 0.9 per cent/year for aspirin, and 0.7 per cent/year for placebo. In addition there is about a 0.6 per cent annual incidence of fatal bleeds, and 10 per cent incidence of minor bleeds for patients on warfarin (Landefeld and Beyth 1993). Anticoagulants used outside of trials are associated with higher rates of bleeding. Both age and the presence of stroke are risk factors, and some risk assessment scores have been produced (Landefeld and Beyth 1993; Stroke Prevention in Atrial Fibrillation Investigators 1996).

It is not clear how soon anticoagulation should be started after an acute stroke. The International Stroke Trial provides evidence that there is no overall benefit from starting anticoagulation (or aspirin) in the first few days after a stroke, as the number of ischaemic strokes avoided was offset by an equal number of haemorrhagic strokes caused (International Stroke Trial Collaborative Group 1997).

More trials comparing directly the effects of aspirin with warfarin in patients with non-rheumatic atrial fibrillation following TIA and stroke would be helpful if they also examined costs and patient preferences. At present, if safe anticoagulation can be assured, and the patient is willing to accept the risks, the evidence supports use of anticoagulation.

Antiplatelet therapy

Platelets are known to be involved in clotting and thrombus formation, so inhibiting their function is also a logical target for prevention. Aspirin has become a widely used treatment for secondary stroke prevention among both TIA and completed stroke patients (Bucknall *et al.* 1986; Lindley *et al.* 1995). There is still uncertainty amongst doctors about who to treat, what dose to use, whether to use alternative agents or combinations of drugs, and how long to continue. Very low doses (30 mg or 75 mg daily), or 300 mg given weekly, or up to 1.2 g given daily can all be supported from laboratory or clinical trial evidence. Low doses are given in the hope that inhibition of vessel wall prostacyclin will be minimal and of platelet prostaglandin maximal, thus optimizing its antithrombotic effects (Hart and Harrison 1996; Patrono and Roth 1996) (or at least, providing equivalent efficacy while minimizing adverse effects).

Choosing the right dose has been difficult. At the time the early clinical trials were set up, the recommended dose was based on that required for analgesic and anti-inflammatory effects. Preliminary results in small series were encouraging. Laboratory studies then suggested that the inhibition of platelet thromboxane synthesis by cyclo-oxygenase is achieved with doses as low as 30 mg/day. The UK-TIA trial compared 1.2 g with 300 mg aspirin and placebo, although it was stated that doses were determined to enable a urine ferric chloride test of compliance with treatment to be used (UK-TIA Study Group 1988). The study designers should not be criticized for using the 'wrong' dose of aspirin. Trials take a long time to do whereas test-tube experiments may advance understanding of pathogenesis very rapidly, apparently making the results of trials of little relevance to up-to-date clinical practice. Laboratory studies are of value in deciding which drugs are worth investigating in human studies, but applying laboratory results to humans directly without trial evidence is most unwise. Person-to-person variation in responses to set doses of aspirin are very large; even 1.2 g may not be sufficient to inhibit *in vitro* platelet aggregation in some subjects (O'Brien 1980; Hanley *et al.* 1981), which may make the blanket use of low, or even medium, doses of aspirin suboptimal (Dyken *et al.* 1992; Barnett *et al.* 1995, 1996). Clinicians should remember when deciding what to offer patients that the best test of efficacy is obtained by doing trials on people, not extrapolating from studies of isolated vessel walls and platelet suspensions.

Unfortunately, interpreting clinical trials can be difficult as well. Most clinical trials are set up to have enough power to demonstrate that the difference between one treatment and another would have been unlikely to occur by chance. There is often a considerable degree of uncertainty surrounding the size (or precision) of the effect. For instance, in a comparison of 75 mg/day of aspirin and placebo amongst 1360 patients who had a TIA or minor ischaemic stroke, the relative risk of stroke or death over the next 5 years was reduced by 18 per cent (relative risk, 0.82; 95 per cent CI, 0.67–0.99) (SALT Collaborative Group 1991). This means that the real relative risk reduction is between 1 and 33 per cent, and that in 1 out of 20 similar trials the observed reduction might have occurred with a real effect more extreme than this (i.e. higher or lower)—hence 95 per cent confidence intervals. While a 33 per cent reduction is very worthwhile, 1 per cent is trivial, and the real reduction (based on this trial data alone) may be even smaller—the chance of this is 1 in 40 (and not 1 in 20) as we are only considering the lower confidence interval. Larger trials are needed to improve precision, which is related to the standard error of the relative risk, and decreases as the square root of the number of trial subjects. Thus another trial (ESPS-2) with 6602 subjects, comparing 50 mg of aspirin against placebo, recorded a relative risk reduction for stroke or death of 12 per cent (95 per cent CI, 3.2–20.8 per cent; Diener *et al.* 1996). This study had five times as many participants and produced an approximate halving of the range of uncertainty. The sample sizes required to compare two active treatments, such as two different drugs (aspirin versus warfarin), or two doses of the same drug, are even greater, unless it is important to detect only sizeable differences in treatment effects (INJECT Group 1995; CAPRIE Steering Committee 1996).

With so much variability in what we can be sure about, resulting from trials of a size which are reasonably practicable, it is not surprising that differing entry and outcome criteria for trials, and subgroup analyses of special populations within them, have generated many hypotheses about the indications for antiplatelet treatment, and groups (e.g. women, elderly people, diabetics) that respond more (or less) than others.

Meta-analysis of antiplatelet trials

One of the most important enterprises in modern cardiovascular epidemiology has been a collaboration to identify, collate, and re-analyse all antiplatelet randomized trial data (Antiplatelet Trialists' Collaboration 1988, 1994*b*). The conclusion of this group was that, across a very wide range of patients at high risk of occlusive vascular disease, aspirin doses from 75 to 1500 mg/day were effective in reducing non-fatal myocardial infaction, non-fatal stroke, or vascular death, with a relative risk reduction of about 25 per cent, regardless of aspirin dose, clinical population (by age, sex, hypertension or diabetes, or risk defined by prior myocardial infarction (MI), acute MI, previous stroke or TIA, or other high risk), or outcome (non-fatal MI, stroke, or vascular death). The effects of other antiplatelet agents, alone or in combination with aspirin, were identical. Effects were also the same when non-fatal MI, non-fatal stroke, or vascular death were considered separately.

Considerable efforts were made to find all the available published and unpublished trials (available by March 1990), thus avoiding the tendency of reviewers to consider trials that support a particular view. One hundred and forty-five trials involving 70 000 high-risk patients and 30 000 low-risk (primary prevention) patients were included; 12 000 had experienced a prior stroke or TIA. Thirty-two trials involving 13 600 subjects compared different drug regimens. Individual patient data were submitted from 32 trials involving 74 000 participants. In the rest, additional summary information was sought from the investigators. The group recorded 11 000 vascular events (MI, stroke, or vascular death), including 500 fatal and 2000 non-fatal strokes. Updating of these trials continues and currently over 400 trials have been found and a further round of analyses is under way (C. Baigent, personal communication).

The remarkable finding was of the consistency of effect between all the different subpopulations examined, once the results from all available trials had been pooled. The trials did not give exactly the same results, but the variation between them was no more than would have been expected by chance from trials of their size. In statistical language, there was no significant 'heterogeneity' between trials. The only major exception to the overall conclusion was that low-risk (primary prevention) patients may benefit less in terms of relative risk reduction (including a 20 per cent increased risk of stroke), but this conclusion was statistically uncertain.

The authors even suggested that their results were so powerful that a general statistical principal (Stein's paradox) could be invoked to conclude that the approximate benefit of any particular therapy might be better estimated by extrapolation from the general effect than that observed directly in small, and therefore, unreliable subgroups.

Specific results for stroke prevention
The odds reduction for non-fatal stroke was 25 per cent (95 per cent CI, 17–33 per cent). Amongst the high-risk groups (excluding the primary prevention trials), the effect was 31 per cent (95 per cent CI, 21–41 per cent), with no difference between categories of patient (prior MI, acute MI, prior stroke or TIA, other high risk). There was probably a small increase in haemorrhagic strokes (0.3 per cent compared with 0.2 per cent), which were more likely to be fatal, and may explain why the effect on fatal stroke (15 per cent reduction) was less than that on non-fatal stroke (25 per cent reduction). Fewer trials (14) had data on disabling strokes, so the estimates of size of

effect are more uncertain, but these showed a 24 per cent reduction (95 per cent CI, 6–42 per cent) in fatal or disabling strokes.

Specific results for patients who had a prior stroke

Amongst the 10 000 patients with a prior history of stroke or TIA, the relative risk reduction was 22 per cent (95 per cent CI, 14–30 per cent) with a NNT (for about 2 years) of 27 for all events and NNT of 50 for recurrent stroke. There was no difference between the effect on patients with a TIA and those with a completed stroke in the 10 trials for which these data were available.

Different aspirin doses and different drugs

Numbers randomized in direct comparisons between different regimens have so far been too small to draw reliable conclusions. There were no significant differences between high- and medium-dose aspirin, aspirin plus dipyrida-mole and aspirin, sulphinpyrazone and aspirin, and ticlopidine plus aspirin, although differences as large as a 20 per cent odds reduction either way could not be excluded. Indirect comparisons can be made by comparing the size of effect in placebo-controlled studies for different doses and agents. There is potential for bias in such comparisons (Bucher *et al.* 1997), but they are generally reliable and may represent the best available evidence. There were no significant differences between the effects of high (500–1500 mg), medium (160–325 mg), and low (75–150 mg) aspirin doses, nor any different effect of different agents or combinations (statistical tests for heterogeneity were not significant). Where events could be categorized by duration of therapy, additional benefit continued to be observed into the second and third years.

More recent trials

Since 1990 several further trials have been completed. These increased to 6000 the number of patients randomized to low-dose regimens, including 5000 given 75 mg/day (which together give a pooled odds ratio reduction of 29 per cent (95% CI,15–43 per cent)). The Swedish Aspirin Low-dose Trial demonstrated a relative risk reduction of 17 per cent (95 per cent CI, 0–30 per cent) for stroke, MI, or vascular death for 75 mg of aspirin compared with placebo for patients after TIA or minor ischaemic stroke (SALT Collabora-tive Group 1991). The Dutch TIA Trial directly compared 30 mg and 283 mg of aspirin in 3131 similar patients, and found no difference for the same outcome (relative risk reduction for lower dose, 9 per cent; 95 per cent CI, 24 to −9 per cent; Dutch TIA Trial Study Group 1991).

The Second European Stroke Prevention Study claims to have demon-strated independent and additive effects for aspirin 50 mg/day and dipyr-idamole 400 mg/day. The study had a 2 × 2 factorial design, randomizing 6602 patients post-stroke or TIA between aspirin or placebo and dipyridamole and placebo (so a quarter received each of the four possible combinations of active treatment and placebo). The outcome used was stroke or (all-cause) death (with stroke, MI, or 'sudden death' being a secondary end point). The primary analysis in such a design is aspirin against placebo (regardless of whether patients were given dipyridamole or not) and dipyridamole against placebo (regardless of whether aspirin was given or not). Factorial 2 × 2 design trials give, in effect, two trials for the price of one. The aspirin effect (reconstructing the secondary end point of combined stroke, MI, and sudden death from the published data for comparability) was an 18 per cent relative risk reduction, while the dipyridamole effect was a 17 per cent reduction. The effect of the combination (compared with the 'double' placebo group—those who did not receive either active drug) was a 33 per cent reduction. The risk reductions were somewhat larger for non-fatal stroke considered alone (21 per cent for aspirin), and smaller for the stroke plus all-cause mortality end point (12 per cent for aspirin) (Diener et al. 1996).

Does this demonstrate conclusively an additional effect for dipyridamole? Unfortunately not. Forty-three previous trials had evaluated aspirin plus dipyridamole combinations, with a total of 1750 events in 14 000 patients. The relative odds reduction for these trials was 28 per cent, identical to that for aspirin alone. Adding the new data increases the pooled relative odds reduction to 32 per cent (95 per cent CI, 25–38 per cent), still consistent with an identical effect to that of aspirin alone. Similarly, for the meta-analysis of the direct comparison studies, where previously 5300 patients had been randomized with no overall difference between regimens. Adding the new data gives a relative odds reduction in favour of the combination of 13 per cent (95 per cent CI, −2 per cent to 26 per cent), again consistent with the hypothesis that the combination is no more effective than aspirin alone. The apparently dramatic results in this single trial are probably the results of two factors. Factorial designs make an assumption of no interactions between treatment effects and, therefore, the main effects of treatments can be assessed by comparing those who received one treatment with those who received placebo or the other treatment. To examine the combination of two drugs compared with double placebo in a 2 × 2 factorial design is essentially a subgroup analysis, a procedure that tends to give undue prominence to extreme results. Also, the effect of aspirin in this trial was somewhat smaller than that found in the Antiplatelet Trialists Collaboration overview (21 per cent compared with 31 per cent), probably a chance phenomenon, but conceivably related to the very low aspirin dose (50 mg/day). Finally, an unrelated issue is to question why, as late as 1995, patients having suffered a TIA or minor stroke were still being randomized to placebo? The Helsinki Declaration governing the ethics of human research state that an individual subject must not be put at disadvantage by taking part in the research, regardless of the scientific importance of the question under study.

A further trial compared a new agent, clopidogrel, with 325 mg/day of aspirin in 19 185 patients at high vascular risk (including 6431 with ischaemic stroke) (CAPRIE Steering Committee 1996). A small but significant relative risk reduction of 8.7 per cent (95 per cent CI, 0.3–17 per cent) for stroke, MI, or vascular death in favour of clopidogrel over aspirin was found. The size of this trial illustrates what is required to demonstrate which of two active drugs is better. Clopidogrel is less toxic than ticlopidine, and is an alternative (along with dipyridamole) for patients intolerant of aspirin.

William of Ockham (1280–1349) suggested that for any given set of observations, the simplest explanation was most likely to be correct. The simplest explanation here is that there is a single effect of platelet inactivation produced by all these different drugs, despite their action on different physiological mechanisms concerned with platelet function. For now, all high-risk vascular patients should be given 75 mg/day of aspirin, enteric-coated if not otherwise tolerated, unless specifically contraindicated. Future evidence may show that even lower doses are as effective, but demonstrating this, or that any alternative combination or drug regime is more effective, will be very difficult statistically. Moreover, the marginal benefit (i.e. over that already achievable with 75 mg aspirin) of alternative regimes will likely be small. The much lower cost of aspirin compared with these alternatives makes it unlikely that it will ever be displaced as first-line treatment for the prevention of recurrent vascular disease unless a vastly more effective antiplatelet agent is found. The onus is on proponents of alternative regimens to demonstrate superiority beyond reasonable doubt.

Finally, if a patient suffers a stroke while taking aspirin, should it be assumed that aspirin has 'failed' and dipyridamole or clopidogrel be substituted? While this is a very worrying problem for both clinician and patient, we have very little evidence to guide us. It is obvious from the trials of antiplatelet agents that they are not 100 per cent effective and that strokes will still occur despite treatment with any agent. In fact, the risk of a vascular event (i.e. stroke or myocardial infarction) or death on antiplatelet drugs is 18.4 per cent over an average of 33 months of treatment, and for non-fatal strokes or myocardial infarctions, about 10 per cent over the same time period. Very similar event rates occur in those on aspirin and on other antiplatelet drugs—all of these drugs have a 'failure' rate. If the policy of switching drugs were adopted, for every 100 patients treated with aspirin for 3 years, 10 would suffer a non-fatal vascular event and be switched. Since recurrence rates are very similar in those treated with alternative antiplatelet agents, a similar 'failure' rate will arise too, presumably demanding a switch back to aspirin. It would be worth finding out whether these patients had taken their aspirin regularly, as adherence to medication may explain failure and be remediable. As a trial of use of alternative antiplatelet drugs among aspirin 'failures' is not likely to be feasible, the only rationale for switching is pathogenesis arguments which suggest that these drugs differ in their sites of action and further trial evidence showing benefit of one type of antiplatelet drug over another.

Lowering blood pressure

Patients who have experienced a stroke or TIA are at high risk for further events, and theoretically have most to gain from blood pressure reduction, even at levels which are not normally considered 'hypertensive'. This view is inadequately tested in randomized trials, but the strong graded relationship between stroke risk and blood pressure persists after a TIA or minor stroke, and is of approximately the same strength as the relationship between blood pressure and first stroke (Rodgers et al. 1996).

Randomized trials

Only two randomized trials of the effects of treating high blood pressure after stroke have been published. The first randomized patients under 80 years old suffering a clinically diagnosed ischaemic stroke (Carter 1970). Patients with pressures over 110 mmHg diastolic (phase unmentioned but probably phase IV at this time in the UK) or a systolic pressure of 160 mmHg or more for over 2 weeks while in hospital were randomized. Forty-nine patients were treated with various antihypertensive drugs and 48 were left untreated. The patients were followed up for 4 years on average and during this time 44 per cent of the controls and 20 per cent of the treated patients suffered a major or fatal stroke. Deaths from heart failure and myocardial infarction were no different between the groups. The 95 per cent confidence intervals of this 24 per cent difference were 6–42 per cent, indicating a significant effect. Patients over 65 years did not share this very beneficial effect but numbers were too small to accept or refute the null hypothesis.

The second randomized controlled trial (Hypertension Stroke Co-operative Study Group 1974) was multi-centre, and randomized 452 patients, 80 per cent of whom were black, and only 9 per cent over 70 years. Four-fifths had suffered a completed stroke and the remainder a TIA. Although active treatment did lower pressures by about 25 mmHg systolic and 12 mmHg diastolic (from an average of 167/100 (phase V) at entry), no significant difference in stroke recurrence was observed. The cumulative 5-year incidence of recurrent stroke was 21 per cent and 24 per cent in the treated and control groups, respectively. The 95 per cent confidence limits of this difference are about –5 to 11 per cent, so the study was able to rule out a true treatment effect of more than 11 per cent. However, the observed recurrence rates were very low and suggest that under-reporting of events might have occurred, with a bias towards those on therapy (with its side-effects) seeking out their physicians and reporting more events, thus leading to the small observed difference. Pooling the results of these two trials by meta-analysis suggests a 38 per cent reduction in risk, but with wide confidence intervals.

An uncontrolled comparison

An observational study by Beevers and colleagues (Beevers *et al.* 1973) is often quoted as evidence of the effectiveness of treating high pressures after stroke. The starting point of this study was a clinic series of 162 patients with a past history of both a stroke and hypertension. An imaginary control group was assembled from a review of the literature. Beevers concluded that a recurrence rate of about 40 per cent over 4 years could be expected. He interpreted the observed recurrence rate of 29 per cent in his series as a favourable effect of therapy when compared with the imaginary control group. Those patients with the best control of their pressures (mean diastolic below 100 mmHg) had fewest recurrences (16 per cent) whereas the patients with the worst control (mean diastolic 110 mmHg or more) had the highest risk (55 per cent) of recurrence. It is quite possible that the observed recurrence rates depended as much on selection effects, non-blind counting of events, changing criteria for an event, and different lengths of follow-up as a true effect of treatments.

A common error when analysing observational data is to ignore the effect of duration of follow-up when making comparisons between subgroups. In clinical trials this may not make too much difference, since randomization will ensure that follow-up will be more or less equal between treated and control groups. In Beevers' series the patients with 'poor' control may have been attending the clinic longer than those with 'good' control. Indeed, in routine practice the main reason for attending a hospital clinic is difficulty in reducing the blood pressure. Thus these badly controlled patients may have been around for a longer time than newer well-controlled patients. Allowance for length of follow-up must be made and is usually done by using life-table methods or patient-years at risk rather than patients as the denominator when calculating rates of recurrence (Peto *et al.* 1976, 1977). In Beevers' study it is impossible to make this allowance because insufficient data were reported. Uncontrolled observations are difficult to interpret even if analysed appropriately and should not be taken at their face value as supporting the case for treatment.

The observations of recurrence and survival among stroke patients in Rochester, Minnesota are interesting because the effects of pre-stroke blood pressure (within 1 year of the initial stroke) and treatment for high blood pressure during the first year after the initial stroke were related to subsequent events (Meissner *et al.* 1988). Diastolic (but not systolic) pre-stroke blood pressure was related to subsequent mortality, especially in the first 3 years after the stroke. Treatment aimed at controlling blood pressure after the stroke had no effect on either survival or stroke recurrence over a 10-year period.

Dangers of antihypertensive treatment

Sudden lowering of the blood pressure in acute stroke patients may lead to disastrous lack of perfusion of the brain, particularly around the lesion, which may worsen the stroke. Furthermore it is suggested that lowering the blood pressure too much may precipitate a myocardial infarction (Cruickshank *et al.* 1987). The dangers of lowering blood pressure in the acute phase of a stroke have been documented by case histories (Jansen *et al.* 1986*b*) but not from the two randomized trials in which no evidence of therapy causing strokes or other serious problems was reported (Carter 1970; Hypertension Stroke Co-operative Study Group 1974). A more recent trial, examining the possible neuroprotective effects of β-blockers compared with placebo, demonstrated that even low doses had the potential to lower blood pressure in the acute phase of stroke and that this was harmful (Barer *et al.* 1988*a*).

In a study of 100 consecutive hospital admissions for acute stroke or TIA (Jansen *et al.* 1986*a*) a relationship between starting diuretics and the onset of symptoms was found in four cases. Ideally, the authors should have collected a series of control patients admitted to the same hospital but without stroke and documented their therapy over the 3 weeks prior to admission, as they did with their series of stroke patients. This case-control method would have given an estimate of the relative risk of suffering a stroke associated with starting antihypertensive therapy. The findings as reported do not demonstrate that starting antihypertensive drugs is associated with an increased risk of stroke.

Massive falls from admission blood pressures over the first 2 months were demonstrated by Adams (1965), using blood pressure data from a subgroup of 35 of 729 patients admitted to hospital with acute stroke. The average falls observed were 50 mmHg and 20 mmHg in systolic and diastolic pressures, respectively. The reasons for this fall include acute effects of the stroke, regression to the mean (a tendency for very extreme values of a continuously distributed variable to become less extreme with repeated measurement), and adjustment of patients to their environment. The implication for therapy is that repeated measurements are needed to define which patients may need treatment.

The easy way out of the 'treat or not to treat' dilemma is to use the substantial amount of evidence that treatment is effective in primary prevention trials of people who have not yet had a stroke (Collins and MacMahon 1994). Certainly, patients who have had TIAs or mild strokes but have diastolic pressures over 100 mmHg (phase V) should be treated if the wisdom of the MRC and European Working Party on High Blood Pressure in the Elderly trials is followed (Amery et al. 1985; Medical Research Council Working Party 1985). The questions of how they should be treated, for example with newer rather than older, riskier drugs (Wilcox et al. 1986), and how far pressures should be lowered remain open.

Patients with major strokes and the very old stroke patient are not very typical of subjects recruited into any of the major primary prevention trials and it is therefore difficult to generalize trial results to these groups. Setting up a trial of antihypertensives for elderly stroke patients would be problematic. Although recurrence rates are likely to be high in such patients, to detect a 50 per cent relative treatment effect (i.e. an absolute difference of about three recurrences prevented per 100 patient-years of treatment) would require over 1000 patient-years of observation in both the treated and control groups. A large trial of blood pressure reduction after stroke is, however, in progress (Rodgers et al. 1996).

In the absence of trial data, it is sensible to act on the existing evidence and treat any patient with persistently raised blood pressure (over 95 mmHg (V), or 160 mmHg systolic) in the non-hemiplegic arm, taken with the patient standing, if possible. In patients at high risk, consideration should be given to reducing lower levels of systolic pressure (perhaps greater than 140 mmHg), possibly after discussing the uncertainties with the patient. Until there is better evidence of the effects of treatment in patients over 80 years, the best option is to include them in this recommendation, providing that care is taken to monitor adverse side-effects. Thiazide diuretics should be used as first-line treatment (Amery et al. 1985), and since ischaemic heart disease is so common in stroke patients, a case can be made for using β-blockade as an alternative (Peto 1982).

Carotid endarterectomy

Following the completion of two large randomized trials, the heated debate about the indications for this operation, which characterized the previous decade (Warlow 1984), has been substantially resolved.

The European Carotid Surgery Trial (ECST) studied patients with TIA, minor ischaemic stroke, or retinal infarct within the previous 6 months, and ipsilateral carotid artery stenosis. Participants were randomized to carotid endarterectomy plus best medical management or medical management alone, and according to the degree of carotid stenosis estimated from an angiogram. Outcome events were death or stroke within 30 days of surgery, disabling or fatal ipsilateral stroke, and any stroke lasting longer than 7 days. For 374 patients with stenosis of 0–29 per cent, 2.3 per cent of patients died or had a disabling stroke within 30 days of operation, but after that there was only one ipsilateral stroke in the next 3 years (in the surgical group). There were a few contralateral, vertebrobasilar, and non-disabling strokes, with no difference between groups. Therefore, after 3 years, the only difference between the groups was the surgical mortality and morbidity, and the procedure is clearly not beneficial (European Carotid Surgery Trialists Collaborative Group 1991).

The 1599 patients with ipsilateral stenoses of 30–69 per cent had a rate of death or major stroke of 7.9 per cent within 30 days of surgery. Over 8 years of follow-up, stroke-free survival was worse for the surgical group up to 3.4 years if carotid stenosis was 30–49 per cent, and up to 2.3 years for stenosis of 50–69 per cent. After that survival curves converged. Clearly, for this group too, surgery is not indicated (European Carotid Surgery Trialists Study Group 1996).

The group with symptomatic carotid stenoses of 70–99 per cent ($n = 778$) did show a benefit from surgery (European Carotid Surgery Trialists Collaborative Group 1991). The benefit was concentrated in patients with stenosis greater than 80 per cent, although this varied slightly with the age and sex of the patient (European Carotid Surgery Trialists 1998). Surgical mortality and morbidity was 7.5 per cent (3.7 per cent fatal or disabling stroke). Over the next 3 years the risk of ipsilateral ischaemic stroke was 12.8 per cent (8.4 per cent disabling) in the control group and 2.8 per cent (1.1 per cent disabling) for the surgical group (odds ratio 0.16; upper 95 per cent confidence limit 0.42). There was also a small reduction in other strokes, presumably a chance finding. Risk of stroke in the control group was greatest in the first year after randomization, and a net benefit for surgery was evident after about 6–9 months. The benefit for surgically treated patients persisted for 3 years, after which the ongoing risk in the two groups became the same (European Carotid Surgery Trialists 1998). In this patient group, and with these surgeons, 20 endarterectomies will cause one stroke and prevent two (over 3 years). These results were repeated in a similar North American trial of 659 patients with severe symptomatic stenosis (with stenosis severity defined slightly differently)(North American Symptomatic Carotid Endarterectomy Trial Collaborators 1991). Surgical mortality and stroke rate was 5.8 per cent. After 2 years' follow-up, relative risks for surgical compared with control patients were 0.35 for ipsilateral stroke, 0.46 for any stroke, and 0.49 for any stroke or death. In both trials, there was a gradient of increasing benefit with increasing severity of stenosis.

It is sometimes difficult to decide what to measure in evaluating a procedure. If carotid endarterectomy is going to do anything, it is going to be a reduction in ipsilateral ischaemic stroke. This gives the most sensitivity, and is useful in comparing surgical techniques or surgeons' skills. There is a potential for bias if patients who die are excluded in these analyses. Series with higher death rates might then appear to have lower morbidity. From the patient's perspective, it matters little if a stroke is in the vascular territory of an operated carotid artery or not. Counting all strokes and deaths, or all disabling strokes and deaths, puts the risk reduction from operation in context. Vascular or all-cause mortality broadens the context further (although of course, avoiding strokes is a reasonable objective regardless of any effect on mortality). The size of the benefit will vary greatly according to which outcome is chosen. In the ECST, 3-year absolute differences varied from 5 per cent to 14 per cent, depending on which outcome was chosen.

The North American trial attempted to measure an overall outcome of relevance to patients and unbiased by selective attrition through death by using a disability scale based on the Katz ADL Index, expanded to 10 items plus two 'instrumental' activities, shopping and visiting outside the home. Each item was scored according to degree of difficulty in performing it, on a 1 to 7 scale. Individual items and an overall score were analysed, the overall score having a range of 10 (no problem) to 70 (maximum difficulty with all items). Patients who died were assigned a notional score one point worse than the most disabled possible on the scale. Scores were closely related to the numbers of strokes recorded. Mean scores for medical and surgical groups diverged over the whole of the 24-month follow-up period, when the mean difference in scores was 3.6 points (i.e. half the range of difficulty on one item). Benefits for surgery were observed in each of the items considered, including vision, language, swallowing, limb function, shopping, and visiting. Relative risk reductions for 'major impairment' (defined in terms of the amount of difficulty in achieving the task) varied from 50 to 90 per cent, and the NNT to avoid one major impairment was 10–25 (Haynes et al. 1994).

Some of the issues that were highlighted before these trial results were published remain current. In the USA, operation rates climbed steadily to reach 100 000 in 1985 before declining slightly. The UK-TIA Study Group (1983) demonstrated that investigation, referral, and operation rates varied dramatically throughout the UK. The same variation was found in the USA, although the operation rates were about twice as high (Haerer et al. 1977). Differences in the type of patient seen did not explain this variation, but the beliefs of physicians and surgeons about the effectiveness of the operation were the most plausible explanation. Professional practice was examined by asking a panel to rate the appropriateness of indications for carotid endarterectomy, and then these criteria were applied to three geographical sites in the USA during 1981 (Winslow et al. 1988). The proportions of appropriate, inappropriate, and equivocal carotid endarterectomies performed at each site were compared, together with outcomes of operation. Overall, 32 per cent of 1302 operations assessed were for equivocal and 32 per cent for inappropriate indications. The main reasons for inappropriate operation were operations for less than 50 per cent stenosis, and operations on patients not suffering carotid distribution transient ischaemic attacks. Moreover, it was surprising that almost a fifth of patients were not being treated with antiplatelet or anticoagulant therapy, and only 16 (1.2 per cent) of the patients operated on were black, perhaps implying that economic and social, rather than medical, criteria were determining use of the operation.

Of great concern were the operative risks, which were extremely high; 9.8 per cent suffered a major complication (stroke with residual deficit at the time of discharge from hospital or death within 30 days of operation). The authors concluded that carotid endarterectomy was substantially overused, and in the hands of most surgeons, operative risks were too high to lead to any net benefit of the procedure. The authors stated that only patients with appropriate indications should be offered surgery, and that complication rates should be monitored. However, it has been noted that because many surgeons, especially in the UK, do fewer than 30 operations a year, it could take from 5 to 15 years before a surgeon with an unacceptable operative risk realized it (Michaels 1988). The operative risk was very high in the UK-TIA series, with a quarter of patients suffering a peri-operative stroke. It is unacceptable to operate when the annual risk of a stroke is of the order of 10 per cent (possibly lower with current medical management) and the operative risk is more than twice this. It is becoming clearer that the clinical freedom of surgeons to decide on whom they will operate, and the number of operations they will perform, is not consistent with good-quality practice for patients. The operation's future lies in centralization with highly experienced surgeons, probably doing little else.

The question of relative risk and benefits is even more vexed for asymptomatic patients found to have carotid stenosis. There appears to be a small benefit for surgical over medical treatment (in a trial with a 2.3 per cent surgical mortality/morbidity rate), but the risk of stroke is low in these patients, and absolute net benefit is small (Asymptomatic Carotid Atherosclerosis Study 1995). Consequently, the cost-effectiveness of operation in asymptomatic people is low, with a marginal lifetime (i.e. 30 years) cost-effectiveness of US$120 000 per quality adjusted life year (Lee et al. 1997). These estimates compare with a cost-effectiveness in symptomatic patients of between US$4000 and US$53 000, depending on the assumptions made (Kuntz and Kent 1996).

A further line of important research which may improve the use of carotid endarterectomy is to identify TIA patients (using prognostic models) who are, or are not, at risk of subsequent stroke, and who might therefore benefit more or less from surgery. Although high- and low-risk groups can be identified, these have not yet proven robust enough to assist in counselling individual patients (Hankey et al. 1993b; Dippel and Koudstaal 1997). None the less, any information that increases the likelihood that operation is offered to higher-risk TIA patients may help improve the low cost-effectiveness and high 'number needed to treat' of this procedure. Alternative carotid percutaneous transluminal angioplasty (PTA) procedures are currently under study in a randomized controlled trial (Brown and CAVATAS Investigators 1998) with clinical event outcomes, which cannot be substituted for by pathophysiological intermediate outcomes (Markus *et al.* 1996). However, concerns have been voiced about the selection of patients for trial entry which may compromise the generalizability of the trial and the early publication of interim findings, and may mean that the trial ceases to recruit patients if harm is demonstrated in these preliminary underpowered analyses (Naylor *et al.* 1997).

Extracranial–intracranial bypass surgery

It is easy to forget that persuasive management strategies based on first principles and presumptions about pathogenesis must be tested experimentally in trials before they are adopted. The heated discussion in the *British Medical Journal* following a trial of extracranial–intracranial bypass surgery for stroke patients (EC–IC Bypass Study Group 1985) illustrated some of the misunderstandings between trialists and clinicians that should be remembered, and hopefully avoided in the new generation of PTA trials.

Anastomosis of the superficial temporal artery to the middle cerebral artery (EC–IC bypass) has been described as 'an elegant procedure without a clinical indication' (Wade 1987). The Canadian-initiated international randomized controlled trial of EC–IC bypass was set up in 1977 to measure the rates of stroke recurrence in a group treated with this novel operation and a control group treated medically. The trial randomized 1377 patients—714 to medical treatment and 663 to surgery—and followed them up for 56 months on average. The patients were young (mean age 56 years), four-fifths were men, and over 90 per cent had minimal or no functional impairment. A third had only had a TIA but many had other problems: half were hypertensive, nearly a fifth had diabetes, and 10 per cent had had a previous myocardial infarction. Both groups were actively treated with aspirin (75 per cent of patients) and antihypertensives.

Surgery did not reduce the risk of recurrence despite being competently performed (96 per cent of anastomoses were patent at final angiographic review). During the peri-operative period stroke occurred in more than 3 out of every 100 operations. By the end of the study the cumulative risk of stroke recurrence was about 30 per cent in both groups. There were no differences in death rates or functional disability either. The results might have occurred by chance, but the probability of accepting the null hypothesis of no benefit when in fact a benefit existed (i.e. a type II error) was less than 1 in 100. The trial was designed and carried out in an exemplary way: it was large, the follow-up was long, patient groups were fairly homogeneous and well balanced, there were no follow-up losses, event criteria were applied by 'blind' adjudicators, similar 'background' therapy was used between both groups, and the surgical technique was effective.

The recurrence rate reported in the EC–IC trial was similar to other less selected series, although with the supposed benefits of modern medical therapy (aspirin and antihypertensives) they might have been expected to do rather better. The trial patients were comparatively young, had minimal or no obvious impairments at randomization, but most had other evidence of arterial disease. These facts help in deciding to whom not to recommend surgery. It is this very group who are most at risk of well-intentioned but possibly harmful effects of this operation.

One weakness of the study was in documenting what happened to non-randomized but eligible patients. This led to a contentious article (Dudley 1987) suggesting that the trial results could not be generalized because 'the trial was biased' due to the exclusion of possibly half to three-quarters of eligible patients. 'Biased' and 'partial' randomization were referred to, which are worrying concepts implying that the method of randomization was at fault, permitting patients to enter the control or treatment group in a non-random way. This would, of course, seriously affect the validity of the trial. The main criticism of the trial was not its validity (which was not in serious doubt) but the question of its generalizability to other settings. Professors Warlow and Peto (1987) considered this question and pointed out that the trial applied to patients who were 'reasonably similar' to those randomized. There is no scientific way of determining what this means but common sense and judgement should be used. Baum (1987) highlighted the 'Catch 22' of generalizability and validity. Having accepted that a trial has given a valid result which is disliked, the last ditch stand to take in refuting its results is to claim that it lacks generalizability. This ruse permits clinicians to continue backing their hunches and pursuing their freedom to go on offering the treatment. Such an approach defies both common sense and medical judgement.

Summary

1. Specific treatments that should be offered to patients with TIAs or strokes (any severity) are aspirin in moderate dose (75–300 mg daily) and antihypertensives to those with systolic pressures over 160 mmHg or diastolic phase V pressures above 90 mmHg.

2. Anticoagulation after a stroke is not associated with any net benefit. In patients with non-rheumatic atrial fibrillation who have suffered a TIA or stroke, anticoagulation appears to be a better option than aspirin in avoiding recurrence, provided risks of bleeding are low.

3. Carotid endarterectomy surgery reduces the risk of disabling stroke or death within a year for symptomatic stenoses of between 70 and 99 per cent, so long as operative mortality and morbidity is low. It is ineffective for lesser stenoses. Extracranial–intracranial bypass surgery is not effective.

4. Information on final level of ability and quality of life is badly needed to complement recurrence rates as outcome measures in trials, together with an economic appraisal of treatment effects (e.g. days spent in hospital, use of community services) and patient preferences, particularly where treatment is risky.

PART 4 PROGNOSIS

- Mortality

- Recurrence

- Effects of stroke

- Recovery

12 Mortality

Why should doctors bother to understand the pattern and predictors of death after a stroke? Knowing when death is most likely and what causes it should help decide where to concentrate effort and lead to innovations in treatment. Perhaps the devastating nature of some strokes leads doctors to feel that death is not a bad outcome, and indeed preferable to a lengthy period of rehabilitation leading to a nursing home bed. This gloomy outlook is far from the truth for the majority of patients (see Chapter 15). Information about prognosis is useful for the following reasons:

- patients and relatives need information to plan their lives;
- to permit triage of patients with different prognoses, thus allowing rationing of resources and balanced comparisons in treatment trials;
- to identify patients with a poor prognosis who may benefit from special efforts, including palliative care;
- to find predictors of poor prognosis that may be amenable to change, and thus possibly improve prognosis.

Risk of dying

The risk of dying after a stroke has been widely studied, but perhaps the most surprising fact is how variable reported case-fatality rates are, ranging from 7 per cent to 67 per cent dead by 1 year (Marshall and Shaw 1959; Stevens and Ambler 1982). The most obvious explanation is that selection bias is responsible for much of the variation. However, even when a standardized protocol was used in a World Health Organization (WHO) multi-centre study, almost twofold variation in 1-year case-fatality rates occurred between participating centres (Aho *et al.* 1980), and 28-day case-fatality varied threefold in the WHO MONICA study (Thorvaldsen *et al.* 1995).

The variation in case fatality is marked in both hospital and community series (Table 12.1). This is because the studies differ in age composition and stroke severity, which together with differences in ascertainment of cases of stroke, have a marked effect on subsequent mortality. The quality of hospital management may also have an important effect on mortality (Stroke Unit Trialists Collaboration 1997). In Weddell and Beresford's study (1979), every effort was made to register cases occurring in a defined population, and many cases were derived from death certificates, which almost certainly accounts

Table 12.1 Variation in cumulative mortality among hospital and community series of stroke patients

Source	1 week	1 month	3 months	6 months	1 year	5 years
			Cumulative mortality (%)			
Community patients						
Eisenberg et al. (1964)		56*				85
Weddell and Beresford (1979)	34	45*	54			80***
Aho et al. (1980)	25	33*	40		50	
Herman et al. (1980)	19		26			
Sacco et al. (1982)		22				35***
Stevens and Ambler (1982)		45			67	
Bonita et al. (1984)	23	34			48	
Harmsen and Wilhelmsen (1984)	22	27*			36	
Wade and Hewer (1987)				34		
Scmidt et al. (1988)		37*	44		52	72
Bamford et al. (1990a),						
Dennis et al. (1993)	12	19			31	53
Wolf et al. (1992)			23			
Bonita et al. (1993)		24				
Anderson et al. (1994a)		24			38	
Feigin et al. (1995b)		31				
Thorvaldsen et al. (1995)		15–57				
Brown et al. (1996)		21			33	
Korv et al. (1996)		30				
Numminen et al. (1996)		23	29		34	
Stegmayr and Asplund (1996)		13				
Hospital patients						
Marshall and Shaw (1959)					7	
Droller (1960)					24	
Adams and Merrett (1961)					20	
Carter (1964)					37	
Marquardsen (1969)		35	46			59
Sheikh et al. (1983)		28*			49	
Kotila et al. (1984)			35		40	
Henley et al. (1985)				30	44	
Barer (1987)		32		46		
Viitanen et al. (1987a)		14*	23		31	68
Terent (1989)		23	25		34	45**
Candelise et al. (1991)		17		24		
von Arbin et al. (1992)		13*				58
Kalra et al. (1993b)	16					
McGovern et al. (1993)	8	14	21	25	27	46
Gompertz et al. (1994b)				39		
Weir et al. (1997)			22		30	

* Three weeks; ** 3 years; *** 4 years.

for the high 1-week case-fatality rate reported. In the study by Herman and co-workers (1980), patients had to be seen by a doctor before registration, which may account for the rather low case-fatality, since early deaths were not registered.

It is probable that patients admitted to hospital have worse strokes and worse survival. In Weddell and Beresford's study, 3-week case fatality among men, but not women, was three times higher in those admitted to hospital (75 per cent died). In the Oxford Community Stroke Project, patients with impaired consciousness were almost four times more likely to be admitted to hospital (Bamford et al. 1986, 1990a), which should lead to improved overall case fatality of those kept at home, due to selective admission of those with the worst prognosis.

Longer-term survival of stroke patients is worse than that of the general population. Annual risks of dying of about 10 per cent for stroke patients under 60 years, 15 per cent at ages 60–69, 25 per cent at ages 70–79, and 50 per cent for those over 80 years were reported by Marquardsen (1969). These rates are about 18–24 times the expected rates in the general population for those under 60, and about twice the expected rates for those over 70 years. Over two decades later, the Oxfordshire Community Stroke Project reported risks after the first year of 2.5 per cent/year for patients under 65, 5.5 per cent/year for patients aged 65–74, 9 per cent/year for patients aged 75–84, and 11 per cent/year for those over 84 (with low numbers and high mortality in the first year in this last group). The relative risk of death compared with the general population after the first year was about twofold (Dennis et al. 1993). Age-adjusted gender differences were small. Similar findings have been reported by others (Viitanen et al. 1987a).

The consistent finding in these studies is that the majority of deaths occur within the first 3 weeks, further deaths occur over the first year, and then deaths continue at a constant, age-dependent but increased rate compared with the general population.

Time trends in case fatality

Case fatality has fallen markedly over recent decades (Hurwitz and Adams 1972; Haberman et al. 1978; Garraway et al. 1983; Harmsen et al. 1992; Korv et al. 1996; Numminen et al. 1996; Stegmayr and Asplund 1996; Thorvaldsen et al. 1997). This factor, as much as decreased incidence, is responsible for the downward trend in stroke mortality (see Chapter 3). For example, in the Minnesota Heart Survey, from 1970 to 1985, age- and sex-adjusted 28-day case fatality fell by 45 per cent (from 26 to 16 per cent), and the improvement was apparent from day 2 of the admission onwards (McGovern et al. 1993). Trends in case fatality are particularly prone to changes in hospital admission rates and the age structure of the population, so the most reliable estimates of this trend come from community-based studies with almost complete ascertainment. In Minnesota, the proportion admitted unconscious fell from 22 to 15 per cent over this period, although the reduction in mortality remained after statistical correction for known prognostic factors. Some studies found improvements for patients with minor, but not major, neurological deficits in cerebral infarction (Shahar *et al.* 1995; Stegmayr and Asplund 1996). Amongst community-based studies, Bonita *et al.* (1993) reported a decline in case fatality between 1981 and 1991, from 27 to 22 per cent in men and 38 to 26 per cent in women. Other studies have not found a decline in case fatality (Terent 1989; Wolf *et al.* 1992; Feigin *et al.* 1995*a*; Brown *et al.* 1996). Results for patients with cerebral haemorrhage are even less consistent. Some studies report large decreases in mortality, but some of this may be due to better detection of small bleeds by CT scanning.

It is unlikely that improved ascertainment of less severe cases wholly explains the data for cerebral infarction, at least. The two alternative explanations are that stroke severity has decreased (due, perhaps, to better risk-factor management, and supported by some evidence that stroke severity has changed; Wolf *et al.* 1992; Bonita *et al.* 1993; Stegmayr and Asplund 1996), or that acute hospital management has improved (suggested by experimental stroke unit evidence; Langhorne *et al.* 1993). Longer-term survival has also improved. Between 1977 and 1985 in Sweden 3-year survival improved from 40 to 55 per cent despite an increase in the average age of patients (Terent 1989), and the Minnesota study found a 30 per cent decrease in 2-year mortality amongst 28-day survivors between 1980 and 1990 (McGovern *et al.* 1993; Shahar *et al.* 1995). It is noteworthy that these changes in mortality, if genuine, are large, have occurred over a relatively short period of time, and are probably larger than will ever be achieved by any, yet to be discovered, acute drug treatment for stroke. Understanding the driving forces behind these trends remains a major priority for epidemiological research as these forces, if they can be manipulated, hold the prospect of further reducing the burden of stroke, particularly in those countries where mortality trends are increasing.

Causes of death after stroke

Even if every patient had a post-mortem examination, it would be impossible to resolve the 'what did this patient die from?' and the 'what did this patient die with?' dilemma. The findings at necropsy in a small hospital series, where virtually all early deaths were examined, were: brain swelling, pulmonary emboli, and recent myocardial infarction (Oxbury *et al.* 1975). A larger series with a high necropsy rate found the stroke to be the cause of death in 90 per cent of first-week deaths. In weeks 2–4, pulmonary embolism (30 per cent), pneumonia (23 per cent), heart disease (20 per cent), and the acute stroke itself (27 per cent) were the causes. Older and immobile patients were more susceptible to pneumonia, but pulmonary embolism was still common amongst patients able to walk 10 days after their strokes (Viitanen et al. 1987b). The Oxfordshire Community Stroke Project found the majority of deaths in haemorrhagic stroke to be due to neurological sequelae (74 per cent) and to occur very early (35 per cent within 12 hours). A few later deaths may be associated with the development of cerebral oedema around day 5. Twenty-eight per cent of patients with infarcts who died, did so of direct neurological sequelae, mainly between days 2 and 6. Forty per cent of these deaths were in patients with brainstem infarcts, and 16 per cent were due to trans-tentorial herniation. Deaths from the complications of immobility were concentrated in weeks 2–4 (Bamford et al. 1990a).

When hospital patients were followed-up for 6 months, the percentage of deaths attributed to each cause was as follows: primary brain death (16 per cent); pneumonia (44 per cent); pulmonary embolism (25 per cent); heart failure, myocardial infarction, or arrhythmia (12 per cent); renal failure (2 per cent); other causes (2 per cent) (Barer 1987). Follow-up to death gives a different picture: recurrent stroke (23 per cent); myocardial infarction (10 per cent); heart failure and/or bronchopneumonia (30 per cent); pulmonary infarction (5 per cent); uraemia (3 per cent) (Marquardsen 1969). The preponderance of ischaemic heart disease deaths during the later phases of follow-up is confirmed by other studies, and continues for several years (Viitanen et al. 1987a; Scmidt et al. 1988; Dennis et al. 1993).

Predictors of early mortality

Conscious level

Predictors of early mortality after stroke noted over 100 years ago were impaired conscious level, breathing abnormalities, bilateral neurological signs, and hypothermia followed by pyrexia (Marquardsen 1969). Impaired consciousness has stood the test of time as an adverse prognostic sign for survival. In the WHO stroke registration project (Aho et al. 1980) and the Minnesota Heart Study (McGovern et al. 1993), 3-week case fatality was 15 times higher in comatose compared with alert patients. The strength of this association varies from four- to fivefold in most studies (Rankin 1957; Marquardsen 1969; Oxbury et al. 1975; Bonita et al. 1988) falling as low as just over twofold in one retrospective hospital series (Lowe et al. 1983) and one large Russian cohort (Scmidt et al. 1988). Most studies have found a stepwise gradient of risk of death with decreasing level of unconsciousness. However, a few initially comatose stroke patients do eventually make a good recovery.

Type of stroke

Although early studies were not able to diagnose type of pathology adequately, most studies have reported very high case fatality for haemorrhagic stroke; from sevenfold increased first-day mortality (Marquardsen 1969), to twofold increased 1-month mortality (Eisenberg et al. 1964; Herman et al. 1982a; Sacco et al. 1982; Garraway et al. 1983; Harmsen and Wilhelmsen 1984). One-month mortality is around 30–60 per cent (Ward et al. 1988; Bamford et al. 1990a; Daverat et al. 1991; von Arbin et al. 1992; Sarti et al. 1993; Anderson et al. 1994a; Brown et al. 1996).

The major problem with clinical diagnosis of cerebral haemorrhage is that an adverse prognostic variable—unconsciousness—is one of the clinical criteria for diagnosing haemorrhagic stroke (see, for example, Tanaka et al. 1982) which confounds the relationship between pathology and mortality. Neuroradiology is required to permit accurate diagnosis and avoid linking unconsciousness, a prognostic indicator, with the means of making the diagnosis. The Oxford Community Stroke Project was able to make a neuroradiological diagnosis in a very high proportion of patients and found a fivefold higher case fatality in haemorrhagic stroke than ischaemic stroke (Bamford et al. 1990b). This difference is very similar to that for clinically diagnosed Framingham patients where 30-day mortality was 82 per cent for haemorrhagic and 15 per cent for thrombotic stroke (Sacco et al. 1982). Various studies with CT verification have recorded similar relative risks (Harmsen et al. 1992; Numminen et al. 1996).

Although clinical diagnostic criteria are too inaccurate to classify individual patients, they appear sufficiently accurate to compare survival in groups of patients, especially if standardized assessments are made (Sandercock et al. 1985b). Ideally, the impact of possible predictors of case fatality should be examined separately for ischaemic, haemorrhagic, and lacunar stroke but this information is not yet available. In practice, mortality after the first few weeks is likely to be among patients with ischaemic stroke, whereas haemorrhagic stroke will tend to weight the early mortality.

Clinical stroke subtypes

Even when CT head scanning is fairly readily available, it is still useful to be able to subdivide strokes clinically into those with a good or bad outlook. The OCSP classification (Bamford et al. 1991), and classifications based on presumed aetiology (Anderson et al. 1994a), provide information that is prognostically useful (Table 12.2). The Perth Community Stroke Study undertook a validation of the OCSP system by measuring 1-year mortality. Findings were broadly similar and the differences may have been caused in part by clinical misclassification, but the confidence intervals were wide and chance could equally well have been responsible (Anderson et al. 1994b).

Table 12.2 Clinical stroke subtypes and mortality

	1 month (%)	1 year (%)
Oxford Community Stroke Project		
Total anterior circulation infarct	39	60
Partial anterior circulation infarct	4	16
Lacunar infarct	2	11
Posterior circulation infarct	7	19
Haemorrhages	52	62
Perth Study		
Total anterior circulation infarct		49
Partial anterior circulation infarct		16
Lacunar infarct		10
Posterior circulation infarct		36
Perth aetiological classification		
Lacunar infarct	0	14
Boundary-zone infarct	0	0
Large-artery thrombosis	11	25
Emboli	26	41
Haemorrhages	30	39

These classifications give a reasonable indication of the prospects for survival, which provides further external validation of the classifications themselves.

Other predictors

Predictors of early mortality (within the first 3 weeks) include high blood pressure on admission to hospital (Rankin 1957; Marquardsen 1969; Aho *et al.* 1980; McGovern *et al.* 1993), age (Marquardsen 1969; Herman *et al.* 1982*a*; Sacco *et al.* 1982; Bamford *et al.* 1990*a*; Candelise *et al.* 1991; McGovern *et al.* 1993), raised blood glucose (Power *et al.* 1988; Weir *et al.* 1997), raised haematocrit (Lowe *et al.* 1983), atrial fibrillation (Lowe *et al.* 1983; Sandercock *et al.* 1986; Candelise *et al.* 1991; Lin *et al.* 1996), pupil changes, gaze paresis, extensor plantar responses, abnormal breathing, abnormal body temperature and meningeal irritation (Rankin 1957; Marquardsen 1969), dysphagia (Barer 1987, 1989*a*; Gordon *et al.* 1987; Kalra *et al.* 1993*b*), and pre-stroke dependency (Bamford *et al.* 1990*a*; Kalra *et al.* 1993*b*; Numminen *et al.* 1996). Table 12.3 lists predictors of early (within 1 month) and late mortality, together with a indication of how strongly they are associated with mortality.

Blood glucose measured after the stroke appears to be a prognostic marker for mortality in case series (Power *et al.* 1988; O'Neill *et al.* 1991; Weir *et al.* 1997). However, in a much larger study, capable of distinguishing between stroke subtypes, very large differences were found in blood glucose and

Table 12.3 Relative risk estimates of the strength of association of predictors with early and late mortality after stroke

Factor	Early mortality	Late mortality
Pre-stroke dependency (Rankin 3–5)	2–3	2.5
Alert versus not alert	2.3–15	2.6–4
Haemorrhagic versus thrombotic stroke	2–5.5	
Dysphagia	5	3.6
Pupil abnormality	1.6–3	
Gaze paresis	1.8	
Extensor plantars	2.2–2.6	
Pyrexia	1.9	
Abnormal breathing	2.2–2.9	
Haematocrit 50%+	2	
Blood glucose >7 mmol/l	1.9	1.4–3.8
Meningeal irritation	1.4	
Barthel <5 out of 20		4.5
Incontinence of urine		4–5
Blood pressure (240+ mmHg)	2	4
Pre-stroke hypertension		2–5
Heart disease/hypertension	3–5	1.7
Age over 70	2	2
Atrial fibrillation	1.5–2	1.5–2
Past stroke		2
Depression		3.4

survival for haemorrhagic strokes only, among Hong Kong Chinese (Woo *et al.* 1988, 1990). Elevated blood glucose may be simply a marker of stroke severity mediated through acute stress hormones, or may contribute to pathogenesis through increasing ischaemic damage (Helgason 1988).

Some of the predictors listed in Table 12.3 tend to be associated with each other as well as with mortality. Combinations of predictors that predict survival and death more accurately have been sought. Any combination of unconsciousness, gaze paresis, and dense hemiplegia was said to be a better predictor of early death in a series of patients with clinically diagnosed cerebral thrombosis (Oxbury *et al.* 1975). As is shown in Table 12.4, adding gaze paresis and dense hemiplegia to conscious level actually reduces the accuracy of the prediction of death compared with using conscious level alone.

Another attempt to produce an overall score (level of consciousness, orientation, speech, gaze paresis, facial weakness, motor strength, disability, spasticity, and sensation) achieved higher predictive accuracy, around 66 per cent, but this was only slightly better than the 50 per cent accuracy of subjective predictions made by the admitting doctor (Britton *et al.* 1980).

Sheikh and colleagues (1983) have tried to unravel the independent contributions of several prognostic variables using multiple regression. Impaired

Table 12.4 Predictive accuracy of conscious level, gaze paresis, and dense hemiplegia for early mortality after stroke (data from Oxbury *et al.* 1975)

Factor	Dead	Alive	Factor	Dead	Alive
Not alert	15	26	Any present	15	38
Alert	0	52	None present	0	40
Predictive value for death = 15/(15 + 26) = 37%			Predictive value for death = 15/(15 + 38) = 28%		

consciousness, conjugate deviation of eyes, age, and severity of motor deficit correctly predicted 73 per cent of deaths within the first 3 weeks. The effects of a history of heart disease, previous stroke, and pupil abnormalities were not important. However, haematocrit, heart rhythm, temperature, and blood pressure, among other known predictors of death, were not included in the multivariate model.

Predictors of late mortality

Mortality beyond 6 months is probably increased by pre-stroke high blood pressure (Sacco *et al.* 1982), although blood pressure measured immediately after the stroke does not predict mortality well (Merrett and Adams 1966). More recent data show a clear gradient of stroke risk with increased blood pressure (Rodgers *et al.* 1996). Age remains a good predictor of late mortality (Marquardsen 1969; Aho *et al.* 1980; Bonita *et al.* 1984), together with indicators of severity of stroke (Wylie 1962; Marquardsen 1969; Aho *et al.* 1980; Anderson *et al.* 1994a) and past history of stroke (Aho *et al.* 1980; Bonita *et al.* 1984). Depression is strongly associated with 10-year mortality, although this may be associated with stroke severity (Morris *et al.* 1993). Initial conscious level probably continues to have some predictive value even 1 year after the stroke (Christie 1981; Anderson *et al.* 1994a). The strength of these associations is shown in Table 12.3.

Multiple regression has been used to predict late mortality. Level of consciousness, age, combined neurological deficits, sensory deficit, and gaze paresis each contributed independently to improving the prediction at 1 year (Sheikh *et al.* 1983). Another model, including coma, urinary incontinence, cardiac failure, severe paresis, and atrial fibrillation achieved a sensitivity of 0.94, specificity 0.62, and positive predictive value of 68 per cent (Anderson *et al.* 1994a).

Despite the enthusiasm for predictive models, two studies have concluded that they perform little better overall than simple variables such as level of consciousness and incontinence (Barer and Mitchell 1989; Gladman *et al.* 1992).

Table 12.5   Accuracy of predicting death and survival at 6 months, comparing urinary incontinence and loss of consciousness (data from Wade and Hewer 1985b)

Consciousness	Dead	Alive	Urinary incontinence	Dead	Alive
Lost	94	60	Present	138	92
Not lost	84	281	Absent	42	251
Predictive value for death = 138/(138 + 92) = 61%			Predictive value for death = 94/(94 + 60) = 60%		
Predictive value for survival = 281/(84 + 281) = 77%			Predictive value for survival = 251/(42 + 251) = 86%		

Disability

In a selected group of patients receiving rehabilitation and followed for 2 years, a score comprising age, walking ability, a past history of myocardial infarction (both measured at variable times up to 3 months after the stroke) predicted 74 per cent of deaths and 79 per cent of survivors (Wade *et al.* 1984). In a community series of patients, poor activities of daily living alone (Barthel score less than 5 out of 20 during the first week) gave similar accuracy, correctly predicting 67 per cent of 6-month deaths and 85 per cent of survivors (Wade and Hewer 1987). The powerful predictive effect of activities of daily living scores on subsequent mortality has also been shown by others (Wylie 1967; Ebrahim *et al.* 1985; Bamford *et al.* 1990a; Kalra *et al.* 1993b; Numminen *et al.* 1996).

Urinary incontinence

Of patients with urinary incontinence after stroke in Copenhagen, 52 per cent were dead within 6 months, compared with 7 per cent of patients who remained continent (Nakayama *et al.* 1997). In another study, incontinence of any cause after stroke was associated with a risk ratio for death within a year of 3.9 (95 per cent CI, 1.4–10.6) (Anderson *et al.* 1994a). Urinary incontinence in the first week of a stroke is claimed to be a better predictor than conscious level for late mortality (Wade and Hewer 1985b). However, direct comparison of these two variables shows that they have very similar predictive ability, as shown in Table 12.5.

Triage

Since conscious level makes such a large impact on both early and late survival prospects, swamping the contribution of other predictors (e.g. gaze paresis, sensory and motor deficit, etc.), it is of great use in triage of patients for specialist rehabilitation. Conscious level is also much easier to measure than many predictors. It has been used successfully with walking ability and pre-stroke disability to allocate patients to a stroke unit (Garraway *et al.* 1981). Refining severity factors into an overall score is not really worthwhile since a more complicated system for deciding on place of treatment would be time consuming and difficult to standardize. Prognostic indicators are not sufficiently accurate to be used to decide on whether or not to withhold supportive treatment in the acute phase (Barer and Mitchell 1989). Repeated application of such prognostic measures (either on their own or as multi-variate scores) over time might result in greater accuracy, but new studies are required to examine this question.

Modifying predictors

It is disappointing that factors which reflect initial stroke severity continue to have such a large effect because this implies that improved late survival may only be achieved by reducing the initial severity of the stroke. However, assessment of causes of death indicates diseases which ought to be avoidable or treatable (pneumonia, pulmonary embolism). The best evidence that risk factors for mortality are modifiable comes from stroke unit trials, which were set up to examine disability outcomes, but which, fortuitously and somewhat surprisingly, turned out to reduce mortality as well (Langhorne *et al.* 1993; Stroke Unit Trialists Collaboration 1997). It is not clear exactly which risk factors were being modified so successfully, but early attention to swallowing problems and feeding, avoidance of venous thrombosis and pressure sores, early detection and treatment of pneumonia, careful attention to co-morbidities, and early mobilization and rehabilitation may contribute.

Of predictors and causes of late mortality, a history of hypertension and heart disease suggest that treatment of these problems may lead to improved survival. Treating hypertension after a stroke may be beneficial (see Chapter 11), as will giving aspirin (Antiplatelet Trialists Collaboration 1994b), and treating moderate to severe heart failure improves survival in other groups (Cooperative North Scandinavian Enalapril Survival Study 1987). Prevention of deep-vein thrombosis and pulmonary emboli by subcutaneous heparin may produce a small improvement in survival (McCarthy and Turner 1986; Turpie *et al.* 1987) but these are almost certainly offset by greater harms due to intracerebral bleeding (International Stroke Trial Collaborative Group 1997). Urinary incontinence and disability may be simply markers of stroke severity, and hence little may be done to modify them, although positive effects of treatment on morale and mood may reduce mortality (Barer 1989b).

More attention should be given to looking for predictors of early and late mortality that are independent of stroke severity or conscious level. For example, dysphagia among alert stroke patients on the first day is associated with a fourfold increased risk of death in the first month (Barer 1987). It is possible that dysphagia merely reflects stroke severity, but among alert patients it is equally possible that preventable complications (such as aspiration and dehydration) lead to death (Norton *et al.* 1996). Similarly, hyperglycaemia may be a 'stress response' reflecting severity of the neurological insult, but may also be an adverse prognostic factor because of a neurotoxic, or oedema-related, effect, and restoration of euglycaemia with insulin in the acute phase is a strategy that is being tested in trials (Weir *et al.* 1997).

Summary

1. Between a quarter and a half of deaths occur in the first 3 weeks after a stroke, and between a third and two-thirds by 1 year. After the first year death rates are about twice those expected in the general population for patients over 70 years but very much higher than this for younger patients.

2. Level of consciousness on admission is the single best predictor of early death. Only marginal improvements can be made by including other predictors. Better prediction may be achieved by examining survival in pathologically defined groups, as haemorrhagic stroke has such a high early case fatality.

3. Hypertension, heart disease, pneumonia, and pulmonary emboli are important treatable causes of death. Prevention, active detection, and treatment are needed.

4. Triage for rehabilitation (and randomization for acute treatment trials) should use conscious level as the simplest and most discriminating predictor of outcome.

5. Late mortality is still influenced by level of consciousness at onset, but potentially modifiable predictors (independent of stroke severity) such as dysphagia, hyperglycaemia, poor activities of daily living, and urinary incontinence require interventions trials.

13 Recurrence

'Will it happen again, doctor?' The stroke patient is asking one of the most difficult questions to answer clearly, and is expecting a straight 'yes' or 'no'. The clinician may toss a mental coin, and say 'no', realizing that this answer will be wrong some of the time but right most of the time. The response may be justified by the paternalistic notion that the patient really does not need negative ideas to ponder during the difficult period of recovery. An alternative is to give a probability of a further stroke. Depending on the optimism of the doctor this may be stated as a per cent chance of having a stroke or a much bigger chance of not having a stroke. The figure usually quoted is around 10 per cent/year (Allen 1984a; Wade *et al.* 1985*b*) but leads to a series of questions: A 10 per cent chance of what and for how long? To which of the diseases that comprise stroke does this figure apply? Does it mean the same level of risk for all types of people—men and women, old and young, severely and mildly affected?

The clinician should be able to give a specific answer that helps both himself and the patient to weigh a risk of further stroke against possible preventive treatments (with their own potential risks), rehabilitation efforts, social, and family affairs.

The chances of a recurrent stroke

Marquardsen's early retrospective study (1969) of 769 patients admitted to hospital from 1940 to 1952 is a most important natural history study as it followed patients for up to 23 years and gave great detail about recurrence of stroke. The criteria used to define stroke recurrence were 'a definite worsening of the neurological sequelae from the primary stroke, if occurring abruptly'. Events were recorded not as they occurred but retrospectively during home visits by Marquardsen himself. This had the virtue that no variation between observers could have occurred, but a single investigator could have changed his rules over such a long time period, and the patients' memories for events might be unreliable.

He found that risk of further stroke (including all subsequent strokes) was 8.9 events per 100 patient-years for men, and 10.6 events per 100 patient-years for women. This risk did not decline as time passed but was higher amongst people over 80 years.

In the Oxfordshire Community Stroke Project recurrent strokes were ascertained prospectively by nurse and neurologist visits. Amongst the 675 patients there were 180 recurrent strokes, including 135 first recurrences, after 2–6.5 years of follow-up. Risk of (first) recurrence decreased progressively with time. In the first year, absolute risk amongst survivors was 13 per cent (95 per cent CI, 10–16 per cent), a relative risk of 15 compared with people who had not already had a stroke. Thereafter, the average annual risk was 4.3 per cent. Overall, the chance of suffering a recurrence within 5 years was 30 per cent. Two-thirds of these were severe. Five-year risk of death or recurrent stroke was 63 per cent. Smokers were at greater risk of recurrence. In this study, from the 1980s, use of secondary preventative measures was quite low: only 6 per cent were taking aspirin; 1 per cent, warfarin; and 17 per cent were treated with antihypertensive drugs (Burn et al. 1994).

The Framingham Study has collected data on stroke recurrence among 394 patients suffering first strokes from 1949 to 1975 in a defined population but found no increased risk with age (Sacco et al. 1982). Men had about twice the risk of recurrence of women, with a male 5-year cumulative risk of recurrence of 42 per cent (an annual risk of about 9 per cent), which is very similar to Marquardsen's hospital series. Women had a 5-year risk of 24 per cent, equivalent to an annual risk of 5 per cent. The better prognosis of women is unexplained, but was thought to be due to their higher compliance with treatment. It is possible that Marquardsen's higher female risk of recurrence resulted from women admitted to hospital being older, and having more heart disease. Recurrence rates from Rochester, Minnesota were of the same order; 10 per cent in the first year but tended to fall over the next 4 years to about 4 per cent/year (Whisnant et al. 1971; Matsumoto et al. 1973). Other studies have not found a decline in recurrence rates after the first year, but this could be explained by higher mortality (from both stroke and ischaemic heart disease) among those at highest risk of recurrence, leading to a somewhat 'fitter' survivor group.

Further observation of stroke patients in Rochester, Minnesota from 1950 to 1979 has demonstrated a low recurrence rate of less than 5 per cent/year, with a 5-year recurrence rate of 19 per cent. Recurrence rates have not changed much over this 30-year time span (Meissner et al. 1988). This suggests that the increased use of antihypertensive and antiplatelet drugs has either not been sufficiently widely applied, or its relatively small effect is insufficient to produce a measurable impact on population burdens of recurrent stroke.

Several other studies have produced similar results. The Stroke Data Bank registered 1273 patients with cerebral infarction admitted to hospital. Four-teen per cent had a recurrence over the next 2 years. In this study lacunar strokes were as likely to recur as were embolic strokes, although strokes presumed to be due to large-vessel atherothrombosis had the highest

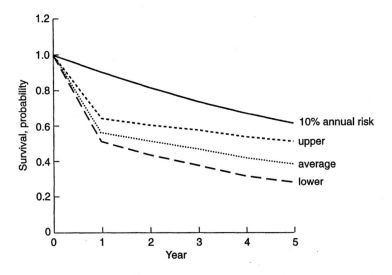

Fig. 13.1 Cumulative survival free of stroke recurrence (Oxford Community Stroke Project data with upper and lower 95% CI).

recurrence rate of all (Hier *et al.* 1991). Von Arbin and colleagues reported a 5-year recurrence rate of 21 per cent in their hospital series of 388 patients, and noted that the case fatality amongst these recurrent strokes was 50 per cent (von Arbin *et al.* 1992). A hospital-based series of 322 non-disabling ischaemic strokes in relatively young patients demonstrated a 10-year mortality of 32 per cent. Risk of disabling recurrent stroke was 14 per cent, despite vigorous investigation and secondary prevention (Prencipe *et al.* 1998). The Dutch TIA trial (which studied both TIAs and minor ischaemic strokes) reported a recurrence rate of 3.6 per cent/year (Kappelle *et al.* 1995).

The cumulative risk of recurrence or death over 5 years is high, ranging from about a half to almost two-thirds affected. As shown in Fig. 13.1, this risk is highest in the first year and it is constant for the following years. A constant hazard of recurrence or death of 10 per cent/year gives a very different picture and is shown in the figure for comparison. The better survival free of further stroke indicated by the constant 10 per cent/year estimate fails to take into account the much higher attrition during the first year, resulting in fewer survivors affected by somewhat lower rates thereafter. The confidence intervals associated with small numbers of events as time passes among those included in the Oxford Community Stroke Project affect the precision of these estimates.

The great strengths of the population-based data, such as the Oxford Community Stroke Project and the Framingham data, are that the estimates of recurrence rate are not affected by selection bias. Increasingly, there is interest in using data from large trials to define epidemiological relationships between risk factors and outcomes, for example the important work defining the relationship between blood pressure and mortality in TIA patients (Rodgers *et al.* 1996). In some circumstances, such trials provide the only large datasets available, but while risk factor–outcome associations are unlikely to be affected by selection bias, great caution must be taken in using such data to define incidence rates, where selection effects of taking part in trials may make participants at very different (usually lower) risk compared with more typical patients. For example, the annual risk of death among participants in the UK-TIA trial was 3.6 per cent/year, compared with 7.2 per cent/year in the unselected OCSP series (Hankey *et al.* 1993*b*). By contrast, but equally difficult to interpret, are the recurrence rates reported in the first 14 days in the International Stroke Trial (1997)—a fatal and non-fatal stroke recurrence rate of 3.9 per cent, which is extraordinarily high. This high rate may reflect difficulty in applying diagnostic criteria in the acute phase of stroke, where extension of an infarct or intercurrent illness may mimic a recurrent event.

Cohort studies, rather than stroke registries, also have the additional advantage that relationships between risk factors and recurrent events can be evaluated both in terms of baseline, pre-stroke levels, and also levels measured after the stroke. Thus, the effects of having the stroke can be disentangled from the direct effects of exposure to the risk factors of interest. This may be particularly important in studying the effects of blood pressure, blood coagulation factors, and nutritional factors, where the stroke itself may alter the risk factor if it is measured after the stroke has occurred. Ideally, studies of recurrence should be nested within population-based cohort studies, and this is becoming increasingly possible with new approaches to pooling of data from a large number of cohort studies, thus increasing the numbers of stroke patients available for study (e.g. Prospective Studies Collaboration 1995).

Blood pressure

Marquardsen highlighted the very poor prognosis of patients with high diastolic blood pressure at the time of the original stroke. Men with diastolic pressures over 120 mmHg (phase and arm used were not reported) on admission had a 4.7-fold increased risk, and women a twofold risk, of further stroke compared with those with diastolic pressures below 99 mmHg. These blood pressure readings were taken on admission and will tend to be higher than pressures taken a few weeks after the stroke (Adams 1965). Several studies reporting recurrence rates have noted hypertension to be a risk factor (Hier *et al.* 1991; Kappelle *et al.* 1995; Prencipe *et al.* 1998).

Johnston and colleagues (1981), using a group of stroke patients attending a blood pressure clinic, found higher first-visit blood pressures among those suffering a recurrence. The lowest recorded systolic pressure during follow-up was 20 mmHg lower in the group without a recurrent stroke. This study appears to support the notion that high blood pressure is associated with recurrent stroke, but it is quite possible that those with higher pressures stayed under follow-up for longer and thus had more time to suffer another stroke. Incidence rates for recurrent stroke, using patient-years of follow-up as a denominator, categorized by level of blood pressure and treatment, should have been calculated so that the risk of recurrent stroke could have been compared in each group.

The relationship between blood pressure and stroke after TIA was examined in the UK-TIA trial (Rodgers *et al.* 1996). The trial included 2435 subjects followed for an average of 4 years, during which time there were 230 strokes, a recurrence rate of about 2.4 per cent/year. These data were analysed according to person-years at risk in each of four blood pressure categories. There was a strong, and graded, relationship between stroke risk and both diastolic and systolic blood pressure. Each 5 mmHg lower (usual) diastolic blood pressure and 10 mmHg lower systolic pressure was associated with 34 per cent and 28 per cent fewer events, respectively. There was no evidence of a J-shaped curve, and the strength of relationship was about the same as that in subjects without previous cerebrovascular disease, although absolute stroke risks were much greater (MacMahon *et al.* 1990). A randomized trial of blood pressure reduction after TIA and minor stroke (the 'PROGRESS' trial) was initiated on the basis of these results.

Type of stroke

In Marquardsen's study, because of the difficulty in diagnosing the pathological process causing a stroke, no separate risk factors were defined for thrombotic, haemorrhagic, or embolic stroke. The recurrence rate for patients suffering transient ischaemic attacks (TIA) and very mild strokes is probably lower than after more severe strokes, about 4 per cent/year in a community series (Heyman *et al.* 1984). An attempt to follow-up a diagnostically 'clean' group of patients with occlusion of the middle cerebral artery suffered from the effects of marked selection (Sacquegna *et al.* 1984). Seventy patients with an average age of 55 years, who had had cerebral angiography between 1970 and 1980 were studied at an Italian Neurology Institute. A cumulative 5-year incidence of recurrent stroke of 10.4 per cent was found. It is likely that this estimate is too low, for two reasons. First, any group of tertiary referral patients is highly atypical. They survived long enough to be investigated and may therefore be less severely affected than more typical cases. Secondly, the method of counting recurrent strokes by interview or telephoning the family doctor was of doubtful accuracy and might underestimate recurrences.

It has been noted that the survival prospects after cerebral haemorrhage are so poor that any study of recurrence is almost the same as a study of recurrence after cerebral infarction (Sacco *et al.* 1982). Risk of recurrence by clinical (and by inference pathological) subtype has been examined amongst patients with cerebral infarctions in the Oxfordshire Community Stroke Project. Nine per cent of patients with lacunar strokes had a recurrence within a year, spread evenly throughout the follow-up period, reflecting the presumption that these represented occlusion of a further small artery. Partial anterior circulation strokes had high early recurrence rate, 17 per cent over the first year, almost entirely concentrated in the first 6 months, reflecting an 'active' cardiac or arterial embolic source. Twenty per cent of posterior circulation strokes suffered recurrence. There were few recurrences in the total anterior circulation stroke group, but survival was low, and damage near-maximal on the affected side, so there was less scope for new damage (Bamford *et al.* 1991).

Large population series of neuroradiologically diagnosed stroke patients provide the best estimates of the true recurrence rates among thrombotic, haemorrhagic, and embolic strokes. As more stroke patients are investigated with CT scans, we will be able to give a more specific and precise prognosis for recurrence.

Atrial fibrillation

A study of stroke recurrence (Sage and Uitert 1983) among 59 patients with atrial fibrillation (AF) but no evidence of valve disease, reported a recurrence rate of 20 per cent/year, equivalent to a 67 per cent chance of a further stroke over 5 years. This is about twice the rate expected and compares with Marquardsen's finding of a 1.6- to 1.8-fold increased risk among men and women with atrial fibrillation.

Including early recurrent stroke deaths in figures for recurrent stroke (usual practice) tends to overemphasize the prognostic importance of factors that have their major impact early on, and often lead to death rather than disability. Such factors may not be as relevant to the prognosis of survivors of the early phase. In the Framingham Study, recurrence within the first year after a stroke was three times as common in patients with AF compared with those without AF (risk ratio 3.1; 95 per cent CI, 1.3–7.7). However, most of these occurred within 30 days of the initial stroke (Lin *et al.* 1996). Data from 30-day survivors in the Oxfordshire Community Stroke Project (Sandercock *et al.* 1986, 1992) have been analysed separately. Among 30-day survivors there was no impact of atrial fibrillation on subsequent risk of recurrent stroke over the following 2 years. The recurrence rate among 30-day survivors with and without atrial fibrillation was about 13 per cent within 2 years. This is lower than the figures obtained by Marquardsen, which may be because of chance, the exclusion of early recurrent stroke deaths, the wider community coverage in the Oxford study, the method of counting recurrences, and perhaps even the effect of modern medical treatment.

The final piece of evidence in establishing a causal relationship between recurrent stroke and AF (see Chapters 2 and 11) is experimental intervention. The European Atrial Fibrillation Trial randomized 1007 patients to aspirin, warfarin anticoagulation, or placebo, and followed them for up to 55 months. Warfarin reduced the risk of stroke from 12 to 4 per cent (risk ratio 0.34; 95 per cent CI, 0.20–0.57) (European Atrial Fibrillation Trial Study Group 1993).

Other factors

Primary polycythaemia certainly increases the risk of strokes (Pearson and Wetherley-Mein 1978). Whether secondary polycythaemia is associated with an increased risk of recurrent stroke is debatable and the effectiveness of treatment was to have been the subject of a trial (Wetherley-Mein et al. 1987), which unfortunately was never completed. Advice to stop smoking (a cause of polycythaemia) in these and other patients can be justified for other reasons despite a lack of randomized trial evidence that it will reduce recurrence.

The Stroke Data Bank Study found diabetes to be a risk for both early and late recurrence (Sacco et al. 1989; Hier et al. 1991). Heart failure apparently increases male, but not female, risk of recurrence by 2.6 times (Marquardsen 1969). The Framingham male recurrence rates (Sacco et al. 1982) were also greatly increased by the presence of 'cardiac comorbidity'—which meant high blood pressure, heart failure, and coronary heart disease. Male 5-year recurrence rates fell from 45 per cent to 28 per cent after removing patients with pre-stroke heart disease and hypertension from analysis. Comparable 5-year female recurrence rates only fell from 24 to 19 per cent, with most of this fall due to the effect of hypertension.

The highest recurrence rate found by Marquardsen was 53 per cent/year, among patients with both atrial fibrillation and an average diastolic blood pressure of $100+$ mmHg (a fivefold increased risk). This suggests that risk factors for recurrent stroke (as in first stroke) are likely to be multiplicative when their combined effects are assessed; for example a man with a diastolic blood pressure of over 120 mmHg on admission, atrial fibrillation, and heart failure might be expected to have a $4.7 \times 2.6 \times 1.6 = 11.7$-fold increased risk of a recurrent stroke.

Further work examining the interactive effects of different risk factors in increasing risk of stroke is required. A better understanding of the ways in which changes in smoking and exercise habits, in weight and dietary intake, and in psychological factors affect stroke recurrence risk would be invaluable in developing better secondary prevention services for stroke patients. In myocardial infarction, the approach to secondary prevention includes both pharmacological and non-pharmacological interventions, which are based on an understanding of the epidemiology of recurrence (Ebrahim and Davey Smith 1996). We need more data in stroke to determine whether we should be making similar investments.

Summary

1. The risk of having a recurrent stroke is high in the first year at about 10–16 per cent, and may be very much higher in the first month. This risk falls over the ensuing years to about 2–7 per cent/year. The cumulative risk of death or recurrent stroke over 5 years is high, at about 60 per cent.

2. These risks are affected by stroke type and the presence of risk factors. The main factors known to increase the risk of a recurrent stroke are male sex, raised blood pressure (before and after the stroke), atrial fibrillation, diabetes, coexisting ischaemic heart disease, and increased age. These factors increase risk of recurrence independently and may operate in a multiplicative fashion.

14 Effects of stroke

Many of the effects of stroke are not obvious for weeks or months, and by this time the patient is often at home without the support of specialist care. Follow-up by rehabilitation teams, hospital, and family doctors after a stroke is patchy, and certainly not related to need—if impairments and disability are accepted as indicators of need (Ebrahim *et al.* 1987*b*)—so it is likely that many complications may go undetected. Avoidable complications of stroke are common and have been reviewed (Mulley 1982). Painful hemiplegic shoulders, spasticity, contractures, and constipation would benefit from more research examining their causes and management options. In the areas of depressed mood, cognition, dysphasia, urinary incontinence, dysphagia, deep-vein thrombosis and pulmonary embolism, quality of life, falls and fractures, and stress affecting carers, much more is now known about occurrence and causes than a decade ago, but more attention is still needed to find practical solutions to these problems.

What problems are common? Table 14.1 lists some of them. Documentation of complications in case records is inadequate, as shown by a review of 607 hospital-admitted stroke patients (Davenport *et al.* 1996*b*); no complications due to dysphagia or urinary incontinence were reported despite their important practical and prognostic significance. The extent of some of these specific complications, their importance, and management will be considered next.

Mood change

Depressed mood has long been known to occur after a stroke (Bleuler 1924) and is of concern, not just because of the human misery involved, but also because it may be a barrier to successful rehabilitation (Adams and Hurwitz 1963). It has been demonstrated that amongst patients with a relatively good spontaneous recovery, depressed mood is associated with a longer hospital stay, although the importance of depression as a barrier to recovery in more severe strokes is doubtful (Ebrahim *et al.* 1987*a*; Parikh *et al.* 1990; Morris *et al.* 1992).

Diagnosing depression

Measurement of the frequency of mood disorder after stroke is beset with problems, particularly of case definition (House 1987*a*). Diagnosis is difficult

Table 14.1   Adverse effects of stroke

- Dysphagia
- Dysphasia
- Urinary incontinence
- Epilepsy
- Infections: chest, urine
- Cognitive impairment
- Mood changes
- Skin breaks/pressure sores
- Deep-vein thrombosis
- Pulmonary embolus
- Cardiac arrhythmias
- Cardiac failure
- Pain: shoulder and elsewhere
- Falls and fractures
- Carer stress

in cases of dysphasia and cognitive impairment, and as with many physical illnesses, symptoms such as fatigue, sleep disturbance, or constipation are as likely due to the stroke as to depression. Mood rating scales have been widely used, but in many cases screening tools have been used to reach definitive diagnoses, there has been much variation in the cut-off points for defining cases, and control groups have rarely been employed. Attempts to use the dexamethasone suppression test as a biological marker of depressed mood have shown that it has limited validity when compared with psychiatric interview (Lipsey *et al.* 1985). Interestingly, it has better validity 3 years after a stroke (sensitivity, 0.7; specificity, 0.97; likelihood ratio, 23), than at 1 week and 3 months post-stroke (likelihood ratios, 1.3 and 1.5). Early 'non-suppressors', however, have a high incidence of depression over the next 3 years (odds ratio, 14; 95 per cent CI, 3–76) (Astrom *et al.* 1993), suggesting that the dexamethasone suppression test may have useful predictive value. Further investigation of the dexamethasone suppression test in dysphasic or cognitively impaired patients also needs to be investigated, as such patients present diagnostic difficulties.

The General Health Questionnaire (GHQ) is a widely used self-completed questionnaire of affective problems and has been used to measure mood in patients with physical illness (MacGuire *et al.* 1974; Knights and Folstein 1977; Glass *et al.* 1978; Hawton 1981) and after stroke (Robinson and Price 1982; Ebrahim *et al.* 1987*a*). Since 7 out of 28 GHQ questions are to do with physical difficulty in carrying out daily tasks, many physically ill people will respond positively to them, thus appearing to be depressed. The usual threshold to distinguish those with a high chance of depression from the rest is 5 or more out of 28 (Goldberg and Hillier 1979) but amongst patients with neurological disability a higher threshold of 12+ is more valid (Bridges and Goldberg 1986).

Several studies have attempted to validate mood rating scales against the 'gold standard' of a structured psychiatric interview (such as the Present State Examination, PSE). House and colleagues (1989a) used both the PSE and the American Psychiatric Association's Diagnostic and Statistical Manual (DSM-III) criteria, administered by a psychiatrist, to validate the Beck Depression Inventory (BDI), a visual analogue mood scale (intended to allow dysphasic or cognitively impaired subjects to respond), a carers' rating, a nurses' rating (made during routine follow-up visits for a research study), and GP records. An immediate problem was that there was not complete concordance between the two 'gold standards'. The PSE method identified more severe cases, and there were also differences in the way that concomitant anxiety was classified. In fact, the BDI had a likelihood ratio of about 1 (i.e. no diagnostic information) throughout its range for diagnosing DSM-III depression, while having good validity for PSE depression. The BDI scores were continuously distributed, indicating that, like blood pressure or cholesterol, the idea of 'diagnosable depression' as a separate entity is not sustained, rather depression is at one end of a range of mood experience.

The visual analogue scale was neither easier to complete than the BDI nor at all valid in making diagnoses. The nurses only managed to make ratings on 77 per cent of patients, and only identified 6 of 15 patients with DSM-III major depression, along with four patients with adjustment disorders and one with dysthymic disorder, and a further five patients who did not have a DSM diagnosis (but who were lonely or had chronic pain). It was concluded that nurses were sympathetic to emotional problems, but without special training their opinions were insufficiently valid to be used for screening. Carers were available for interview for only half the patients. They identified all the patients with major depression, and three with other diagnoses. GPs identified two-thirds of patients with major depression as having psychological problems. Benzodiazepines were prescribed to four and low-dose antidepressants to five, but none was followed-up adequately for response (House et al. 1989a).

The same team compared the Hospital Anxiety and Depression Scale (HADS) with a structured psychiatric interview 3–5 years after a stroke. The HADS places less emphasis on physical symptoms, making it more suitable in physically ill subjects. Compared with any DSM-III depressive diagnosis, diagnosis by HADS was good (sensitivity, 0.73; specificity, 1.0), and for major depression it was excellent (sensitivity, 1.0; specificity, 0.94), although a non-standard cut-off was used (Sharpe et al. 1990). The HADS and GHQ-30 (a version of the GHQ stripped of somatic items) were compared with standardized psychiatric interview in another study of 6-month survivors of hospital-discharged stroke patients who were entered into a family support worker trial. Good validity was found for both these instruments, with the optimal (non-standard) cut-off having sensitivity and specificity about 0.8 (O'Rourke et al. 1998).

Rating scales can give a valid indication of mood disturbance, but they are relatively crude, and completion rates are rarely better than 80 per cent. In clinical use they should be followed up by a clinical mental state examination to make a precise diagnosis.

Nabarro (1984) has drawn attention to the hidden problem of depression in medical patients who have made good physical recoveries, arguing for increased psychiatric referral. A better policy would be the routine use of a depression questionnaire, such as the GHQ, and referral of those with high scores. Others have questioned the very nature of post-stroke 'depression', preferring instead to use the term 'post-stroke misery', to capture its multi-faceted nature and multi-factorial causes. Indeed, with any psychiatric sequelae of physical illness, it is necessary to consider the general meaning of the disease (e.g. stroke is life-threatening), its specific meaning for the individual (e.g. a stroke may be the last straw in a conflict-laden relationship), and the pathology-related factors (e.g. associated cognitive deficits) in coming to a formulation of the psychological problems experienced by patients (House and Ebrahim 1991).

Frequency of mood disturbance

Depressed mood after stroke seems common. One of the problems in saying how common, is variation in the populations from which cases are drawn, leading to selection bias. Robinson and Price's early study (1982) found that 23 per cent of patients had GHQ scores of five or more, which they equated with a high prevalence of depression. However, the study group was not typical of hospital or community practice. The GHQ cut-point may have been inappropriately low, and some patients had their strokes many years previously. Ebrahim et al. (1987a), using a threshold of 12 or more on the GHQ, reported a 6-month mood disorder prevalence of 23 per cent (95 per cent CI, 16–30 per cent) among a consecutive series of patients admitted to hospital with acute stroke. Follow-up losses were only 5 per cent, and only those with expressive dysphasia and cognitive impairment were excluded, and all were at home at the time of completing the GHQ. Other examples of this type of study have yielded prevalences of depression between 14 and 61 per cent (House 1987b).

Structured psychiatric interviews offer the opportunity for much greater precision in characterizing psychiatric syndromes, their severity, and to some extent their origins and interpretation. A lower prevalence of psychiatric disorder (19 per cent with an abnormal score on the PSE) was found in the Oxford Community Stroke Project (House 1987a; House et al. 1991). By 1 year after the stroke this had fallen to 11 per cent, of whom half had DSM-III defined depression and half adjustment disorders. Using similar methods in the Perth Community Stroke Study, Burvill et al. (1995a) reported 15 per cent major depression and 8 per cent minor depression 4 months post-stroke. Eight months later nearly half these cases had resolved. The hospital-derived series of O'Rourke and colleagues revealed major depression in 13 per cent and any depression in 19 per cent (O'Rourke *et al.* 1998).

Depressed mood is quite common in people who have not had a stroke. In the UK up to 13 per cent of women aged 65–74 years report depressive symptoms (Ebrahim *et al.* 1988), so it is important to use a control group of unaffected subjects. Depressive symptoms are about twice as common in stroke patients (6 months after the event) compared with age- and sex-matched controls (Ebrahim *et al.* 1986). By contrast, the distribution of BDI scores 1 month after a stroke are little different from that in a control group (House *et al.* 1991). However, only 10 per cent had PSE diagnoses, 8 per cent DSM major depression, and 1 per cent dysthymic disorder. The Perth Study found slightly lower rates of depression in controls: 5 per cent major and 3 per cent minor depression (Burvill *et al.* 1995*a*). This variation between studies probably represents differences in the patients studied, the instruments used, and timing of assessments after stroke.

Anxiety and other minor psychiatric syndromes

Various psychological and emotional symptoms occur after stroke, and there has been a tendency to lump then all together as 'depression'. Moreover, current psychiatric classifications subsume anxiety under the manifestations of depression, and its prevalence is under-recorded. In the early phase, physical tension, insomnia, and restlessness are described, along with anxiety, frustration, irritability (or even aggression), poor concentration, and sadness. These are probably part of an understandable psychological reaction to acute illness, a so-called 'adjustment reaction'. Some patients respond to failure in the performance of previously achievable tasks with 'catastrophic reactions' (temper or evasion) or apathy (Starkstein *et al.* 1993). Emotional inappropriateness may have a specific (non-dominant hemisphere) neurological explanation. Together, these phenomena contribute to what many relatives of stroke patients call 'personality changes', which is another source of confusion, because these are not what psychiatrists would call 'personality disorders' (House 1987*b*).

Anxiety disorders are probably almost as common as depression after stroke, in particular agoraphobia (going beyond an understandable fear of recurrence, falls, or the stigma of abnormal movement). The Oxford study found 15 per cent to have agoraphobia, anxiety, or anxious adjustment disorders 1 month after stroke, compared with only 3 per cent of controls (House *et al.* 1991). Only the adjustment disorders appeared to abate over the first year, and diagnosable anxiety was present in 20 per cent of patients re-examined 3–5 years after their strokes (Sharpe *et al.* 1990). In Perth, similar high levels of anxiety were found, especially agoraphobia, and particularly in women. Some of this was accounted for by pre-stroke problems, but the prevalence was much greater than in control subjects (Burvill *et al.* 1995*b*).

Emotionalism

Emotional lability is the sudden, uncontrollable, onset of socially and emotionally inappropriate crying or laughter. It is common after stroke, but only one study has examined its frequency and causes (House *et al.* 1989*b*). Lability or 'emotionalism' affected 1 in 5 patients at 6 months and 1 in 10 patients at 1 year after their first stroke in the Oxfordshire Community Stroke Project. Although lability is thought to be common after bilateral strokes, it is clearly also common after a single stroke. Lability was also strongly associated with the size of lesion on CT scanning, and with high mood scores, suggesting an association with depressed mood. Several studies have shown that antidepressants are effective in ameliorating emotionalism, including both tricyclics and selective serotonin re-uptake inhibitors (Andersen *et al.* 1993).

Causes of depression

Depression in old age is strongly associated with losses and life events (Murphy 1982) and post-stroke depression may well be a reaction to the loss of physical health and function. A small study comparing 20 stroke patients and 10 orthopaedic patients with similar levels of disability found that depression was more than four times as common in those with stroke (Folstein *et al.* 1977). A better comparison might have been with patients suffering a disease with an acute onset and an unpredictable prognosis. Mood disorder was strongly associated with both the extent of motor impairment and functional disability, and was worst in those whose disability increased over the first 6 months (Ebrahim *et al.* 1987*b*; Burvill *et al.* 1997).

In a general elderly population, disability, and especially handicap, were very strongly associated with risk of depression (Prince *et al.* 1997). This association with severity was found in the Oxford Community Stroke Project (Sharpe *et al.* 1994), and as a higher proportion of less severe strokes was included, this may explain the lower prevalence of psychiatric disorder compared with other hospital studies.

Lesion location

Robinson and co-workers have claimed that the site of the stroke lesion is an important determinant of depressed mood; left hemisphere, more anterior lesions shown on CT scan were most strongly associated with depression

(Robinson *et al.* 1984). However, their correlation was very dependent on two subjects with very bad depression and anterior lesions, and the group included was only a small fraction of their total series. Attempts to replicate Robinson's work have failed (Sinyor *et al.* 1986; House *et al.* 1990*b*; Sharpe *et al.* 1990), and no laterality effect was found in Ebrahim *et al.*'s study (1987*b*), suggesting that the observation may be a spurious result caused by selection bias. The original findings may be an example of Berkson's bias: in a hospital series a spurious association may arise if a risk factor is associated with hospital admission (dysphasic patients are more likely to be admitted), and the outcome (depression) is also associated with hospital admission (which it will be if patients with more severe strokes are more likely to be depressed) (Sackett 1979). An alternative explanation is that left anterior lesions are associated with emotionalism, which was mistakenly classified as depression (House *et al.* 1989*b*).

Treatment

The majority of patients with depressed mood do not receive antidepressants when discharged from hospital (Ebrahim *et al.* 1987*b*), but are antidepressants of any use? Few trials of antidepressant therapy after stroke have been published. The first from Johns Hopkins University (Lipsey *et al.* 1984) used a double-blind, randomized design but suffered from a 33 per cent withdrawal rate among the 39 patients randomized. This was compounded by an analysis of those remaining on treatment, rather than an intention-to-treat analysis (Schwartz and Lellouch 1967; Hampton 1981). The study was small, with only 17 given the tricyclic antidepressant, nortriptyline, and 22 on placebo, included relatively young patients, and was concluded after only 6 weeks. Mood, but not functional ability, showed an improvement in both groups, but a much bigger change in those on active treatment. This was interpreted as a benefit from treatment but it is quite likely, because of losses to follow-up and treatment withdrawals, that those with only mild to moderate depression at the start of the study were the only ones still remaining on treatment at the end of the study. One correspondent pointed out that the only thing shown with any certainty in Lipsey's study was that nortriptyline is a toxic drug to give patients after a stroke (Agerholm 1984)!

A second treatment trial was reported by Reding and colleagues (1986) in which patients with and without depression (categorized in a variety of ways, including a dexamethasone suppression test) were randomized to either placebo (22 patients) or trazadone hydrochloride (25 patients). Treated patients were followed up for a week longer than placebo patients, with an overall trial length of about 1 month, thus treated patients had longer to improve. These investigators used the Barthel ADL Index as their outcome measure but were only able to show a significantly improved Barthel score in seven patients with an abnormal dexamethasone suppression test. The investigators stated that they studied a consecutive series of patients, yet the majority (89 per cent) had some evidence of depression. Although the anti-depressant used was meant to have fewer side-effects than older tricyclic compounds, a quarter of the patients were withdrawn because of side-effects. This study was unethical in concept since active, toxic treatment was given to patients who did not have any clinical indication for treatment. Sadly, the study does not contribute any useful information about the role of antidepressant therapy after stroke.

Two more recent randomized controlled trials of selective serotonin re-uptake inhibitors have shown greater improvements in mood among those patients on active treatment, but both trials were small, suffered with drop-outs and large spontaneous recovery in the control groups, and were far too short at only 6 weeks (Andersen et al. 1994; Dam et al. 1996).

The preventative effect of early and structured rehabilitation on post-stroke mood disorder has been demonstrated in a study of 315 patients randomized to a stroke unit or general wards. GHQ scores were identical 3 and 6 months after the stroke, but significantly lower amongst those treated on the stroke unit after 12 months (mean scores 20 versus 17). Psychological adjustment was also better after stroke unit treatment, although differences were small (Juby et al. 1996). Two British and one Canadian trial of post-discharge support and counselling have failed to provide evidence of improved psychological outcomes (despite making measurements on the GHQ, HADS, and a social adjustment scale) (Friedland and McColl 1992; Forster and Young, 1996; Dennis et al. 1997), whereas an American trial of counselling did find some evidence of improved adjustment but did not measure mood (Evans et al. 1988). In view of the obvious toxicity of drug therapy in brain damaged people, these approaches should be pursued, most obviously by performing a randomized trial of multi-disciplinary assessment and treatment based on community psychiatric nurses, as has been shown to be effective in depressed elderly people without stroke (Waterreus et al. 1994) .

A small but properly designed trial of about 50 subjects in each group would be powerful enough to detect a treatment effect of about 50 per cent relative improvement in mood and ADL scores, assuming a similar measure-ment variance to that reported in earlier trials. Much less toxic and probably lower doses of antidepressant should be used in any further drug trials. Follow-up should be for much longer than a few weeks—most antidepres-sants take at least 2 weeks to even begin to work. In the meantime, it is sensible to detect impaired mood using a questionnaire, refer patients with problems for a psychiatric opinion, and if drug treatment is recommended, to use low initial doses of antidepressants together with a supportive and encouraging rehabilitation programme.

Cognitive impairment

Adams and Hurwitz (1963) first drew attention to the poor rehabilitation prospects of patients suffering with cognitive impairment after a stroke. The size of this problem depends on the type of assessment of cognitive ability used. There is no general agreement about what abilities should be included under the heading of cognition. Most of the standard techniques used to assess 'cognition' focus mainly on short- and long-term memory, and orientation. All currently available assessment methods have been criticized because of failure to include items such as constructional apraxia, agnosia, verbal recall, nominal aphasia, auditory comprehension, and concept formation, and for their conceptual inadequacy (Ritchie 1988).

Most methods share common threads of short- and long-term memory and orientation in time, place, and person. Short assessments agree with longer tests reasonably well (Hodkinson 1972) and are widely used. Despite its conceptual inadequacy (e.g. one of the items 'write a sentence' requires motor, psychomotor, visuo-spatial, visual scanning, and language skills), the Mini-Mental State Examination (MMSE; Folstein et al. 1975) has some particular virtues: it covers a wide range of cognitive ability (orientation, registration, attention, calculation, recall, language, ability to follow a complex command, writing, and copying a drawing) than the shorter tests; it is easy to use with stroke patients; and patients may not find it as demeaning as the short tests (which include naming the Queen or Prime Minister). It shares some of the problems of any pencil-and-paper test: it cannot be used with some dysphasic patients and it requires an attention span of at least 10 minutes.

The dilemma of where to draw the cut-off point between 'normal' and 'impaired' has been tackled, at least in part. The MMSE was validated by comparisons with a physician's independent clinical assessments and with the Weschler Adult Intelligence Scale. The MMSE is meant to 'separate patients with cognitive disturbance from those without such disturbance'. In fact the MMSE discriminates well between diagnostic groups but does not classify individuals so well.

Examination of the range of scores in each group gives an indication of the sensitivity and specificity of the MMSE, the appropriate measurements for assessing the ability of a test to classify individuals. Normal subjects never scored below 24, and clear-cut demented subjects never scored above 21. A threshold of 24 or more would clearly separate out normal subjects. In practice, the clinical task is more subtle than this and tests are needed that will discriminate between dementia and depression. Depressed subjects scored anywhere from 8 to 30, the maximum. A threshold of 21 and below would pick up demented and depressed subjects with a specificity of 100 per cent; it would not permit discrimination between demented and depressed subjects. The MMSE is of some use in describing the amount of cognitive impairment present but is not a diagnostic test. It must be supplemented with clinical observations and examination over a period of time.

In a consecutive series of 189 6-month survivors of an acute stroke, 12 per cent (95 per cent CI, 7–17 per cent) of subjects had an MMSE score below 22 out of 30, and in a third of these patients there was no prior evidence of dementia, cerebrovascular disease, or depression (Ebrahim 1985). In the subjects whose cognition declined between 1 and 6 months an association with depressed mood was found. Stroke severity was strongly associated with cognitive impairment, which supports the view that the major determinant of cognitive impairment is the amount of brain damage (Tomlinson et al. 1970). A study among patients less than 65 years old reported a very similar level of 12 per cent suffering some impairment, with 6 per cent severe enough to satisfy DSM-III criteria for mild dementia (Kotila et al. 1986b). Finnish and American hospital series reported rates of 26 per cent diagnosed clinically according to DSM-III-R criteria, although this proportion was less when other classifications were used (see Chapter 4), and increased with age (Tatemichi et al. 1993; Pohjasvaara et al. 1997). In the Oxford Community Stroke Project, cognitive impairment was common (21 per cent affected) and similar relationships were seen with markers of stroke severity (House et al. 1990c).

Symptoms and signs of memory disturbance after stroke have been studied. Subjective complaint of memory impairment was more common amongst stroke patients than orthopaedic patients (Tinson and Lincoln 1987), and performance on story and picture memory was impaired in 29 per cent and 14 per cent, respectively, 3 months after a stroke (Wade et al. 1986b), although comparative data for these tests were not available. This leads to difficulty in deciding on a threshold for abnormality, consequently these prevalence estimates are arbitrary.

Fisher (1982) has reported six patients suffering a specific disorientation for place associated with right hemisphere parieto-occipital lesions, and in Ebrahim's study (1985) an excess of recall difficulty was found in patients with left-hemisphere stroke. These observations suggest that the type of cognitive impairment may well depend on the site of the brain damage.

Clinicians should assess cognition routinely, using the MMSE (Folstein et al. 1975) rather than the shorter, and less informative, memory and orientation tests. They should consider the possibility of depressive illness in patients with impairments. The effects of subjective memory impairment and learning difficulties on recovery require further study, and the impact of memory retraining for those with less severe problems is not yet known but may hold some hope (Wilson 1982). The importance of advice and support for carers of cognitively impaired stroke patients and appropriate resettlement for badly affected patients should be obvious but, as with many aspects of stroke management, is often neglected (Ebrahim et al. 1987b).

Dysphasia

The frequency of dysphasia among early survivors varies from 10–16 per cent in community series (Hopkins 1975; Legh-Smith *et al.* 1987) to 33 per cent in hospital series (Marquardsen 1969; Pedersen *et al.* 1995). The prognosis for recovery among patients still dysphasic at 10 weeks is not good, with the majority of patients only making small improvements by 6 months (Lendrum and Lincoln 1985; Pedersen *et al.* 1995). Type of aphasia, age, and sex do not influence recovery. Overall, full recovery is expected in about 30 per cent, but of patients with severe aphasia on admission, half will die in hospital, 12 per cent will recover fully, and another 12 per cent will regain reasonable language function.

Treatment

At least three trials of speech therapy have been done, two making comparisons between professional and volunteer treatment (Meikle *et al.* 1979; David *et al.* 1982) and one with an untreated control group (Lincoln *et al.* 1984). The scale of improvement in all three trials was modest; scores on a Functional Communication Profile and the Porch Index of Communicative Ability rose by only a few points, with no difference between speech therapy and volunteers or untreated controls. Drop-outs and those who recovered early were not included in the analyses, which may tend to underestimate the true effects of therapy, but is unlikely to make a major change to the trial results. A curious finding in the Bristol trial (David *et al.* 1982) was that nine patients taken on long after the stroke (3 months to 2.5 years) showed exactly the same pattern of improvement as the rest. This has been interpreted as a genuine benefit of treatment since spontaneous recovery is very unlikely to occur by this time. However, it is quite possible that patients simply did better on the communication tests as they got used to them. The two baseline assessments for both early and late referrals showed an increasing trend prior to starting therapy, which supports this interpretation.

As with any negative trial, it is useful to examine the confidence intervals of the difference observed between comparison groups. The Bristol trial (David *et al.* 1982) compared 48 patients in each group and observed a difference of about 2 per cent in the Functional Communication Profile which has a standard deviation of about 20 per cent. The 95 per cent confidence intervals of this 2 per cent difference ranged from −6 per cent to 8 per cent. The Nottingham trial (Lincoln *et al.* 1984) had similar confidence intervals. Despite the relatively small size of these trials, it is unlikely that an important treatment effect has been missed because such a precise measure of outcome was applied to every subject. A Cochrane review of speech therapy is planned and should be available in the next year (Greener *et al.* 1998).

Speech therapists have responded, particularly to the Nottingham trial, claiming that the treatment given was too little and started too late (after 10 weeks); that patients might have been unable to benefit because of deafness, dementia, or other problems; and that the real questions are what methods and regimens of speech therapy are successful with which patients (Howard 1984; Williams *et al.* 1984). However, providing and attending intensive speech therapy is difficult; in Bristol only 5 per cent of those referred and 1 per cent of all cases of stroke were suitable for treatment 5 days a week (Legh-Smith *et al.* 1987). A case for the continued involvement of speech therapists with stroke patients has been made (Wade *et al.* 1985*b*) but with an emphasis on assessment; advising relatives, patients, and staff; provision and instruction in use of communication aids; and organization of group activities for patients and relatives. There is no doubt that the withdrawal of speech and language therapists from the management of dysphasic stroke patients in many stroke services has been an unfortunate consequence of these trials which, in retrospect, were too narrowly focused on impairment outcomes.

Urinary incontinence

Urinary incontinence after a stroke is a bad prognostic feature, both for survival and functional recovery (Lorenze *et al.* 1959; Marquardsen, 1969; Hurwitz and Adams, 1972; Anderson *et al.* 1994*a*; Taub *et al.* 1994; Nakayama *et al.* 1997). If patients survive their stroke, however, continence tends to improve (Barer 1989*b*; Nakayama *et al.* 1997). The World Health Organization stroke project (Aho *et al.* 1980) measured the occurrence of incontinence among a large but variably collected group of stroke patients. They found that 8 per cent were incontinent before the stroke, 25 per cent at 3 weeks, 14 per cent at 3 months, and only 10 per cent at 1 year. A New Zealand study of 151 hospital-admitted patients also found a high prevalence of incontinence; 60 per cent at 1 week, 42 per cent at 1 month, and 29 per cent at 3 months after the stroke (Borrie *et al.* 1986). A similar pattern of falling prevalence after stroke was found by Brocklehurst and co-workers studying a selected group of patients (Brocklehurst *et al.* 1985). In a community series (Wade and Hewer 1987) a lower prevalence was found; at 1 week, 3 weeks, and 6 months, 44 per cent, 24 per cent, and 11 per cent, respectively, were incontinent of urine, which is remarkably similar to the WHO series. Amongst people with incontinence, a history of stroke is seven times more common than in the rest of the population (Wetle *et al.* 1995). Some of the variability in prevalence comes about because of the problem of definition. Some have advocated the inclusion of all urinary symptoms, such as frequency and nocturia, as frank incontinence is only the extreme end of a spectrum (Sakakibara *et al.* 1996; Brittain *et al.* 1998).

The prospect of recovering continence after stroke depends on the severity of the incontinence at 1 month. In Borrie's series (Borrie *et al.* 1986) two-thirds of those with only mild problems got better by 3 months, under a fifth of those with more severe incontinence had improved by this time, and an equal proportion had died. Incontinence before the stroke was not a bar to improvement in continence afterwards. The reduction in incontinence after a stroke is a result of spontaneous recovery among the mildly affected and death of the more severely incontinent.

Urinary incontinence is a common enough problem, but what underlying mechanisms are responsible? Borrie's study (1986) used cystometry on those suffering with moderate or severe incontinence, although only 19 patients were investigated. Detrusor instability (termed 'hyperreflexia' in the presence of neurological disease) was the most common abnormality found, but this is common in old age and it may be a coincidental finding in stroke patients. Since a control group was not studied concurrently, it is difficult to comment on the importance of the cystometric results observed. It is quite possible that patients without incontinence have detrusor instability and that other factors (such as immobility, cognitive impairment, depression, site of lesion, prostate enlargement) must be present before incontinence results. Future studies should concentrate on examining urodynamics in both continent and incontinent patients, with consideration of these other important factors that may hinder achieving continence. Other studies, again without controls, and in addition to unstable bladders, identified minorities with detrusor hypotonia, and normal bladders, and pointed out that this latter group were all aphasic, demented, or severely disabled (i.e. simply could not communicate a need or get to a toilet) (Gelber *et al.* 1993; Burney *et al.* 1996; Sakakibara *et al.* 1996).

Treatment

Treatment of incontinence depends on its cause. Algorithms can be used to define specific causes (Hilton and Stanton 1981), leaving a residual group who may be assumed to have detrusor instability, although this may be unwarranted on present evidence. Since the numbers of patients with persistent incontinence are relatively small, urodynamic studies should probably be used more often so that a precise diagnosis is reached, especially if empirical or first-line treatment has failed (Nitti *et al.* 1996). No specific treatment trials of incontinent stroke patients have been carried out, so experience among other types of patients with detrusor instability must be used. Several studies have shown benefits from habit retraining, in which patients are taken to the toilet and encouraged to urinate regularly (initially every 30–60 minutes), with the duration of time being extended as control improves. This may be augmented by use of anticholinergic drugs (Castleden *et al.* 1986). In institutional settings 'prompted voiding' (usually every 2 hours) may be undertaken.

A major problem with anticholinergics is their toxicity, especially in brain-damaged people. Several agents are available, including oxybutinin, imipramine, and tolterodine, and although these have a greater effect on bladder function than does placebo treatment, the effect is still relatively small (Rentzhog *et al.* 1998). Single-case study designs (*n*-of-1 trials) may well be helpful in assessing the use of various drugs for an individual patient if habit retraining is unsuccessful. A double-blind design is feasible and incontinence may be recorded using a visual analogue scale or by nursing staff using the gradings of Castleden *et al.* (1986). The dangers of precipitating acute urinary retention are always present (especially as another important cause of detrusor instability is prostatic hypertrophy; Nitti *et al.* 1996), and patients should be assessed carefully before starting anticholinergic therapy. This has been made much easier with the introduction of simple ultrasound devices for estimating post-void residual bladder volumes.

Patients with incontinence are often catheterized. During a randomized trial Kalra *et al* (1995) found that the rate of catheterization on general medical wards was more than twice that on a stroke unit. This probably accounted for a doubling in incidence of urinary infection. It is said that there is no such thing as a catheter without problems, and in the absence of urinary retention every effort should be made to avoid their use.

Dysphagia

Choking on food and drink in the acute phase of both brainstem and hemisphere stroke is common. Up to 45 per cent of hospital-admitted patients may have some evidence of dysphagia (Gordon *et al.* 1987) and among conscious patients about a third are affected initially (Barer 1984, 1987). Management of this serious complication varies from mandatory use of 'some alternative method of giving fluids' (Hewer 1987), 'swallowing therapy' (Barrett *et al.* 1987), to a 'wait and see' policy (Barer 1984). The presence and prognosis of dysphagia after hemisphere stroke probably depends on stroke severity, which should influence management. In the Bristol series (Gordon *et al.* 1987) 73 per cent of dysphagic patients also had some degree of impaired consciousness, with an associated poor prognosis; overall almost half the patients were dead within 6 weeks. Most survivors were able to swallow by 2 weeks. Maintaining hydration in drowsy, dysphagic patients may lead to survival of patients with a very poor prospect of improvement, and their high early death rate suggests that brain death, rather than complications of dehydration, is more important.

In a series of 121 conscious, acute stroke patients, Smithard and colleagues (1996) found half their patients to have an unsafe swallow clinically, and 21 per cent aspirated during videofluoroscopy (having excluded those unfit for the procedure). Patients with a clinically unsafe swallow were more likely to get a chest infection (33 per cent; odds ratio, 2.7), die (37 per cent; odds ratio, 9.1), or suffer the combined poor outcome of death or institutional care (65 per cent; odds ratio, 5.4). Length of stay was doubled. Aspiration on video-fluoroscopy was less strongly associated with these outcomes, but the patients most likely to suffer them had been excluded because they were unfit for the procedure. Biochemical and anthropomorphic indices of nutrition deterio-rated over a month in patients with dysphagia. Dysphagia remained a poor prognostic feature even after statistical adjustment for other indices of stroke severity. This poor functional outcome confirmed the earlier work of Barer (1989a).

Barer's two hospital series are of interest since his patients had a relatively good prognosis (all unconscious patients were excluded) and were seen within 48 hours, the majority on the day of admission. One week after the stroke, almost a half had recovered, a quarter had died, and the rest were still affected to some degree (Barer 1984). In Barer's second series (1987) of 357 stroke patients, an analysis of the mortality of dysphagic patients, allowing for level of consciousness, showed that even alert dysphagic patients had an increased chance of dying (33 per cent dead by 6 months) compared with other alert stroke patients (7 per cent dead by 6 months). A further case series with aspiration defined by videofluoroscopy found the prevalence to decrease from 42 to 8 per cent between 3 days and 3 months post-stroke (Kidd et al. 1995).

It is not clear whether dysphagia during the acute phase causes significant dehydration leading to complications among survivors. Barer (1987) reported that changes in haematocrit and blood urea from admission to 1 week after the stroke were independent of dysphagia (and patients were not treated with intravenous fluids or naso-gastric tubes). Gordon and colleagues (1987) found that chest infections in the first week were more common among dysphagic patients (an 11 per cent difference; 95 per cent CI, 3 to 25 per cent) but did not allow for impaired consciousness which might also make infection more common. They asserted that naso-gastric tubes or intravenous fluids would prevent dehydration and chest infections, although there is no evidence to support the claim. It is quite possible that both of these practices could prove harmful, or lead to a reduced mortality but increased disability. Kidd's study found that parenteral fluids without oral intake had no impact on the incidence of chest infection (Kidd et al. 1995). In Barer's study (1987) pneumonia as a cause of death was equally common amongst those with and without dysphagia, and dysphagic patients were twice as likely to suffer a primary brain death, which probably reflects a simple association with stroke severity. Furthermore, the Italian and Scandinavian trials of haemodilution (Scandinavian Stroke Study Group 1987; Italian Acute Stroke Study Group 1988) did not produce any benefits and did not reduce the incidence of chest infections.

Treatment

Starvation is unpleasant, depresses mood and the immune system, and leads to muscle catabolism which might later hinder rehabilitation. Tube feeding is often tried for patients with persistent dysphagia. Selley (1985) makes a strong case against the use of naso-gastric tubes for stroke patients: first, patients have to swallow, aspirate, or drool about a litre of saliva a day and a naso-gastric tube is an effective method of increasing salivation; secondly, a naso-gastric tube causes pharyngeal irritation which produces a peristaltic wave in the wrong direction, hence counteracting the feedback needed for involuntary swallowing; thirdly, the tube can cause vomiting and aspiration; and fourthly, patients do not like naso-gastric tubes. Percutaneous endo-scopic gastrostomy (PEG) is increasingly available and is widely used as an alternative.

Management of dysphagia in the first 2 weeks is likely to remain controversial, with the nihilists using a wait-and-see approach and interven-tionists giving fluids, or instituting tube feeding. There is insufficient information to make a sound judgement on the issue, but a large-scale randomized controlled trial (FOOD trial, planned by the Edinburgh stroke research team) examining several management options to cope with the wide range of clinical practices and beliefs may clarify clinical practice in future. Naso-gastric tubes have many theoretical problems, therefore intravenous or subcutaneous hydration may be preferable in the small group of alert patients who have a relatively good prognosis but suffer with persistent difficulty in swallowing. Unconscious patients will continue to present a dilemma, although it is likely that maintaining hydration in badly affected patients does not influence their outcome.

Patients with persistent swallowing difficulty may be considered for long-term naso-gastric feeding. A study which examined the indications and outcomes of such management (Ciocon et al. 1988) demonstrated a very high complication rate. The major problems were aspiration pneumonia and the need for restraint to keep a naso-gastric tube in place. Tube feeding did not prevent weight loss and was associated with a high mortality. PEG feeding, on the other hand, is very easy to manage, permits the delivery of almost all the intended feed, and improves nutritional indices. One small (30 patients), randomized trial has demonstrated considerable practical and mortality (odds ratio, 0.21) advantages for PEG over naso-gastric feeding, but it is unclear how well balanced the groups were at randomization (Norton et al.

1996). Even in the absence of a substantial change in mortality associated with this treatment, PEG feeding might reasonably be considered part of palliative or terminal care.

Deep-vein thrombosis and pulmonary embolus

Several series of stroke patients have been investigated for deep-vein thrombosis (Warlow *et al.* 1972; Denham *et al.* 1973; McCarthy *et al.* 1977). The common conclusion from these studies is that deep-vein thrombosis (DVT) is very common, with an incidence of DVT in the first 2 weeks after a stroke of up to 75 per cent. Clinical diagnosis alone is not very sensitive, about 60 per cent in Warlow's series of 30 patients (Warlow *et al.* 1972), and although false-positive diagnoses are not likely to be common, the chances of correctly diagnosing DVT are around 50 per cent (Whitehouse 1987). This predictive value can be improved by a further clinical examination performed by a radiologist (Charig and Fletcher 1987).

Detecting clinically silent DVT can be difficult but investigation by non-invasive tests such as liquid crystal thermography or Doppler ultrasound (Whitehouse 1987) which have much higher sensitivity than clinical examination, and hence a greater negative predictive value, will increase the overall accuracy of diagnosis from around 60 per cent to 98 per cent, which is a major advance. In settings without ready access to diagnostic imaging, such as rehabilitation hospitals or general practice, plasma D-dimer (a fibrin degradation product) has been evaluated as a diagnostic test. At its point of maximum accuracy, the test has specificity of 0.79, specificity 0.78, for a modest likelihood ratio of 3.5. A lower cut-off had 100 per cent sensitivity, and so could be used to exclude DVT, but the poor specificity would mean a lot of confirmatory investigations for those who screened positive, as the positive predictive value was only 30 per cent (Harvey *et al.* 1996). The consequences of recognizing this extra pathology are increased numbers of patients considered for anticoagulation, the risks of bleeding, and the need for neuroradiology to exclude haemorrhage as the cause of stroke prior to starting therapy.

Preventing DVT

Prevention is a much better option than diagnosing and treating established DVT. Prevention of DVT and pulmonary emboli by use of prophylactic low-dose heparin is effective after surgery, the risk of each being about halved (Collins *et al.* 1988). This led McCarthy and Turner (1986) to investigate whether prophylaxis was effective after a stroke. Since the risk of DVT is highest in the first week after a stroke, treatment must begin early to stand any chance of success. They randomized any patient (without contraindication to anticoagulation) seen within 48 hours of a stroke to subcutaneous calcium heparin given 8-hourly for 14 days, but did not do CT scans to exclude patients with haemorrhages or haemorrhagic infarcts. Heparin reduced the incidence of DVT from 73 per cent amongst controls to 22 per cent (95 per cent CI of difference, 41–61 per cent). Pulmonary emboli diagnosed at post-mortem were reduced from 70 per cent among controls to 29 per cent. The overall 12-week mortality was also reduced from 33 per cent to 22 per cent, with this benefit limited to patients with less severe strokes. There was no excess risk of haemorrhage in those given heparin. The study was too small to detect even a large difference in haemorrhagic complications but, if heparin really is so effective, the balance of benefits and harm would favour use of heparin. A subsequent meta-analysis of 10 small trials showed an 80 per cent relative reduction in the risk of DVT, and a halving of pulmonary embolism (Sandercock *et al.* 1993).

Administration of aspirin is also effective in reducing the risk of DVT (odds ratio, 0.61; 95 per cent CI, 0.51–0.71; numbers needed to treat, about 11) and pulmonary embolism (odds ratio, 0.36; 95 per cent CI, 0.16–0.56; NNT, 59) (Antiplatelet Trialists Collaboration 1994*a*). Most of the trials have been in surgical patients, but eight trials including 814 high-risk medical patients, including stroke, gave exactly the same results. Currently favoured heparinoids are very expensive, and it would appear that aspirin is a cost-effective alternative. Most stroke patients should now receive aspirin early in their clinical course.

In view of the frequency with which pulmonary embolism is associated with death after stroke (see Chapter 12), it was, therefore, surprising that neither the International Stroke Trial (IST) (of aspirin and/or heparin against placebo; risk ratio for death in heparin-treated group, 0.97) nor the Chinese Acute Stroke Trial (of aspirin against placebo; risk ratio for death, 0.85) demonstrated more substantial reductions in mortality after stroke (see Chapter 9). Pulmonary embolism did occur less frequently in heparin-treated patients (in IST 0.8 per cent versus 0.5 per cent; risk ratio, 0.63), but the reported occurrence of pulmonary embolism was extremely low compared with other studies, suggesting that this complication was severely underascertained. Low-dose heparin was associated with a statistically significant lower 14-day death or recurrence rate (compared with placebo 10.8 per cent versus 12.0 per cent; risk ratio, 0.90), with only a very small and insignificant increase in extracranial bleeds, whereas any benefit from higher-dose heparin was offset by more haemorrhagic strokes and extracranial bleeds (Chinese Acute Stroke Trial Study Group 1997; International Stroke Trial Collaborative Group 1997). In the longer term, there was no advantage of even low-dose heparin on deaths and dependency at 6 months. In the face of this evidence, there is a strong case for use of aspirin as a preventive measure for both recurrent stroke and pulmonary embolism, and to make greater use of compression stockings for prevention of deep-vein thrombosis.

Falls, fractures, and arthritis

Elderly people are at high risk of falling even if they have not had a stroke (Overstall 1995). Each year, a person over 65 has a 30 per cent chance of falling, with 1 in 10 of these leading to injury and 1 in 100 leading to hip fracture (Blake *et al.* 1988; Campbell 1996). Paretic limbs become osteopenic (Sato *et al.* 1997), and as stroke patients tend to fall to their paretic side, 80 per cent of post-stroke hip fractures are on this side. Fear of falling is almost as much of a problem as actual injury related to falls, leading to restricted mobility and social disengagement. By definition, agoraphobia represents an irrational or exaggerated fear, but the prospect of falling must provide a fertile substrate for stroke-related neurosis. General risk factors for falling include visual and neurological impairment, polypharmacy, muscle weakness, and postural hypotension, and risk increases with the number of risk factors (Tinetti *et al.* 1988). Efforts to reduce the number of falls should logically be aimed at as many of these factors as possible, and a relatively simple multi-faceted intervention has been shown to reduce the risk of falling by 30 per cent in fairly fit elderly people (Tinetti *et al.* 1994).

Few studies have examined systematically the incidence of falls after stroke, but one which did found that 73 per cent of these patients fell in the 6 months after discharge (Forster and Young 1995). The study was part of a Bradford trial of home physiotherapy compared with day hospital attendance (Young and Forster 1992). Patients were over 60, and were discharged home with some residual disability. Twenty-one per cent reported a fall in the year prior to their stroke, and half fell while in hospital. In all, the 108 patients reported 270 falls, and 47 per cent had two or more falls. Most falls occurred in the day, at home, while walking or transferring. Two-thirds needed help to get up. Four fractures resulted. Subjects who fell twice or more were more likely to have fallen in hospital, had worse balance and disability, were less socially active, more depressed, and their carers were more stressed.

What to do about this state of affairs is less clear. The epidemiological approach is to look for risk factors that are amenable to modification (Tutuarima *et al.* 1997). All the patients in the Bradford trial had had some in-patient rehabilitation, all were receiving one form or another of out-patient therapy, and presumably balance and safety in walking and transferring had been considered. Thirty per cent of patients had been taught techniques for getting up after falling, three-quarters of whom subsequently fell, but most still required assistance to rise. Mechanical hip protectors have been shown to prevent fractures amongst people at risk from falls who do not find them too uncomfortable to wear (Lauritzen *et al.* 1993), and this population would seem to be at high enough risk to warrant their consideration. Vitamin D supplementation has been shown to retard bone loss and decrease the risk of fracture post-stroke (Sato *et al.* 1997). Vigilance by health professionals for potentially reversible factors, and providing the means to summon help if needed (e.g. pendant alarms), would seem sensible.

A small study has documented that 23 of 111 acute stroke patients developed acute arthritis within a median of 8 days of stroke onset. In the majority of cases, arthritis was due to crystals and was on the hemiplegic side, and resolved well with intra-articular steroid treatment (Chakravarty *et al.* 1993). The long-term sequelae of acute arthritis were not considered and further work examining the reasons for such high levels of acute arthritis would be helpful.

Quality of life

One of the major aims of rehabilitation is to increase a patient's quality of life. Indicators of quality of life have not been much used as outcomes of the effectiveness of specific interventions, and yet may be more relevant than improvement in impairments, physical disability or mortality (Seale and Davies 1987). A major problem has been the development of suitable measurement techniques (Walker and Rosser 1988). This, in turn, reflects the difficulty of defining quality of life (Ebrahim 1995). There are many aspects, including disability and handicap, unpleasant symptoms, vigour and well-being, expectations, adjustment to illness, and the attitudes of the rest of society.

Theoretically, all these features can be quantified as the 'utility' of a state of health, which represents its value, worth, or desirability (Solomon *et al.* 1994; Gage *et al.* 1996). There are methods for measuring utility directly, including the standard gamble, and time trade-off techniques, but these are difficult to do. A simpler method, magnitude estimation ('give this health state a score out of 100'), may not be as valid. Interactive computer programs may help (O'Boyle *et al.* 1992). Several health status instruments have attempted to measure utilities indirectly, by putting scale weights on responses to a set of classifying questions, and these include the Quality of Wellbeing scale (Kaplan *et al.* 1976), EuroQol (EuroQol Group 1990; Dorman *et al.* 1998), and London Handicap Scale (Harwood and Ebrahim 1995). Another approach is to consider 'quality of life' as an overtly multi-dimensional entity, and to describe it using a profile of scores (such as 'physical functioning', 'vitality', and 'pain'). Examples include the SF-36 (Ware *et al.* 1993), Sickness Impact Profile (Bergner *et al.* 1981), and Nottingham Health Profile (Hunt *et al.* 1986). These have given interesting results, demonstrating a wide range of problems, some of which were not expected (such as the high prevalence of pain post-stroke) (Ebrahim *et al.* 1986; De Haan *et al.* 1993; Sneeuw *et al.* 1997; Indredavik *et al.* 1998). They are difficult to interpret if used in treatment comparisons as it may be necessary to trade-off improvements in one domain against no improvement or deterioration in another. Their use in cost-effectiveness analyses is therefore limited. Given the problems with definition, it is not surprising that attempts to survey quality of life have been limited (Anderson 1992).

One important concept closely related to (but distinct from) quality of life is that of handicap. There has been much confusion about exactly what this is, and it is often talked of as the 'social consequences' of illness. A reasonable paraphrase of the original definition (World Health Organization 1980) is 'the disadvantage resulting from ill health, compared with what is normal for someone of the same age, sex, and background'. The dimensions of mobility, occupation, independence, social integration, orientation, and economic self-sufficiency were suggested in the original classification. We see it as the manifestation of disability in a social and physical context, in other words, what someone can do (or is permitted or enabled to do), given their resources, relationships, physical environment, wants, and psychological state.

At least six instruments purport to measure handicap (Whiteneck *et al.* 1992; Harwood *et al.* 1994*b*; Harwood and Ebrahim 1995; Segal and Schall 1995). Attempts to measure handicap do appear to give different information from that provided by diagnosis, impairment or disability alone, but the strongest predictors of handicap are impairment and disability. Social and environmental factors are important (if rather difficult to quantify), but their contribution appears to be relatively small compared with health status (De Haan *et al.* 1993, 1995*b*; Harwood *et al.* 1997, 1998). This suggests that efforts to improve stroke-related handicap will be influenced more by prevention, acute treatment, and rehabilitation, than by manipulating the social environment. However, testing these ideas requires a substantial investment in further work examining relationships between social position, severity of stroke and handicap, and intervention trials.

The World Health Organization is currently revising the International Classification of Impairments, Disabilities and Handicaps and favour more positive terms, hence the new classification will be called *Impairments, Activities and Participation* (World Health Organization 1997). The substitution of the term 'participation' for 'handicap' is a worthwhile attempt to avoid stigmatizing people, and more fully emphasizes the social and environmental determinants of peoples' difficulties in achieving full participation in life. The WHO defines participation as 'the nature and extent of a person's involvement in life situations in relation to impairments, activities, health conditions and contextual factors. Participation may be restricted in nature, duration and quality'. The strong emphasis on contextual factors, defined as '. . .

Table 14.2   Domains of partipation

- Personal maintenance
- Mobility
- Exchange of information
- Social relationships
- Eduation, work, leisure, and spirituality
- Economic life
- Civic and community life

objects, structures, human-made organisations, service provision . . . physical, social and attitudinal environment in which people live and conduct their lives', is important as this provides a useful framework for exploring the impact of these factors in a more systematic way. This will require the relevant domains to be determined by systematic interviewing of people with and without chronic diseases, rather than simply relying on the views of 'experts' as shown in Table 14.2. New research initiatives are required to operationalize and test these new ideas of participation among stroke patients. The Nottingham Leisure Scale (Drummond and Walker 1994, 1995), which was developed by occupational therapists who were interested in the wider range of aspirations of the patients they saw, may prove helpful in assessing participation, as suggested by the new World Health Organization classification of participation. An earlier social engagement scale (Morgan *et al.* 1985), developed for use with elderly people in the community, may also be capable of development.

   The London Handicap Scale used with stroke patients demonstrates a very wide range of overall handicap scores, but the median for patients 1 year after a stroke (53/100) was much less than that in a survey of elderly people living at home (83/100) (Harwood *et al.* 1994*a*; Harwood and Ebrahim 1995). Handicap is associated with stroke severity, disability, and mood (Harwood *et al.* 1997). All the dimensions are affected, in particular occupation, physical independence, and mobility.

   A very widely used scale is the modified Rankin, or Oxford Handicap scale (Rankin 1957; Bamford *et al.* 1989; De Haan *et al.* 1995*a*). It is simple, with six levels in ascending order of dependency, reliable (Bamford *et al.* 1989; Van Swieten *et al.* 1988) and practical for use in large studies. It has been used in the Oxfordshire Community Stroke Project (Bamford *et al.* 1988), the UK-TIA trial (Farrell *et al.* 1991), the European Atrial Fibrillation Trial (European Atrial Fibrillation Trial Study Group 1993), the International Stroke Trial (International Stroke Trial Collaborative Group 1997), and other studies (Rodgers *et al.* 1997; Wilkinson *et al.* 1997). It is often grouped, to distinguish independent from dependent patients, allowing analysis of a dichotomized outcome: independent/dead-or-dependent. It has been suggested that the modified Rankin scale is more a measure of disability than handicap (De Haan *et al.* 1995a), but essentially, the scale is concerned with dependency rather than the concept of disadvantage associated with impairment and disability.

Other studies have concentrated more closely on specific aspects of 'quality of life'. Descriptive studies have assessed the impact of stroke on quality of life using a social activities index (the Frenchay Activities Index, FAI) for stroke patients (Wade *et al.* 1985c). This consists of 15 activities, half of which are 'higher-order' activities of daily living (housework, walking, shopping), but also includes going out, gardening, reading, and work. The activities were chosen by a social worker rather than by enquiry from stroke patients or other people of activities done normally. Although the authors consider that the FAI is a 'valid, sensitive, reliable, communicable and relevant' measure, this conclusion stands on shaky ground. Comparisons were not made with other quality of life indicators, or with an age–sex matched control group. Reliability was only assessed in 14 patients, and an overall correlation coefficient of 0.8 was used as an index of agreement, which tends to hide the real extent of disagreement (Bland and Altman 1986). No data were presented on changes over time in individual patients, so the sensitivity to change of the FAI is not known. The FAI did highlight a possible reduction in driving and using public transport and an increase in social outings after the stroke. Despite some of these drawbacks, it has proved popular in a number of studies (Greveson *et al.* 1991; Young and Forster 1992; Forster and Young 1996; Wilkinson *et al.* 1997; Holmqvist *et al.* 1998; Indredavik *et al.* 1998). In intervention studies it has proved difficult to demonstrate differences on the FAI, suggesting that it is not very sensitive to change (or that the interventions do not have much impact on social functioning).

Less structured methods have also been used to investigate quality of life, including interviews and specially designed questionnaires. Themes that have emerged include those of abandonment after hospital discharge, lack of participation in leisure or other occupational activities, social isolation, diminished or absent sexual activity, and prejudice resulting from movement abnormalities or other complications such as incontinence (Greveson *et al.* 1991; Greveson and James 1991; King 1996; Niemi *et al.* 1988).

Studies of the effectiveness of health and social services in improving quality of life probably tell us more about the measurement instruments (i.e. they are imperfect, insufficiently sensitive to change, and need more development) than they do about the interventions tested. The descriptive studies reported do highlight how common problems are, show how such outcome measurements can be made, and also show that much more attention must be given to the targeting of services to those in most need. Problems such as pain and disturbed sleep need much more detailed systematic study to determine their causes and effective treatment.

Routine use of quality of life and disability measurements will undoubtedly increase awareness of the extent of a patient's difficulties. Until there are guidelines from trials of specific rehabilitation techniques, individual goals should be set and progress monitored (using quality of life indicators as well as activities of daily living), and treatment (which may require several different skills) continued until goals are achieved or a plateau is reached.

Many patients' problems will not be solved by health and social services alone. An early pioneering study in Glasgow of the social consequences of stroke found that after discharge from hospital no patients went to the hairdresser, a library, or to places of entertainment (Isaacs *et al.* 1976). Innovative services must be developed aimed at improving various aspects of quality of life, since these studies show that present rehabilitation falls far short of the desired goal of reducing handicap. Many barriers to improving quality of life will only be tackled when widespread social attitudes towards ageing and disability improve.

Carers of stroke patients

The life of many stroke patients is dependent on the person they live with, in most cases a spouse (Wade *et al.* 1986*a*; Ebrahim and Nouri 1987). The questions of how much support and for how long carers can be expected to give support, and how best carers can themselves be helped need to be answered. A small, very selected group of 13 spouses and patients living at home and interviewed at 6 months was reported by Field and colleagues (1983). The patients were not very disabled and this selection bias probably led to the conclusion that carers were 'coping with the practical problems ... but all reported problems with emotional aspects of caring'. Study of a larger, consecutive series of patients living with someone would be a much more appropriate method to describe the extent of the burden of caring and the effects on the carer.

Even large studies of consecutive patients may run into problems if they ignore other sources of bias and do not make appropriate comparisons. A study reported from Bristol (Wade *et al.* 1986*a*) found that 11–13 per cent of carers were depressed (using the General Health Questionnaire) between 6 months and 2 years after the stroke. However, a higher threshold than that recommended (Goldberg and Hillier 1979) was used, which tended to underestimate the frequency of mood disorder. No comparison was made with an age- and sex-matched control group, which was unfortunate because when used in general population surveys the General Health Questionnaire gives a high prevalence of mood disorder, around 27 per cent for people aged 18–64 (Freeling *et al.* 1985). Even clinical assessments by doctors yield high percentages (around 14 per cent) with psychiatric problems (Wilkinson *et al.*

1985). It might be concluded that carers of stroke patients had less mood disorder than expected!

The Bristol study may well have estimated the extent of carers' mood problems unreliably because of response bias. Although no response rates are reported, of 302 carers that could have been interviewed at 1 year after the stroke, 74 per cent were seen at 6 months, 78 per cent at 1 year, and 44 per cent at 2 years. Response bias may lead to those with fewest problems not being available for interview (perhaps because they were out working at the time), thus inflating the proportion with difficulties. A further source of bias in this study is due to selective survival of patients with less severe disability. This probably led to the lack of association between the patient's disability and the carer's mood at 2 years. Bereaved carers were not contacted, which was a missed opportunity. The emotional needs of bereaved people may be met through counselling, but whether any impact can be made on their increased mortality (McAvoy 1986) is not known.

A smaller study done in Nottingham (Ebrahim and Nouri 1987) suffered less from selection and response bias. However, the patients studied had all been admitted to hospital initially and carers were only seen once, 6 months later. A response rate of 98 per cent was achieved. Over two-thirds of carers had to give more care than before the stroke. Perhaps not surprisingly wives did more caring for more dependent spouses than husbands. Only a third of patients had been left unattended for all or part of the day prior to interview, and almost one in five required help every night. Two-thirds of carers felt that this burden had had an adverse effect on their lives. Inventories of problems, such as the Caregiver Strain Index, have been used to suggest that 30 per cent of carers are under 'severe strain'. Care is required in interpreting these studies (the parents of young children also score in the 'severe strain' category), but qualitative investigation of the factors underlying carer strain highlight unpredictability, changed 'personality', practical annoyances (such as difficulties with incontinence pad supplies), and the uncertain future, as well as the tiredness and physical effort associated with looking after a dependent relative (Greveson et al. 1991; Wilkinson et al. 1997).

The limited role of health and social services in supporting carers has been demonstrated among elderly people in Wales (Jones and Vetter 1985), and this appears to be the case for stroke patients. Relief care (admission to an institution for a break, together with opportunity for rehabilitation, medical, and social therapy) tends to be offered to carers of less, rather than more, disabled people, and in the Nottingham series of patients, none had had a relief admission. Despite many patients being in touch with a 'service', patients and carers with bad problems were not picked up and referred. Recovery in some series of stroke patients is related to the amount of social support available (Glass et al. 1993), although it may be both amount and quality of support that matters (Glass and Maddox 1992). Hospital departments discharging patients should adopt some sort of follow-up and the family doctor must take a much more active role in the assessment and referral of those patients kept at home.

Summary

1. Mood disorder, usually depression, including a number of subtypes, and anxiety, affects about a quarter of 6-month survivors. It frequently goes unrecognized. Treatment with antidepressants is hazardous and of unproven value. Alternatives to drug therapy should be sought.

2. Cognitive impairment affects about 12 per cent of 6-month survivors but underlying depressive illness may be responsible rather than dementia. Specific treatment for milder memory and learning problems must be evaluated.

3. Dysphasia affects between 10–16 per cent of early survivors. Individual speech therapy does not lead to greater improvements than can be expected from spontaneous recovery alone.

4. Urinary incontinence is common early on (24 per cent affected at 3 weeks), but gets less common (11 per cent at 6 months) because of the combined effects of increased mortality and spontaneous improvement. The effectiveness of habit retraining and anticholinergic drugs has not been tested in stroke patients.

5. Dysphagia affects 45 per cent of acute stroke patients initially, falling to about 1 in 10 affected by 2 weeks. The importance of maintaining nutrition is increasingly recognized, and percutaneous endoscopic gastrostomy used more freely in the acute phase. Its value, and that of naso-gastric tubes, parenteral hydration, and prophylactic antibiotics, in reducing mortality and complications is not known.

6. Deep-vein thrombosis affects up to three-quarters of hospital stroke patients, usually within the first 2 weeks of onset. Prevention with subcutaneous heparin is feasible but has no overall benefit in reducing long-term mortality or dependency. Use of aspirin and compression stockings are reasonable and safer alternatives.

7. Three-quarters of patients with residual disability after stroke, who are discharged home, fall within 6 months. It is unclear what can be done therapeutically to reduce this, but mechanical hip protectors may afford some protection from hip fracture.

8. Quality of life is poor in many patients despite good physical recovery. More innovative programmes of social and psychological rehabilitation are needed.

9. Informal carers provide most of the support for patients and many do not get appropriate support despite being in touch with various health

and social services. More systematic methods of routine follow-up are needed, together with improvements in the type and amount of support provided.

15 Recovery

Giving a prognosis for recovery is of obvious importance to patients and relatives. Prognostic information is also needed for deciding who should continue to have rehabilitation and should help in planning services and policy. Highlighting the problems of patients who make a poor recovery should make us look for new solutions and treatments. Indicators of recovery may also be used as a yardstick to audit the work done during rehabilitation.

Measuring recovery

The first question is what is meant by recovery? The conceptual framework previously discussed in earlier chapters—the *International Classification of Impairments, Disabilities and Handicaps* (World Health Organization 1980)—developed by Wood and Badley (1978), is the most useful way of thinking about recovery. To recap, impairment is the physical or psychological lesion (e.g. hemianopia, hemiplegia); disability is the functional consequence of an impairment (e.g. inability to walk or dress); handicap is the disadvantage that occurs as a result of impairments and disability (e.g. social isolation because of inability to get outdoors). The virtues of this model are that it accommodates the heterogeneous impact of chronic diseases, with an almost limitless combination of impairments, disabilities, and handicaps. However, many diverse impairments in stroke may lead to equally diverse types and degrees of handicap, but the number of possible disabilities is relatively small, especially if only ability for self-care is considered. Measurement of disability can therefore be applied to individuals with heterogeneous impairments and handicaps to produce relatively homogenous groups of people with a much more limited range of disabilities. Estimates of recovery have to be made from pooling the experience of groups of patients, so the most commonly used indicator of recovery after stroke, achieving independence in self-care, is helpful for this purpose.

Impairments

Interestingly, while the early research on recovery focused largely on disability, more recent publications have been dominated by recovery in specific impairments associated with stroke. In part, this is due to the greater availability and accuracy of the latest neuroimaging techniques, which permit serial examinations of anatomical and functional activity in the brain over the time. However, there can be little doubt that the seductive romance of technology is at work here, which tends to promote a view that 'proper science' is concerned with that which can be measured most accurately and precisely. Fortunately, there are sufficient researchers who are interested in those aspects of recovery that interest patients and society at large (i.e. disability, dependency, handicap), and importantly, the links between changes in anatomical and physiological factors and disability. It is this latter area that holds great promise for understanding which aspects of pathophysiology might be most amenable to intervention and would result in improvements in ability to return to as normal a life as possible.

Pathology

The underlying pathological factors are important in determining whether recovery will occur. The beneficial aspects of pathophysiological changes following the acute event might be augmented to improve recovery prospects.

Cerebral haemorrhage

Cerebral haemorrhage is caused by bleeding from small micro-aneurysms (Charcot–Bouchard aneurysms) associated with changes in arterial walls (lipohyalinosis) due to long-term hypertension (Russell 1975). In older patients, amyloid angiopathy is the most common cause of haemorrhagic stroke (Shuaib and Hachinski 1991) and results from weakness in arterial walls infiltrated with amyloid. Binswanger's disease may cause strokes and is diagnosed from CT scan appearances of diffuse white matter changes around the lateral ventricles (Caplan 1995). In Binswanger's disease the underlying pathology may be related to amyloid angiopathy and small white matter lacunes are found in association with lipohyalinosis (Allen *et al.* 1988). Subarachnoid haemorrhage is uncommon in older patients and is associated with berry aneurysms occurring largely in the anterior cerebral circulation.

Bleeding into the brain parenchyma results in haematoma formation with raised intracranial volume, reduction in cerebral compliance, and the potential for raised intracranial pressure and reduced cerebral perfusion (Diringer 1993). Sometimes decompression occurs by extension of the haematoma into the ventricular system. Many large haemorrhages are rapidly fatal due to these direct effects but in the case of smaller haemorrhages, resolution does occur through invasion of the haematoma with phagocytic glial cells, new blood vessel formation, and breakdown of haemoglobin by macrophages over several weeks. The prospects for finding interventions that will enhance recovery do not seem good.

Thrombo-embolism

Occlusion of arteries often occurs at sites of atheroma where the endothelium has been damaged (Davies and Woolf 1993), leading to the activation of platelets which become sticky, leak ADP and thromboxane A2, which both cause more platelets to clump together. Activated platelets also switch on the coagulation cascade, with the conversion of prothrombin to thrombin, which results in the formation of a platelet thrombus. Endothelial cells also have a counterbalancing role, converting arachidonic acid to prostacyclin via the cyclo-oxygenase pathway, which leads to platelet disaggregation and vasodilatation (Allen et al. 1988).

Following occlusion of the cerebral circulation, a series of complex inter-related mechanisms come into play, initially in attempts to maintain delivery of oxygen and glucose to neurones, and subsequently to reduce the metabolic demands of neurones by reversible reduction in electrophysiological activity, and, finally, an irreversible phase associated with failure of calcium home-ostasis and cell death occurs (Pulsinelli 1992). The speed with which cell death occurs depends on the severity of occlusion and typically evolves over a period of a few hours. The area of brain immediately around the occluded artery is the first to undergo cell death, and areas more distant from the centre form an ischaemic 'penumbra' (Heiss and Graf 1994) in which reversible infarction has occurred, opening the possibility of salvage of neurones by maintenance of cerebral blood flow or drugs preventing extension of infarction to the penumbra (Siesjo 1992), thus enhancing recovery. Cellular processes of lactic acidosis, free-radical damage, excitatory neurotransmitter release, and calcium influx into neurones are of particular importance in the 'ischaemic cascade' (Collins et al. 1989). These steps in the ischaemic cascade have generated substantial research interest as they offer the possibility of new neuroprotective therapeutic approaches (see Chapter 9) to reducing acute cellular damage (Pulsinelli 1992).

Of considerable research interest are recent findings that, in experimental animal models of stroke, acute ischaemia results in induction of a wide range of genes responsible for survival (e.g. heat-shock proteins) and growth of neurones (e.g. trophic growth factors) (Kawamata et al. 1997). However, the major result of ischaemia appears to be a general reduction in gene expression which is associated with neuronal death, suggesting that biological responses to ischaemia comprise both beneficial and harmful effects (Koistinaho and Hokfelt 1997). The search for gene therapies for enhancing recovery will have to contend with the underlying complexity of a homeostatic system under threat.

These fundamental mechanisms must explain some of the inherent plasticity of the brain, although it is interesting that external factors, such as 'environmental enrichment' (i.e. toys and things to do) improve functional recovery among experimental animals subjected to acute ischaemic damage to their brains (Johansson and Grabowski 1994).

Neuroradiology

Not surprisingly, the amount of brain damaged as indicated by CT scanning has an influence on recovery (Hertanu et al. 1984; Brott et al. 1989b; Beloosesky et al. 1995). Positron emission tomography (PET) following stroke is a growing research area with the potential for demonstrating how the brain functions and reorganizes its activity during the recovery process (Stephan and Frackowiak 1997). For example, among recovering dysphasic patients, repeat PET scanning has shown bilateral changes in glucose metabolism, with low levels of metabolism in anatomically normal brain in the contralateral hemisphere (Cappa et al. 1997). By contrast, better motor recovery is associated with increased metabolism in the affected hemisphere motor cortex, and also in the unaffected hemisphere. Those patients who recover least well do not show any increased metabolism in either hemisphere (Di Piero et al. 1992). Less expensive and technically demanding single photon emission computed tomography (SPECT) scanning, which measures regional cerebral blood flow as an index of function, shows some correlation with recovery in abilities of daily living (Rupright et al. 1997), but the notion that SPECT scanning 'could be useful to help determine patient placement for rehabilitation' is rather unrealistic, and alternatives (such as talking to patients and their carers, and assessing ability) hold very much greater promise! PET and SPECT scanning are technically difficult to perform and inevitably require careful selection of patients, so not surprisingly the numbers of patients studied are small and the general relevance of such findings remain in doubt. Coupling PET scanning to randomized controlled trials of specific interventions would be a promising way forward in understanding the extent to which changes seen on PET or SPECT can be modified by external factors. Such an approach would be of greater relevance for clinical practice than focusing on understanding of mechanisms, which may only come from animal studies in primates (Stephan and Frackowiak 1997).

Specific impairments

Some impairments show a similar pattern of recovery as disability. For example, upper arm paresis shows most recovery between 3 and 6 weeks, depending on initial severity, and by 3 months no further recovery can be expected (Nakayama et al. 1994). Similarly, visual hemianopia and motor impairment (assessed by the MRC scale) tend to recover fairly quickly, with a plateau approached by 28 days, which unfortunately was the limit of both of the reports on the same cohort of patients (Gray et al. 1989, 1990). In a study comparing both upper and lower limb recovery, patterns were similar, with rapid recovery in the first month and a clear plateau reached by 90 days, which rather contradicts the clinical belief that upper limb recovery is less good than lower limb recovery (Duncan *et al.* 1994).

The pattern of recovery of cognitive impairment may be different; long-term changes between 3 months and a year appear to occur (Desmond *et al.* 1996) which is important, as cognitive impairments are usually thought to be permanent, and even progressive, and may interfere with ability in other activities of daily living. This work requires further replication and should be linked with parallel study of changes in functional performance.

In a series of 50 selected patients, changes in the National Institutes of Health stroke scale (indicators of impairment) were monitored at various times up to a mean follow-up of 44 days (Wityk *et al.* 1994), with half showing improvements by follow-up. However, in contrast to other investigators (Samuelsson *et al.* 1996), no relationship between initial severity and follow-up recovery was found, and patients with lacunar stroke did not show improvement. These findings are probably affected by selection bias and failure to conduct recovery assessments at uniform time periods and for a sufficient duration of time.

Disability

Disability has been assessed in different ways: motor ability, dependency on others, capacity for work, and an ability for self- and household care have all been used (Sainsbury 1973). Most methods of disability measurement deal only with self-care, so-called activities of daily living (ADL) scales. Most of the scales currently in use contain similar items (Table 15.1) and there have been attempts to unify them (Donaldson *et al.* 1973; Goble 1976; Jay 1976). This has been unsuccessful because scales are used for different purposes and tend to enjoy periods of popularity. Assessments primarily for individual patients may be very detailed and time consuming, whereas if the purpose of measurement is to examine the outcome of a group of patients, then a short assessment containing key variables will be of more use. For example, it has been shown that walking, making tea, bathing, dressing, and transfer from floor to chair are the activities that explain most of the observed variation in the Northwick Park ADL Score (Sheikh *et al.* 1979).

The International Stroke Trial (1997) developed a very simple pair of questions to define recovery: 'Have you made a complete recovery from your stroke?' and 'Did you require help from another person in day-to-day activities in the last fortnight?' both of which required a yes or no answer (van Gijn and Warlow 1992). For a large-scale international trial, simplicity is essential and even these questions would have presented serious problems in translation. It seems likely that the term 'complete recovery' would be prone to response biases determined by social and cultural differences, and the dependency question would also be biased by social circumstances and

Table 15.1 Comparison of items included in various activities of daily living scales

	Barthel	Northwick	Katz	Kenny	Rivermead
Feeding	+	+	+	+	–
drinking	–	–	–	–	+
eating	–	–	–	–	–
Grooming	+	–	–	–	–
clean teeth	–	+	–	–	+
comb hair	–	+	–	–	+
make-up/shave	–	+	–	–	+
wash face/hands	–	+	–	–	+
Dressing	+	+	+	+	–
undress	–	–	–	–	+
dress	–	–	–	–	+
Transfers lay/sit	+	–	–	–	–
bed/chair	+	+	+	+	+
floor/chair	–	+	–	–	+
Mobility					
indoor	+	+	+	+	+
outdoor	–	+	–	–	+
stairs	+	+	–	–	–
Use of toilet	+	+	+	+	+
Bathing					
wash in bath	+	+	+	+	+
in/out bath	–	–	–	–	+
overall wash	–	–	–	–	+
using taps	–	+	–	–	–
Tea making	–	–	–	–	+
prepare for	–	+	–	–	–
making tea	–	+	–	–	–
Continence	–	+	+	–	–
bladder control	+	–	–	–	–
bowel control	+	–	–	–	–

+ = Included.

attitudes. In large trials, like the International Stroke Trial, these biases are not important as randomization will ensure that similar proportions of people from participating countries and from different social strata are in both intervention and control groups.

Of some interest in both trials and descriptive studies is the relationship between recovery, dependency, and disability. For example, stroke patients who score over 16 out of 20 on the Barthel ADL Index are generally considered to be able to live outside hospital and therefore can be classified as independent, but clearly, they still have measurable disability. Some of them, by virtue of getting home, might consider themselves to have made a complete recovery, whereas others with full marks on the Barthel ADL Index might still consider themselves to have failed to recover fully. These relationships deserve much more detailed enquiry, involving not just further quantitative research, but also in-depth interviews with patients to discover what factors determine apparently inconsistent responses between different aspects of recovery, dependency, and disability.

Despite differences in items and scoring, comparisons between different ADL scales have shown high levels of agreement (Kelman and Willner 1962; Bebbington 1977) and appeared to classify very similar proportions of stroke patients as independent (Gresham et al. 1980).

A case has been made for stroke researchers to use the same indicator of disability so that comparisons may be made more easily. The favoured indicator of some investigators is the Barthel Index (Wade and Hewer 1987; Wade and Collin 1988). The Barthel Index shares the same problems of most ADL scales, which is that the maximum and minimum scores do not represent a patient's best and worst functional condition. Sensitivity to change, particularly at the less disabled end of the scale, is poor, which may lead to problems in detecting any benefits from rehabilitation among relatively fit patients. A further problem is that it is impossible to work out what a patient with a particular Barthel score can and cannot do, unless they score the minimum or maximum.

A ranked or hierarchical scale has the advantage that a scale score indicates which abilities a patient can and cannot do. It also has the advantage that not every item in an ADL assessment has to be tested. If patients cannot do items in the middle of a ranked scale, it is highly unlikely that they will be able to do more difficult activities. Other benefits of ranking are that more information about types of disability is provided, people with the same scores can do the same activities, and it is quicker to administer than a conventional additive scale as not all the items need to be tested. A ranked ADL scale has been developed for stroke patients (Ebrahim et al. 1985) and the Barthel Scale using a different method of scoring from the original has hierarchical properties (Wade and Hewer 1987), but such approaches have failed to gain popular support.

The Rankin grades of disability (Rankin 1957) have been widely used to report functional recovery, particularly among hospital series of patients (Adams and Hurwitz 1963; Marquardsen 1969). The grades range from I to V: I is 'no significant disability', able to carry out all usual duties; II is 'slight disability', unable to carry out some of previous activities but able to look after own affairs without assistance; III is 'moderate disability', requiring some help but able to walk without assistance; IV is 'moderately severe disability', unable to walk without assistance and unable to attend to own bodily needs without assistance; V is 'severe disability', bedridden, incontinent, and requiring constant nursing care and attention. The major problems with Rankin grades are that the groupings, although rather crude, require some subjective judgement when allocating the patient to a grade, and because the grades are broad, it is not a very sensitive indicator of recovery. Furthermore, the Rankin Scale confuses the separate concepts of dependency and disability—the former is affected by the social circumstances in which a patient lives, whereas the latter is an indicator of what the patient can do. Despite these limitations, the Rankin Scale remains popular.

Since rehabilitation is concerned with reducing the degree of handicap patients experience because of disease, it has been argued that stroke rehabilitation involves several different outcomes: physical, functional, social, and emotional dimensions (Seale and Davies 1987). This will give a more complete picture of the effects of rehabilitation but may lead to the question of which outcome is of most importance; for example, quality of life indicators are not coupled with improved physical ability (Ebrahim *et al.* 1986). For the purpose of reporting outcome after a stroke, many studies have simply compared the proportions independent with those dependent for various self-care activities (for example, Garraway *et al.* 1980*a,b*). This makes comparisons and meta-analyses difficult because different self-care activities may be used. It may lead to an inadequate appraisal of the true effects of rehabilitation since the severity of a stroke is the major determinant of subsequent physical ability rather than efforts at rehabilitation. Clinical trials of rehabilitation and natural history studies now tend to measure several dimensions of outcome, which overcomes these problems.

Recovery is essentially time dependent, but in several widely quoted sources the time at which observations were made is not stated (Rankin 1957; Adams and Hurwitz 1963; Marquardsen 1969). Often we are concerned with not whether a patient recovered or not, but how quickly they recovered. Consequently, it is essential that observations be made at specified time points after onset if the observations are to be of any use. When calculating percentage of recovery, the question of whether to include or exclude from the denominator patients who die also arises. An apparent increase in independence may be achieved by the more disabled patients dying, rather than disabled people getting better. It is essential, therefore, when examining the rate of recovery to take account of those who die over the time period. In simple descriptive studies, it is reasonable to consider only patients who survived for the whole time interval, thus ensuring that the denominator stays the same, or alternatively, the proportion dying during each time interval should be stated. In clinical trials of treatment, such simple methods are inadequate. In general, we wish to know not only whether outcomes occurred but when they occurred, and leaving those who die out of analyses runs the risk of biasing comparison groups carefully established by randomization. The classical method of dealing with this is to use some form of survival analysis requiring both the number of outcomes occurring and also the time at which they occurred (Pocock 1983). With this information it is possible to construct survival curves, and in the case of clinical trials, it is generally best to settle for one outcome (e.g. death), but in the case of stroke we are also concerned about dependency and disability, so a combined end point of death or dependency, as used in the International Stroke Trial, makes good sense.

Survival curves are seldom used to report the results of stroke trials, largely because the information on dependency and disability is collected at only a few points in time (e.g. at discharge from hospital and at 6 months), but have been used in descriptive studies (Reding and Potes 1988). Use of simple questions would permit such questions to be asked more frequently and might be augmented by questions about when achievement of recovery or independence had been achieved. Further work would be required to obtain reliable and valid indicators of the timing of these outcomes.

Pattern of recovery

The proportion of patients achieving independence in self-care by 1 year after a stroke ranges from 60 per cent (Aho *et al.* 1980) to 69 per cent (Andrews *et al.* 1981) in community series; from 38 per cent (Stevens and Ambler 1982) to 68 per cent (Kotila *et al.* 1984) in hospital series; and from 60 per cent (Bernspang 1987) to 83 per cent (Skilbeck *et al.* 1983) in rehabilitation patients. Data from these and other studies are shown in Table 15.2.

Why should estimates be so variable? The precision of the estimates shown in Table 15.2 demonstrates that chance alone is not the sole explanation. The community series are less variable probably because of less selection bias in the severity of cases considered. The proportion classified as able will also depend on the activities considered. For example, in Wade and Hewer's study (1987), 85 per cent were able to walk but only 47 per cent were able to do all activities of daily living. Stevens and Ambler (1982) used only four activities (washing, toileting, dressing, and eating) and yet found one of the lowest levels of functional recovery of any published series. Most studies give very little detail about how ability was measured, yet the method used to rate ability will affect the levels found. For example, nurses tend to rate patients as more disabled than formal assessments done by an occupational therapist (Ebrahim *et al.* 1985).

There is much greater agreement in the place of residence after a stroke, which reflects dependency but also availability of institutional care (Table 15.3). Presumably this is because differences in criteria and method do not have an effect. Surprisingly good agreement between community and hospital series is found, with about one in five survivors resident in an institution at 1 year.

The majority of these studies only examined ability levels at a few time points. A more recent large cohort of hospital-admitted acute stroke patients from the Copenhagen Stroke Study provides much more detailed weekly

Table 15.2 The percentage of survivors of stroke achieving abilities in self-care and other activities at various times after stroke

Study	Time since stroke	Percentage able (95% CI)
Community patients		
Aho *et al.* (1980)	3 months	51 (50–52)
	1 year	60 (59–61)
Andrews *et al.* (1981)	6 months	70 (61–79)
	1 year	69 (59–79)
Gresham *et al.* (1979)	6 months to 4 years	68 (60–76)
Wade and Hewer (1987)	6 months	47 (43–51)
in a transfer		81 (78–84)
Weddell and Beresford (1979)	3 months	
in a transfer		71 (63–79)
Hospital patients		
Allen (1984a)	2 months	56 (48–64)
	6 months	66 (58–74)
Garraway *et al.* (1980a)	1 year	57 (47–67)
Henley *et al.* (1985)	1 year	55 (45–65)
Kotila *et al.* (1984)	3 months	62 (54–70)
	1 year	68 (61–75)
Stevens and Ambler (1982)	1 year	38 (29–47)
in walking		67 (58–76)
Rehabilitation patients		
Bernspang (1987)	4-6 years	60 (48–71)
Kinsella and Ford (1985)	4 weeks	32 (16–48)
	8 weeks	58 (41–75)
	12 weeks	71 (55–87)
	1+ years	75 (60–90)
Skilbeck *et al.* (1983)	3 months	71 (62–80)
	6 months	81 (73–89)
	1 year	83 (75–91)

information on recovery patterns, stratified by initial stroke severity (Jorgensen *et al.* 1995*b*,*c*). Recovery in neurological impairments was most rapid and preceded recovery in abilities by about 2 weeks. Recovery in both impairments or disabilities was most rapid in the least badly affected patients. Although this study is described as a community study, at least 12 per cent of stroke patients were not admitted to hospital, but any bias caused by the omission of these patients is likely to affect the recovery patterns for either the very mildest strokes or the most severe, in whom survival will be low. The study confirms earlier work, finding that one in five patients were discharged to a nursing home and that, for the majority, recovery has occurred by 13 weeks, and, importantly, more severely affected patients may continue to recover between 13 and 18 weeks.

Table 15.3 Place of residence after stroke in a range of community and hospital series of stroke patients

Study	Time since stroke	Percentage (95% CI) institutionalised
Community patients		
Aho *et al.* (1980)	3 weeks	65 (63–67)
	3 months	25 (24–26)
	1 year	16 (15–17)
Gresham *et al.* (1975, 1979)	6 months to 4 years	15,16 (10–21)
Weddell and Beresford (1979)	3 months	30 (22–38)
Hospital patients		
Barer (1987)	1 month	60 (56–64)
	6 months	18 (13–23)
Kotila *et al.* (1984)	3 months	31 (24–38)
	1 year	22 (16–28)
Stevens and Ambler (1982)	1 year	22 (14–30)
Rehabilitation patients		
Bernspang (1987)	4–6 years	14 (6–22)
Isaacs and Marks (1973)	1 year	31 (23–39)

The rate of recovery has also been measured in small series of patients seen regularly (Andrews *et al.* 1981; Skilbeck *et al.* 1983; Partridge *et al.* 1987). These studies confirm that the bulk of spontaneous recovery occurs in the first 3 months after the stroke, with some continued improvement up to 6 months and little change after this. This appears to be so for both overall ability in self-care and also for language recovery and motor recovery (Skilbeck *et al.* 1983).

The recovery of very severely affected stroke patients is of great importance because these groups often receive a lot of rehabilitation effort without much apparent benefit (Brocklehurst *et al.* 1978), and even the larger stroke studies (e.g. Copenhagen) can only provide imprecise estimates of recovery. Even in such patients, over half may make some improvement over the first year. While most of this improvement occurs in the first 6 months, with only 6 per cent of survivors improving to the point of walking with aids by 1 year (Andrews *et al.* 1981), these figures hide the fact that if a patient is unable to walk at 6 months the chances of walking by 1 year are 40 per cent. Moreover, more modest improvements such as requiring one helper instead of two have not been studied, and yet have a great impact on possibilities for resettlement. Rationing rehabilitation resources after 6 months has been suggested (Andrews *et al.* 1981) and is widely practised but is not supported by strong evidence. Further research in this area would be fruitful in clarifying the ability to benefit late in the course of stroke.

Recovery of rolling, sitting balance, transfers, and walking among patients referred for rehabilitation appear to follow a very predictable pattern over the first 8 weeks (Partridge *et al.* 1987; Jorgensen *et al.* 1995a). Therefore it may be possible to produce an expected profile against which an individual patient's progress may be compared. This would be of use in identifying patients whose recovery was slower than expected, would allow goals to be set, and should lead to identification of factors limiting progress. Such an approach would be most useful in examining the question of continued rehabilitation for severely affected stroke patients.

The indicators of recovery currently used limit the detection of small-scale but important improvements and also reach a ceiling which does not correspond to maximum ability. These problems could be overcome by using more sensitive grades of dependency and adding more complex activities to the top of the scale. A bigger problem is the need to consider recovery of other dimensions of life, besides physical function. For example, at 6 months post-stroke Nottingham Health Profile scores are about 2–4 times higher than expected, due to social isolation, lack of energy, and emotional upset, and yet most patients are at home by this time, and most are able to do a majority of activities of daily living (Ebrahim et al. 1986). These problems persist for a long time; survivors of stroke in the Framingham study showed decreased interest in hobbies and difficulty using transport up to 4 years after the stroke (Gresham et al. 1979). A study of patients discharged from a stroke rehabilitation unit found that almost two-thirds of patients had decreased life satisfaction (usually concerned with global, sexual, and leisure satisfaction) 4–6 years later (Bernspang 1987). Since rehabilitation aims to improve specific impairments, functional abilities, and handicap, it will be necessary in future to examine the natural history of recovery of not just physical disability but other aspects of quality of life.

The importance of return to leisure activities as goals of rehabilitation is not widely recognized, particularly in patients who appear to have made a good physical recovery. The Nottingham Leisure Scale (Drummond and Walker 1994) provides a systematic means of assessing leisure activities and should prompt more rehabilitation efforts in this area. Since leisure activities are associated closely with quality of life, it is likely that interventions targeted on gardening, going out, handicrafts, and games will result in improved quality of life (Parker et al. 1997). Such work remains to be done and presents a potentially very rewarding area for patients (and researchers).

When considering patterns of recovery, it is tempting to examine activities of daily living data as changes in scores per unit of time (e.g. Barthel points gained per week; Shah et al. 1990, 1991), but this requires the assumption of interval scaling (i.e. the distance between Barthel points on the scale is equal) which is certainly not the case. The better way of analysing ADL data is to consider a specific item of ability, such as walking, and to make estimates of the time taken to walk a set distance, or alternatively, to estimate the time taken to achieve maximum ability, as done in the Copenhagen Stroke Study (Jorgensen et al. 1995a).

Table 15.4 Predictors of recovery

Site and extent of lesion	Other factors	Complications
Severe motor deficit	Age	Urinary incontinence
Sensory inattention	Sex	Pneumonia
Balance/posture	Marital status	Hypotension
ADL in first month	Previous stroke	Mood
Proprioception	Pre-stroke immobility	Poor motivation
Impaired consciousness		
Duration of unconsciousness		
Flaccidity		
Hemisensory loss		
Bilateral signs		
Visuo-spatial impairment		
Memory impairment		
Aphasia		
Right hemisphere lesion		
Gaze paresis		
Nystagmus		

Predictors of recovery

Ideally predictors for types of stroke, different severities, and for a range of indicators of recovery (recovery of impairments, disabilities, and handicap) are needed. In practice there are reports on the predictors of recovery of aphasia only (Lendrum and Lincoln 1985; Pedersen *et al.* 1995) and arm function (Wade *et al.* 1983a). The natural history of hemi-inattention (Kinsella and Ford 1985), of visual neglect (Kotila *et al.* 1986a; Sunderland *et al.* 1987), and of motor function (Skilbeck *et al.* 1983) have been described. Prediction of recovery of impairments has focused on motor recovery, which is the obvious priority. By 6 months, over three-quarters of a community cohort of 384 New Zealand stroke patients had no, or only mild, motor deficits (Bonita and Beaglehole 1988). Both this study and others have confirmed the importance of initial severity of motor deficit in determining recovery (Duncan *et al.* 1992). A more recent report examined the relationship between a psychological factor—sustained attention—and motor (and functional) recovery and found a clear relationship supporting the idea that recovery depends on re-learning of abilities (Robertson *et al.* 1997).

Most work has been done on predicting death (see Chapter 12) and physical ability, using activities of daily living scales. Very little work has been done on predicting the quality of life of stroke patients (Ebrahim *et al.* 1986; Bernspang 1987). Numerous factors have been described which influence the functional ability of stroke patients (Table 15.4). These may be classified as those concerned with the site and extent of the lesion, with complications of the stroke, and with other factors such as mood and morale, pre-stroke morbidity, social factors, and age.

A review of the literature of prediction of disability in stroke concluded that of 78 studies considered, only 10 studies satisfied 8 out of 11 pre-set criteria relating to study quality (i.e. validity and reliability of measurements used; a properly defined inception cohort; adequate and uniform assessment of end points; control for drop-outs; statistical testing of relationships; sufficient sample size; control for correlation between variables; specification of patient characteristics; description of any treatments given; and cross-validation in a second independent sample of stroke patients) (Kwakkel *et al.* 1996). It is surprising that so few studies met most of these requirements as they represent quite modest scientific design characteristics. Of those studies considered not to have substantial methodological flaws, 'age, previous stroke, urinary incontinence, conscious level at onset, disorientation in time and place, severity of paralysis, sitting balance, admission ADL score, level of social support, and metabolic rate of glucose outside the infarct area in hypertensive patients' were considered to be valid predictors.

Prognostic scores

While methodological flaws can be identified and should be overcome, there are limitations in our thinking about prediction and the use of mathematical models. Most of the variables identified by Kwakkel and colleagues (1996) are highly correlated with each other and, under these circumstances, multiple regression models are inadequate to determine so-called 'independent' effects of specific variables. The lack of any underlying conceptual model is also apparent in some approaches to prediction. Fullerton and colleagues simply took a long and disparate list of factors that were significantly associated with outcomes and included those that were significant in univariate analysis in a canonical discriminant function analysis (a form of multivariate analysis) (Fullerton *et al.* 1988). The variables considered important were Albert's test (a 'perceptual neglect' test of crossing out lines on a sheet of paper), leg function, level of consciousness, arm power, mental score, and ECG changes. If the authors had asked themselves whether the variables measured were underpinned by a strong conceptual understanding of recovery, it would be apparent that, however good the statistical fit of the model, it is lacking in important components such as pre-stroke status, physical and social background of the patient, complications associated with the acute stroke, and treatment factors.

By contrast, the prediction of functional recovery in the Functional Independence Measure (FIM) was assessed in terms of living circumstances and social role pre-stroke, age, severity of stroke, and cognition. The resulting prediction equation derived from analysis of 3760 patient records at 96 institutions in the USA appears very robust, prompting the investigators to conclude that the index can be used to predict individual prognosis (Stineman *et al.* 1997). If this is true, it would be a remarkable achievement, but as it stands, the report demonstrates interesting predictive ability using variables measured in various ways that must be replicated in other datasets using prospective and uniform collection of data.

Guy's Hospital prognostic score

The Guy's Hospital prognostic score (Allen 1984*b*) comprises degree of paralysis, 'complicated stroke' (i.e. higher cerebral dysfunction and hemianopia and hemiplegia), loss of consciousness at onset, impaired consciousness for more than 24 hours, and age. It classified correctly 92 per cent of good outcomes and 84 per cent of bad outcomes at 2 months. However, it was developed with patients under 76 years old, did not examine the influence of predictors later in the course of recovery, and included death as a bad outcome. This last point probably explains the importance of impaired consciousness in the score, since 58 per cent of the 'bad' outcomes at 2 months were due to death. Social, emotional, and pre-stroke factors were not considered.

The Guy's prognostic score has now been tested on another series of patients, to replicate the items used, and in a wider age range of patients, over a longer time period (Gompertz *et al.* 1994*b*). The simplified Guy's Score, (termed the G-score), makes use of Bayesian approaches to prediction. If the prior probability of a bad outcome can be estimated, then the additional value of the G-score (given by the likelihood ratio for different score thresholds) can be assessed as the posterior probability. For example, the overall probability of a bad outcome (death or disability) at 6 months is about 60 per cent in most hospital series of patients, so if we know nothing else about a patient, the best estimate of a bad outcome, the prior probability, is 0.60. If the patient was aged over 75 (score 3), drowsy or unconscious at 24 hours (score 1), there was complete paralysis (score 1), and there were higher cortical deficits (score 1), the G-score would be 6, which has a likelihood ratio of 8.05. This is then multiplied by the prior odds (odds = probability/1 – probability = 1.5), that is 8.05×1.5 = post-test odds of 12.07 = posterior probability of 92 per cent for a bad outcome, a large improvement in predictive ability.

The Bristol prognostic score

The Bristol prognostic score (Wade *et al.* 1983*b*) was derived from 83 patients referred for rehabilitation. It comprises age, presence of hemianopia or visual inattention, urinary incontinence, severity of motor deficit in the arm, and sitting balance. Eighty-nine per cent of these measurements were made within the first month, but only 20 per cent within the first week after onset. The score aimed to predict 6-month Barthel scores, but only predicted 38 per cent of the variance and was accurate to ±5 Barthel points in 55 per cent of patients. Although the authors claimed that this was better than any other method, Britton *et al.* (1980) showed that the admitting doctor made a correct functional prognosis in 59 per cent of cases without the aid of any scoring system!

The Bristol system should have been tested in another group of patients, with measurements made at a set time after stroke, before being promoted as a prognostic index. When this was done using data from a community series of patients (Wade and Hewer 1987), different factors were important: urinary incontinence, initial Barthel score, age, and sitting balance measured within 1 week predicted 26 per cent of the variance in 6-month Barthel scores, but incorrectly classified at least a third of patients. At 3 weeks after the stroke IQ, measured using Raven's matrices, and Barthel score, together with urinary incontinence, age, sitting balance, and arm motor function, accounted for 29 per cent of the variance in 6-month Barthel scores, but still incorrectly predicted scores in over a third of the patients. The analyses were restricted to patients with some disability at the time of being seen, so it is uncertain whether the index is capable of predicting deterioration in these patients. Social and emotional factors, and pre-stroke disability should also be considered, and since so little of the variance in Barthel scores was explained, it is quite possible that other, more important, predictors of functional outcome exist.

Heterogeneity of stroke patients makes it very unlikely that any one prediction system will be applicable to mild and severe strokes, lacunar and total anterior circulation strokes, or for elderly and young stroke patients (Barer and Mitchell 1989).

Some recent work has suggested that perceptual factors, long considered to be predictive of a poor outcome (Adams and Hurwitz 1963), are not predictive of disability outcomes (Kalra *et al.* 1997; Pedersen *et al.* 1997), but this may represent differences in the methods of assessing perceptual deficits and the statistical methods used to control for confounding by stroke severity, and the covariates measured (Barer 1990). Indeed, it has been shown that dressing ability, for example, correlates with physical motor ability for dressing the lower half of the body but with cognitive ability in dressing the upper half (Walker and Lincoln 1991). Wider social and economic factors are also likely to be important; a study in northern England showed that locality of residence also had an impact on dependency (Tennant *et al.* 1997). These complexities make it unlikely that general mathematical prediction rules will be found that are clinically more helpful than simple methods.

Other predictors of recovery

Urinary incontinence, age, extensive motor deficit, and combined neurological deficits are important predictors of functional ability at discharge from hospital (Sheikh *et al.* 1983). This study also found that disability from a previous stroke and female sex had an adverse effect, but was only able to account for 18 per cent of the variation in ability at discharge. Arm motor function, proprioception (thumb finding), and 'postural function' (i.e. sitting and standing balance, and walking) were the most important factors among a group of patients admitted to a stroke unit (Prescott *et al.* 1982). In this case the outcome used was 'reaching independence', which could be achieved at any point in time up to 16 weeks. The patients had been triaged initially, so do not reflect the range of severity seen in patients admitted to hospital. Furthermore, the length of follow-up was really too short and variable to be certain that these variables would have a lasting adverse influence.

Among a series of patients admitted to hospital and followed up for 6 months, urinary incontinence, sensory inattention, pre-stroke mobility, severity of motor deficit, and age predicted 58 per cent of the variation in 6-month activities of daily living scores. Addition of 1-month ADL scores improved the prediction to 66 per cent and classified 69 per cent of patients to within one scale point of the activities of daily living score. Half of the variation in 6-month activities of daily living scores was explained by just three factors: persisting urinary incontinence, sensory inattention, and pre-stroke immobility (Ebrahim 1985). These factors are easy to measure and should be applicable to hospital-admitted stroke patients (rather than those referred for rehabilitation, or community patients). Their predictive power has been replicated in another hospital series (Barer and Mitchell 1989).

Predicting independent life outside an institution is an important task. However, the two studies that tried to do this have included measures of disability in the prediction equations. Not surprisingly, independent life is more likely if the patient has a good level of functional ability (DeJong and Branch 1982; Henley *et al.* 1985). These studies do show an important contribution of mood and marital status in determining independence. It would be much more useful to examine predictors of independent life among severely affected patients, or those referred for rehabilitation. Choice of predictors should be guided by considering whether they may be modifiable either by health service or social intervention.

Research into predictors of recovery needs deeper thought; for example the reasons for urinary incontinence may include immobility, cognitive failure, loss of morale, too few toilets, and each could be responsible for a poor prognosis. Alternatively, incontinence may simply reflect stroke severity. Sensory inattention also requires further study. Small studies have shown that even amongst those who recover attention, their ADL recovery is worse than expected (Kinsella and Ford 1985; Kotila *et al.* 1986*a*), and the adverse effects of perceptual impairments are long lasting (Bernspang *et al.* 1987). Perhaps most importantly, the impact of other diseases causing poor mobility and function before the stroke are determinants of recovery and merit diagnosis and treatment. This should not come as any surprise to geriatricians, but it is comforting that standard practice is actually reflected in a multivariate regression!

Summary

1. The pattern of recovery after stroke is very variable, depending on the patients considered, the criteria used to define independence, and the time at which observations are made. Best estimates for survivors from community series are 45 per cent independent at 6 months and about 60 per cent independent at 1 year. Hospital series range from 38 to 68 per cent independent at 1 year. Around 20 per cent of survivors are in an institution at 1 year after the stroke.

2. More standard methods of reporting disability, dependency, and the social and emotional consequences of stroke are needed. Without standard methods it is impossible to compare studies and our understanding of the pattern of recovery will remain limited to physical aspects of disability. This may lead to underestimation of the effects of treatment.

3. The bulk of recovery of physical ability in self-care appears to occur over the first 6 months and is most rapid over the first 3 months. However, among the very disabled, almost half show improvements between 6 months and 1 year. No studies have examined rate of recovery beyond this time, but since these patients are often having rehabilitation, this needs to be done. The rate of recovery of other aspects of life has not been studied.

4. The main predictors of recovery of physical ability for self-care at 6 months are severity of the stroke, urinary incontinence, sensory inattention, pre-stroke mobility, balance, and arm motor deficit measured in the first week. Predictors among severely affected patients and those referred for rehabilitation are needed. Predictors of other aspects of handicap (especially emotional and social outcomes) are needed.

References

Abbott, R.D., Yin, Y., Reed, D.M., and Yano, K. (1986). Risk of stroke in male cigarette smokers. *New England Journal of Medicine*, **315**, 717–20.

Abbott, R.D., Donahue, R.P., MacMahon, S.W., Reed, D.M., and Yano, K. (1987). Diabetes and the risk of stroke. The Honolulu Heart Program. *Journal of the American Medical Association*, **257**, 949–52.

Abbott, R.D., Behrens, G.R., Sharp, D.S. *et al.* (1994*a*). Body mass index and thromboembolic stroke in nonsmoking men in older middle age. The Honolulu Heart Program. *Stroke*, **25**, 2370–6.

Abbott, R.D., Rodriguez, B.L., Burchfiel, C.M., and Curb, J.D. (1994*b*). Physical activity in older middle-aged men and reduced risk of stroke: the Honolulu Heart Program. *American Journal of Epidemiology*, **139**, 881–93.

Abbott, R.D., Curb, D., Rodriguez, B.L. *et al.* (1996). Effect of dietary calcium and milk consumption on risk of thromboembolic stroke in older middle aged men: the Honolulu Heart Program. *Stroke*, **27**, 813–18.

Acheson, R.M. and Sanderson, C. (1978). Strokes: social class and geography. *Population Trends*, **12**, 13–17.

Acheson, R.M. and Williams, D.D.R. (1980) . Epidemiology of cerebrovascular disease: some unanswered questions. In *Clinical neuroepidemiology*, (ed. F.C. Rose), pp. 88–104. Pitman Medical, London.

Acheson, R.M. and Williams, D.D.R. (1983). Does consumption of fruit and vegetables protect against stroke? *Lancet*, **i**, 1191–3.

Adams, G.F. (1965). Prospects of patients with strokes, with special reference to the hypertensive hemiplegic. *British Medical Journal*, **ii**, 253–9.

Adams, G.F. and Hurwitz, L.J. (1963). Mental barriers to recovery from stroke. *Lancet*, **ii**, 533–7.

Adams, G.F. and Merrett, J.D. (1961). Prognosis and survival in the aftermath of hemiplegia. *British Medical Journal*, **i**, 309–14.

Adams, H.A., Bendixen, B.H., Kappelle, J. *et al.* (1993). Classification of subtype of acute ischaemic stroke: definitions for use in a multicentre clinical trial. *Stroke*, **24**, 35–41.

Addington-Hall, J., Lay, M., Altmann, D., and McCarthy, M. (1995). Symptom control, communication with health professionals, and hospital care of stroke patients in the last year of life as reported by surviving family, friends, and officials. *Stroke*, **26**, 2242–8.

Adelman, S.M. (1981). National Survey of Stroke. Economic impact. *Stroke*, **12**, (Suppl. 1), I-69–I-87.

Agerholm, M. (1984). Side effects of nortriptyline treatment for post stroke depression. *Lancet*, **i**, 519–20.

Aho, K., Harmsen, P., Hatano, S., Marquardsen, J., Smirnov, V.E., and Strasser, T. (1980). Cerebrovascular disease in the community: results of a WHO Collaborative Study. *Bulletin of the World Health Organization*, **58**, 113–30.

Aisen, M.L., Krebs, H.I., Hogan, N., McDowell, F., and Volpe, B.T. (1997). The effect of robot-assisted therapy and rehabilitative training on motor recovery following stroke. *Archives of Neurology*, **54**, 443–6.

Alderman, M.H. (1994). Non-pharmacological treatment of hypertension. *Lancet*, **344**, 307–11.

Alderman, M.H. (1997*a*). The great salt war. *American Journal of Hypertension*, **10**, 584–5.

Alderman, M.H. (1997*b*). Modest salt restriction in older people. *Lancet*, **350**, 1702; discussion 170.

Alderman, M.H., Madhavan, S., Cohen, H., Sealey, J.E., and Laragh, J.H. (1995). Low urinary sodium is associated with greater risk of myocardial infarction among treated hypertensive men. *Hypertension*, **25**, 1144–52.

Alderman, M.H., Cohen, H., and Madhaven, S. (1998). Dietary sodium intake and mortality: the National Health and Nutrition Examination Study (NHANES-I). *Lancet*, **351**, 781–5.

Alfredsson, L., von Arbin, M., and de Faire, U. (1986). Mortality from and incidence of stroke in Stockholm. *British Medical Journal*, **292**, 1299–303.

Allen, C.M.C. (1983). Clinical diagnosis of the acute stroke syndrome. *Quarterly Journal of Medicine*, **52**, 515–23.

Allen, C.M. (1984*a*). Predicting recovery after acute stroke. *British Journal of Hospital Medicine*, **31**, 428–34.

Allen, C.M.C. (1984*b*). Predicting the outcome of acute stroke: a prognostic score. *Journal of Neurology, Neurosurgery and Psychiatry*, **47**, 475–80.

Allen, C.M.C., Harrison, M.J.G., and Wade, D.T. (1988). *The management of acute stroke*. Castle House Publications, Tunbridge Wells, Kent.

Altman, D.G. (1996). Better reporting of randomised controlled trials: the CONSORT statement. *British Medical Journal*, **313**, 570–1.

Amar, K. and Wilcock, G. (1996). Vascular dementia. *British Medical Journal*, **312**, 227–31.

Amarenco, P., Cohen, A., Tzourio, C. *et al.* (1994). Atherosclerotic disease of the aortic arch and the risk of ischaemic stroke. *New England Journal of Medicine*, **331**, 1474–9.

American Psychiatric Association (1993). *Diagnostic and statistical manual of mental disorders*, (4th edn). American Psychiatric Association, Washington, DC.

Amery, A., Birkenhager, W., Brixko, P. *et al.* (1985). Mortality and morbidity results from the European Working Party on High Blood pressure in the Elderly trial. *Lancet*, **i**, 1349–54.

Andersen, G., Vestergaard, K., and Riis, J.O. (1993). Citalopram for post-stroke pathological crying. *Lancet*, **342**, 837–9.

Andersen, G., Vestergaard, K., and Lauritzen, L. (1994). Effective treatment of poststroke depression with the selective serotonin reuptake inhibitor citalopram. *Stroke*, **25**, 1099–104.

Anderson, C.S., Jamrozik, K.D., Broadhurst, R.J., and Stewart-Wynne, E.G. (1994*a*). Predicting survival for 1 year among different subtypes of stroke. Results from the Perth Community Stroke Study. *Stroke*, **25**, 1935–44.

Anderson, C.S., Taylor, B.V., Hankey, G.J., Stewart-Wynne, E.G., and Jamrozik, K.D. (1994*b*). Validation of a clinical classification for subtypes of acute cerebral infarction. *Journal of Neurology, Neurosurgery and Psychiatry*, **57**, 1173–9.

Anderson, R. (1992). *The aftermath of stroke: the experience of patients and their families*. Cambridge University Press, Cambridge.

Andrews, K., Brocklehurst, J.C., Richards, B., and Laycock, P.J. (1981). The rate of recovery from stroke-and its measurement. *International Rehabilitation Medicine*, **3**, 155–61.

Anonymous (1983). Why has stroke mortality declined? *Lancet*, **i**, 1195–6.

Antiplatelet Trialists' Collaboration (1988). Secondary prevention of vascular disease by prolonged antiplatelet treatment. *British Medical Journal*, **296**, 320–31.

Antiplatelet Trialists Collaboration (1994a). Collaborative overview of randomised trials of antiplatelet therapy III: Reduction in venous thrombosis and pulmonary embolism by antiplatelet prophylaxis among surgical and medical patients. *British Medical Journal*, **308**, 235–46. [See eratum *BMJ* (1994), **308**, 1540.]

Antiplatelet Trialists Collaboration (1994b). Collaborative overview of randomised trials of antiplatelet therapy I: Prevention of death, myocardial infarction, and stroke by prolonged antiplatelet therapy in various categories of patients. *British Medical Journal*, **308**, 81–106.

Appel, L.J., Moore, T.J., Obarzanek, E., and Vollmer, W.M. (1997). A clinical trial of the effects of dietary patterns on blood pressure. *New England Journal of Medicine*, **336**, 1117–24.

Arboix, A., Marti-Vilalta, J.L., and Garcia, J.H. (1990). Clinical study of 227 patients with lacunar infarcts. *Stroke*, **21**, 842–7.

Aring, G.C.D. and Merritt, M.H. (1935). Differential diagnosis between cerebral haemorrhage and thrombosis. *Archives of Internal Medicine*, **56**, 435–56.

Asplund, K., Tuomilehto, J., Stegmayr, B., Wester, P.O., and Tunstall-Pedoe, H. (1988). Diagnostic criteria and quality control of the registration of stroke events in the MONICA project. *Acta Medica Scandinavica Supplementum*, **728**, 26–39.

Asplund, K., Bonita, R., Kuulasmaa, K. *et al*. (1995). Multinational comparisons of stroke epidemiology. Evaluation of case ascertainment in the WHO MONICA Stroke Study. World Health Organization Monitoring Trends and Determinants in Cardiovascular Disease. *Stroke*, **26**, 355–60. [See erratum in *Stroke* (1995), **26**, 1504.]

Asplund, K., Israelsson, K., and Schampi, I. (1998) . Haemodilution in acute ischaemic stroke (Cochrane review). In *Cochrane database of systematic reviews (disc and CD-ROM). Stroke module*, (ed. C.P. Warlow, J. van Gijn, and P.A.G. Sandercock). Update Software/BMJ Publishing, Oxford.

Astrom, M., Olsson, T., and Asplund, K. (1993). Different linkage of depression to hypercortisolism early versus late after stroke. A 3-year longitudinal study. *Stroke*, **24**, 52–7.

Asymptomatic Carotid Atherosclerosis Study (1995). Endarterectomy for asymptomatic carotid artery stenosis. *Journal of the American Medical Association*, **273**, 1421–8.

Atrial Fibrillation Investigators (1994). Risk factors for stroke and efficacy of antithrombotic therapy in atrial fibrillation. Analysis of pooled data from five randomized controlled trials. *Archives of Internal Medicine*, **154**, 1449–57. [See erratum in *Arch. Int. Med.* (1994), **154**, 2254.]

Atrial Fibrillation Investigators (1997). The efficacy of aspirin in patients with atrial fibrillation. Analysis of pooled data from 3 randomized trials. *Archives of Internal Medicine*, **157**, 1237–40.

Baker, R., Broward, J., Fang, H. *et al*. (1962). Anticoagulant therapy in cerebral infarction: report on cooperative study. *Neurology*, **12**, 823–9.

Balarajan, R. (1991). Ethnic differences in mortality from ischaemic heart disease and cerebrovascular disease in England and Wales. *British Medical Journal*, **302**, 560–4.

Bamford, J. (1992). Clinical examination in diagnosis and subclassification of stroke. *Lancet*, **339**, 400–2.

Bamford, J. and Warlow, C. (1988). Evolution and testing the lacunar hypothesis. *Stroke*, **19**, 1074–82.

Bamford, J., Sandercock, P., Warlow, C., and Gray, M. (1986). Why are patients with acute stroke admitted to hospital? *British Medical Journal*, **292**, 1369–72.

Bamford, J., Sandercock, P., Dennis, M. *et al.* (1988). A prospective study of acute cerebrovascular disease in the community: the Oxfordshire Community Stroke Project 1981–86. 1. Methodology, demography and incident cases of first-ever stroke. *Journal of Neurology, Neurosurgery and Psychiatry*, **51**, 1373–80.

Bamford, J.M., Sandercock, P.A.G., Warlow, C.P., and Slattery, J. (1989). Inter-observer agreement for the assessment of handicap in stroke patients. *Stroke*, **20**, 828.

Bamford, J., Dennis, M., Sandercock, P., Burn, J., and Warlow, C. (1990a). The frequency, causes and timing of death within 30 days of a first stroke: the Oxfordshire Community Stroke Project. *Journal of Neurology, Neurosurgery and Psychiatry*, **53**, 824–9.

Bamford, J., Sandercock, P., Dennis, M., Burn, J., and Warlow, C. (1990b). A prospective study of acute cerebrovascular disease in the community: the Oxfordshire Community Stroke Project–1981–86. 2. Incidence, case fatality rates and overall outcome at one year of cerebral infarction, primary intracerebral and subarachnoid haemorrhage. *Journal of Neurology, Neurosurgery and Psychiatry*, **53**, 16–22.

Bamford, J., Sandercock, P., Dennis, M., Burn, J., and Warlow, C. (1991). Classification and natural history of clinically identifiable subtypes of cerebral infarction. *Lancet*, **337**, 1521–6.

Barer, D.H. (1984). Lower cranial nerve function in unilateral vascular lesions of the cerebral hemisphere. *British Medical Journal*, **289**, 1662.

Barer, D.H. (1987). Dysphagia in acute stroke. *British Medical Journal*, **295**, 1137–8.

Barer, D.H. (1989a). The natural history and functional consequences of dysphagia after hemispheric stroke. *Journal of Neurology, Neurosurgery and Psychiatry*, **52**, 236–41.

Barer, D.H. (1989b). Continence after stroke: useful predictor or goal of therapy? *Age and Ageing*, **18**, 183–91.

Barer, D.H. (1990). The influence of visual and tactile inattention on predictions for recovery from acute stroke. *Quarterly Journal of Medicine*, **74**, 21–32.

Barer, D.H. and Mitchell, J.R. (1989). Predicting the outcome of acute stroke: do multivariate models help? *Quarterly Journal of Medicine*, **70**, 27–39.

Barer, D.H., Ebrahim, S., and Smith, C. (1984). Factors affecting day to day incidence of stroke in Nottingham. *British Medical Journal*, **289**, 662.

Barer, D.H., Cruickshank, J.M., Ebrahim, S., and Mitchell, J.R. (1988a). Low dose beta blockade in acute stroke ('BEST' trial): an evaluation. *British Medical Journal*, **296**, 737–41.

Barer, D.H., Ebrahim, S., and Mitchell, J.R. (1988b). The pragmatic approach to stroke trial design: stroke register, pilot trial, assessment of neurological then functional outcome. *Neuroepidemiology*, **7**, 1–12.

Barer, D.H., Leibowitz, R., Ebrahim, S., Pengally, D., and Neale, R. (1989). Vitamin C status and other nutritional indices in patients with stroke and other acute illnesses: a case-control study. *Journal of Clinical Epidemiology*, **42**, 625–31.

Barker, D.J.P. (1992). *Fetal and infant origins of adult disease*. BMJ Publishing Group, London.

Barker, D.J.P. and Osmond, C. (1987). Death rates from stroke in England and Wales predicted from past maternal mortality. *British Medical Journal*, **294**, 83–6.

Barker, D.J.P., Bull, A.R., Osmond, C., and Simmonds, S.J. (1990). Fetal and placental size and risk of hypertension in adult life. *British Medical Journal*, **301**, 259–62.

Barnett, H.J.M., Eliasziw, M., and Meldrum, H.E. (1995). Drugs and surgery in the prevention of ischaemic stroke. *New England Journal of Medicine*, **332**, 238–48.

Barnett, H.J., Kaste, M., Meldrum, H., and Eliasziw, M. (1996). Aspirin dose in stroke prevention: beautiful hypotheses slain by ugly facts. *Stroke*, **27**, 588–92.

Barrett, J.A., Fullerton, K.J., Wyatt, R., and O'Neill, P.A. (1987). Dysphagia in acute stroke. *British Medical Journal*, **295**, 1137.

Baskin, D.S. and Hosobuchi, Y. (1981). Naloxone reversal of ischaemic neurological deficits in man. *Lancet*, **ii**, 272–5.

Bath, P.M.W. and Bath, F.J. (1998). Prostacycline and analogues in acute ischaemic stroke (Cochrane review). In *Cochrane database of systematic reviews (disc and CD-ROM). Stroke module*, (ed. C.P. Warlow, J. van Gijn, and P.A.G. Sandercock). Update Software/ BMJ Publishing, Oxford.

Bath, P.M.W., Bath, F.J., and Asplund, K. (1998). Pentoxifylline, propentofylline and pentifylline in acute ischaemic stroke (Cochrane review). In *Cochrane database of systematic reviews (disc and CD-ROM). Stroke module*, (ed. C.P. Warlow, J. van Gijn, and P.A.G. Sandercock). Update Software/BMJ Publishing, Oxford.

Baum, M. (1987). Endoscopic coagulation of upper gastrointestinal haemorrhage, one; randomised clinical trials, two. *British Medical Journal*, **295**, 212.

Beauchamp, G.K., Bertino, M., and Engleman, K. (1983). Modification of salt taste. *Annals of Internal Medicine*, **98**, 763–9.

Bebbington, A.C. (1977). Scaling indices of disability. *British Journal of Preventative and Social Medicine*, **31**, 122–6.

Beech, R., Ratcliffe, M., Tilling, K., and Wolfe, C. (1996). Hospital services for stroke care. A European Perspective. European Study of Stroke Care. *Stroke*, **27**, 1958–64.

Beevers, D., Fairman, M., Hamilton, M. *et al.* (1973). Anti-hypertensive treatment and the course of established cerebrovascular disease. *Lancet*, **i**, 1407–9.

Begg, C., Cho, M., Eastwood, S. *et al.* (1996). Improving the quality of reporting of randomized controlled trials. The CONSORT statement. *Journal of the American Medical Association*, **276**, 637–9.

Beloosesky, Y., Streifler, J.Y., Burstin, A., and Grinblat, J. (1995). The importance of brain infarct size and location in predicting outcome after stroke. *Age and Ageing*, **24**, 515–18.

Bereczki, D. and Fekete, I. (1998). Vinpocetine in acute ischaemic stroke (Cochrane review). In *Cochrane database of systematic reviews (disc and CD-ROM). Stroke module*, (ed. C.P. Warlow, J. van Gijn, and P.A.G. Sandercock). Update Software/BMJ Publishing, Oxford.

Berger, K., Kase, C.S., and Buring, J.E. (1996). Interobserver agreement in the classification of stroke in the physicians' health study. *Stroke*, **27**, 238–42.

Bergner, M., Bobbitt, R.A., Carter, W.B., and Gilson, B.S. (1981). The sickness impact profile: development and final revision of a health status measure. *Medical Care*, **19**, 787–805.

Bernspang, B. (1987). Consequences of stroke. Aspects of impairments, disabilities and life satisfaction. With special emphasis on perception and on occupational therapy. Umea University Medical Dissertations NS 202, pp. 1407–9.

Bernspang, B., Asplund, K., Eriksson, S., and Fugl-Meyer, A.R. (1987). Motor and perceptual impairments in acute stroke patients: effects on self-care ability. *Stroke*, **18**, 1081–6.

Berwanger, C.S., Jeremy, J.Y., and Stansby, G. (1995). Homocysteine and vascular disease. *British Journal of Surgery*, **82**, 726–31.

Besson, G., Robert, C., Hommel, M., and Perret, J. (1995). Is it clinically possible to distinguish nonhemorrhagic infarct from hemorrhagic stroke? *Stroke*, **26**, 1205–9.

Bikkina, M., Levy, D., Evans, J.C. *et al.* (1994). Left ventricular mass and risk of stroke in an elderly cohort. The Framingham Heart Study. *Journal of the American Medical Association*, **272**, 33–6.

Blackburn, H., Blomgvist, G., Freiman, A. *et al.* (1968). The exercise electrocardiogram: differences interpretation. Report of a technical group on exercise electrocardiography. *American Journal of Cardiology*, **21**, 871–80.

Blake, A.J., Morgan, K., Bendall, M.J. *et al.* (1988). Falls by elderly people at home: prevalence and associated factors. *Age and Ageing*, **17**, 365–72.

Bland, J.M. and Altman, D.G. (1986). Statistical methods for assessing agreement between two methods of clinical measurement. *Lancet*, **i**, 307–10.

Blauw, G.J., Lagaay, A.M., Smelt, A.H., and Westendorp, R.G. (1997). Stroke, statins, and cholesterol. A meta-analysis of randomized, placebo-controlled, double-blind trials with HMG-CoA reductase inhibitors. *Stroke*, **28**, 946–50.

Bleuler, E.P. (1924). *Textbook of psychiatry*. MacMillan, New York.

Bobath, B. (1970). *Adult hemiplegia: evaluation and treatment*. William Heinemann, London.

Boers, G.H., Smals, A.G., Trijbels, F.J. *et al.* (1985). Heterozygosity for homocystinuria in premature peripheral and cerebral occlusive arterial disease. *New England Journal of Medicine*, **313**, 709–15.

Bogousslavsky, J., Van Melle, G., and Regli, F. (1988). The Lausanne Stroke Registry: analysis of 1,000 consecutive patients with first stroke. *Stroke*, **19**, 1083–92.

Bogousslavsky, J., Vanmelle, G., Regli, F., and Kappenberger, L. (1990). Pathogenesis of anterior circulation stroke in patients with non-valvular atrial fibrillation. The Lausanne Stroke Registry. *Neurology*, **40**, 1046–50.

Boiten, J. and Lodder, J. (1991). Lacunar infarcts: pathogenesis and validity of the clinical syndromes. *Stroke*, **22**, 1374–8.

Bonita, R. (1993). Stroke trends in Australia and New Zealand: mortality, morbidity, and risk factors. *Annals of Epidemiology*, **3**, 529–33.

Bonita, R. and Beaglehole, R. (1986). Does treatment of hypertension explain the decline in mortality from stroke? *British Medical Journal*, **292**, 191–2.

Bonita, R. and Beaglehole, R. (1988). Recovery of motor function after stroke. *Stroke*, **19**, 1497–500.

Bonita, R. and Beaglehole, R. (1989). Increased treatment of hypertension does not explain the decline in stroke mortality in the United States, 1970–1980. *Hypertension*, **13**, (Suppl.), I69–73.

Bonita, R., Beaglehole, R., and North, J.D.K. (1984). Event, incidence, and case-fatality rates of cerebrovascular disease in Auckland, New Zealand. *American Journal of Epidemiology*, **120**, 236–43.

Bonita, R., Scragg, R., Stewart, A., Jackson, R., and Beaglehole, R. (1986). Cigarette smoking and risk of premature stroke in men and women. *British Medical Journal*, **293**, 6–8.

Bonita, R., Ford, M.A., and Stewart, A.W. (1988). Predicting survival after stroke: a three-year follow-up. *Stroke*, **19**, 669–73.

Bonita, R., Stewart, A., and Beaglehole, R. (1990). International trends in stroke mortality: 1970–1985. *Stroke*, **21**, 989–92.

Bonita, R., Broad, J.B., and Beaglehole, R. (1993). Changes in stroke incidence and case-fatality in Auckland, New Zealand, 1981–91. *Lancet*, **342**, 1470–3.

Bonn, D. (1998). Stopping anti-hypertensive drugs raises the risk of intracerebral haemorrhage. *Lancet*, **351**, 1863.

Boon, A., Lodder, J., Heuts-van Raak, L., and Kessels, F. (1994). Silent brain infarcts in 755 consecutive patients with a first-ever supratentorial ischemic stroke. Relationship with index-stroke subtype, vascular risk factors, and mortality. *Stroke*, **25**, 2384–90.

Borrie, M.J., Campbell, A.J., Caradoc-Davies, T.H., and Spears, G.F. (1986). Urinary incontinence after stroke: a prospective study. *Age and Ageing*, **15**, 177–81.

Boushey, C.J., Beresford, S.A., Omenn, G.S., and Motulsky, A.G. (1995). A quantitative assessment of plasma homocysteine as a risk factor for vascular disease. Probable benefits of increasing folic acid intakes. *Journal of the American Medical Association*, **274**, 1049–57.

Bousser, M.G. (1997). Aspirin or heparin immediately after a stroke? *Lancet*, **349**, 1564–5.

Bowen, B.C., Quencer, R.M., Margosian, P., and Pattany, P.M. (1994). MR angiography of occlusive disease of the arteries in the head and neck: current concepts. *American Journal of Roentgenology*, **162**, 9–18.

Boysen, G., Nyboe, J., Appleyard, M. *et al.* (1988). Stroke incidence and risk factors for stroke in Copenhagen, Denmark. *Stroke*, **19**, 1345–53.

Brass, L.M., Isaacsohn, J.L., Merikangas, K.R., and Robinette, C.D. (1992). A study of twins and stroke. *Stroke*, **23**, 221–3.

Brennan, P.J., Greenberg, G., Miall, W.E., and Thompson, S.G. (1982). Seasonal variation in blood pressure. *British Medical Journal*, **285**, 919–23.

Bridges, K. and Goldberg, D. (1986). The validation of the GHQ-28 and the use of the Mini-Mental State Examination in neurological inpatients. *British Journal of Psychiatry*, **148**, 548–53.

Brittain, K.R., Peet, S.M., and Castleden, C.M. (1998). Stroke and incontinence. *Stroke*, **29**, 524–8.

Britton, M., Faire, U.D., Helmers, C., and Miah, K. (1980). Prognostication in acute cerebrovascular disease. *Acta Medica Scandinavica*, **207**, 37–42.

Britton, M., Hultman, E., Murray, V., and Sjoholm, H. (1983). The diagnostic accuracy of CSF analyses in stroke. *Acta Medica Scandinavica*, **214**, 3–13.

Brocklehurst, J.C., Andrews, K., Richards, B., and Laycock, P.J. (1978). How much physical therapy for patients with stroke? *British Medical Journal*, **i**, 1307–10.

Brocklehurst, J.C., Andrews, K., Richards, B., and Laycock, P.J. (1985). Incidence and correlates of incontinence in stroke patients. *Journal of the American Geriatrics Society*, **33**, 540–2.

Broderick, J.P., Phillips, S.J., Whisnant, J.P., O'Fallon, W.M., and Bergstralh, E.J. (1989). Incidence rates of stroke in the eighties: the end of the decline in stroke? *Stroke*, **20**, 577–82.

Broderick, J.P., Brott, T., Tomsick, T., Huster, G., and Miller, R. (1992). The risk of subarachnoid and intracerebral hemorrhages in blacks as compared with whites. *New England Journal of Medicine*, **326**, 733–6.

Brott, T., Thalinger, K., and Hertzberg, V. (1986). Hypertension as a risk factor for spontaneous intracerebral hemorrhage. *Stroke*, **17**, 1078–83.

Brott, T., Adams, H.P., Olinger, C.P. *et al.* (1989*a*). Measurements of acute cerebral infarction: a clinical examination scale. *Stroke*, **20**, 864–70.

Brott, T., Marler, J.R., Olinger, C.P. *et al.* (1989*b*). Measurements of acute cerebral infarction: lesion size by computed tomography. *Stroke*, **20**, 871–5.

Brown, M.M. and CAVATAS Investigators (1998). Results of the carotid and vertebral artery transluminal angioplasty study (CAVATAS). *Cerebrovascular Diseases*, **8**, (Suppl. 4), 21.

Brown, R.D., Whisnant, J.P., Sicks, J.D., O'Fallon, W.M., and Wiebers, D.O. (1996). Stroke incidence, prevalence, and survival: secular trends in Rochester, Minnesota, through 1989. *Stroke*, **27**, 373–80.

Bryan, R.N., Levy, L.M., Whitlow, W.D. *et al.* (1991). Diagnosis of acute cerebral infarction: comparison of CT and MRI. *American Journal of Neuroradiology*, **12**, 611–20.

Bucher, H.C., Guyatt, G.H., Griffith, L.E., and Walter, S.D. (1997). The results of direct and indirect treatment comparisons in meta-analysis of randomized controlled trials. *Journal of Clinical Epidemiology*, **50**, 683–91.

Bucknall, C.A., Morris, G.K., and Mitchell, J.R.A. (1986). Physicians' attitudes to four common problems: hypertension, atrial fibrillation, transient ischaemic attacks, and angina pectoris. *British Medical Journal*, **293**, 739–42.

Bulpitt, C.J. (1995). Vitamin C and vascular disease. *British Medical Journal*, **310**, 1548–9.

Burchfiel, C.M., Curb, J.D., Rodriguez, B.L., Abbott, R.D., Chiu, D., and Yano, K. (1994). Glucose intolerance and 22-year stroke incidence. The Honolulu Heart Program. *Stroke*, **25**, 951–7.

Buring, J.E., Hebert, P., Romero, J. *et al.* (1995). Migraine and subsequent risk of stroke in the Physicians' Health Study. *Archives of Neurology*, **52**, 129–34.

Burn, J., Dennis, M., Bamford, J., Sandercock, P., Wade, D., and Warlow, C. (1994). Long-term risk of recurrent stroke after a first-ever stroke. The Oxfordshire Community Stroke Project. *Stroke*, **25**, 333–7. [See erratum in *Stroke* (1994), **25**, 1887.]

Burney, T.L., Senapati, M., Desai, S., Choudhary, S.T., and Badlani, G.H. (1996). Acute cerebrovascular accident and lower urinary tract dysfunction: a prospective correlation of the site of brain injury with urodynamic findings. *Journal of Urology*, **156**, 1748–1750.

Burvill, P.W., Johnson, G.A., Jamrozik, K.D., Anderson, C.S., Stewart-Wynne, E.G., and Chakera, T.M. (1995*a*). Prevalence of depression after stroke: the Perth Community Stroke Study. *British Journal of Psychiatry*, **166**, 320–7.

Burvill, P.W., Johnson, G.A., Jamrozik, K.D., Anderson, C.S., Stewart-Wynne, E.G., and Chakera, T.M. (1995*b*). Anxiety disorders after stroke: results from the Perth Community Stroke Study. *British Journal of Psychiatry*, **166**, 328–32.

Burvill, P., Johnson, G., Jamrozik, K., Anderson, C., and Stewart-Wynne, E. (1997). Risk factors for post-stroke depression. *International Journal of Geriatric Psychiatry*, **12**, 219–26.

Calandre, L., Arnal, C., Ortega, J.F. *et al.* (1986). Risk factors for spontaneous cerebral hematomas. Case-control study. *Stroke*, **17**, 1126–8.

Camargo, C.A. (1989). Moderate alcohol consumption and stroke. The epidemiologic evidence. *Stroke*, **20**, 1611–26.

Campbell, J. (1996). Falls. In *Epidemiology in old age*, (ed. S. Ebrahim and A. Kalache), pp. 361–8. BMJ Books, London.

Candelise, A. and Cicconi, A. (1998). Gangliosides in acute ischaemic stroke (Cochrane review). In *Cochrane database of systematic reviews (disc and CD-ROM). Stroke module*, (ed. C.P. Warlow, J. van Gijn, and P.A.G. Sandercock). Update Software/BMJ Publishing, Oxford.

Candelise, L., Pinardi, G., and Morabito, A. (1991). Mortality in acute stroke with atrial fibrillation. The Italian Acute Stroke Study Group. *Stroke*, **22**, 169–74.

Caplan, L.R. (1991*a*). Diagnosis and treatment of ischemic stroke. *Journal of the American Medical Association*, **266**, 2413–18.

Caplan, L.R. (1991*b*). Strokes in African-Americans. *Circulation*, **83**, 1469–71.

Caplan, L.R. (1995). Binswanger's disease – revisited. *Neurology*, **45**, 626–33.

Cappa, S.F., Perani, D., Grassi, F. *et al.* (1997). A PET follow-up study of recovery after stroke in acute aphasics. *Brain and Language*, **56**, 55–67.

Cappuccio, F.P., Markandu, N.D., Carney, C., Sagnella, G.A., and MacGregor, G.A. (1997). Double-blind randomised trial of modest salt restriction in older people. *Lancet*, **350**, 850–4.

CAPRIE Steering Committee (1996). A randomised blinded trial of clopidogrel versus aspirin in patients at risk of ischaemic events (CAPRIE). *Lancet*, **348**, 1329–39.

Carter, A.B. (1961). Anticoagulant therapy in progressing stroke. *British Medical Journal*, **2**, 70–3.

Carter, A.B. (1964). *Cerebral infarction*. Pergamon Press, London.

Carter, A.B. (1970). Hypotensive therapy in stroke survivors. *Lancet*, **i**, 485–9.

Casper, M., Wing, S., Strogatz, D., Davis, C.E., and Tyroler, H.A. (1992). Antihypertensive treatment and US trends in stroke mortality, 1962 to 1980 . *American Journal of Public Health*, **82**, 1600–6.

Castleden, C.M., Duffin, H.M., and Gulati, R.S. (1986). Double blind study of imipramine and placebo for incontinence due to bladder instability. *Age and Ageing*, **15**, 299–303.

Celani, M.G., Righetti, E., Migliacci, R. *et al.* (1994). Comparability and validity of two clinical scores in the early differential diagnosis of acute stroke. *British Medical Journal*, **308**, 1674–6.

Cerebral Embolism Task Force (1986). Cardiogenic brain embolism. *Archives of Neurology*, **43**, 71–84.

Cerebral Embolism Task Force (1989). Cardiogenic brain embolism. The second report of the Cerebral Embolism Task Force. *Archives of Neurology*, **46**, 727–43. [See erratum in *Arch. Neurol.* (1989), **46**, 1079.]

Chakravarty, K., Durkin, C.J., al-Hillawi, A.H., Bodley, R., and Webley, M. (1993). The incidence of acute arthritis in stroke patients, and its impact on rehabilitation. *Quarterly Journal of Medicine*, **86**, 819–23.

Charig, M.J. and Fletcher, E.W.L. (1987). Emergency phlebography service: is it worthwhile? *British Medical Journal*, **295**, 474.

Charlton, J., Murphy, M., Khaw, K.T., Ebrahim, S., and Davey Smith, G. (1997). Cardiovascular diseases. In *Health of adult Britain, 1841–1994*, (ed. M. Murphy and J. Charlton), pp. 60–81. Office of National Statistics, HMSO, London.

Chikos, P.M., Fisher, L.D., Hirsch, J.H., Harley, J.D., Thiele, B.L., and Strandness, D.E. (1983). Observer variability in evaluating extracranial carotid artery stenosis. *Stroke*, **14**, 885–92.

Chin, P., Angunawela, R., Mitchell, D., and Horne, J. (1980). Stroke register in Carlisle: a preliminary report. In *Clinical Neuroepidemiology*, (ed. F.C. Rose), pp. 131–43. Pitman Medical, London.

Chinese Acute Stroke Trial Study Group (1997). CAST: randomised placebo-controlled trial of early aspirin use in 20,000 patients with acute ischaemic stroke. *Lancet*, **349**, 1641–9.

Chinn, S. and Burney, P.G.J. (1987). On measuring repeatability of data from self-administered questionnaires. *International Journal of Epidemiology*, **16**, 121–7.

Chodosh, E.H., Foulkes, M.A., Kase, C.S. *et al.* (1988). Silent stroke in the NINCDS Stroke Data Bank. *Neurology*, **38**, 1674–9.

Christie, D. (1981). Stroke in Melbourne, Australia: an epidemiological study. *Stroke*, **12**, 467–9.

Chui, H.C., Victoroff, J., Margolin, D. *et al.* (1992). Criteria for the diagnosis of ischaemic vascular dementia. *Neurology*, **42**, 473–80.

Ciocon, J.O., Silverstone, F.A., Graver, L.M., and Foley, C.J. (1988). Tube feeding in elderly patients. Indications, benefits, and complications. *Archives of Internal Medicine*, **148**, 429–33.

Clark, W.M., Warach, S.J., Pettigrew, L.C., Gammans, R.E., and Sabounjian, L.A. (1997). A randomized dose–response trial of citicoline in acute ischemic stroke patients. Citicoline Stroke Study Group. *Neurology*, **49**, 671–8.

Clarke, R., Daly, L., Robinson, K. *et al.* (1991). Hyperhomocysteinemia: an independent risk factor for vascular disease. *New England Journal of Medicine*, **324**, 1149–55.

Cochrane, A.L., Chapman, P.J., and Oldham, P.D. (1951). Observer errors in taking medical histories. *Lancet*, **i**, 1007–9.

Cohen, J. (1960). A coefficient of agreement for nominal scales. *Educational and Psychological Measurement*, **XX**, 37–46.

Collin, C., Wade, D.T., Davies, S., and Horne, V. (1988). The Barthel ADL Index: a reliability study. *International Disability Studies*, **10**, 61–3.

Collins, R. and MacMahon, S. (1994). Blood pressure, antihypertensive drug treatment and the risks of stroke and of coronary heart disease. *British Medical Bulletin*, **50**, 272–98.

Collins, R., Scrimageour, A., Yusuf, S., and Peto, R. (1988). Reduction in fatal pulmonary embolism and venous thrombosis by perioperative administration of subcutaneous heparin. *New England Journal of Medicine*, **318**, 1162–73.

Collins, R.C., Dobkin, B.H., and Choi, D.W. (1989). Selective vulnerability of the brain: new insights into the pathophysiology of stroke. *Annals of Internal Medicine*, **110**, 992–1000.

Collins, R., Peto, R., MacMahon, S. *et al.* (1990). Blood pressure, stroke, and coronary heart disease. Part 2, Short-term reductions in blood pressure: overview of randomised drug trials in their epidemiological context. *Lancet*, **335**, 827–38.

Consensus Conference (1988). Treatment of stroke. *British Medical Journal*, **297**, 126–8.

Cook, N.R., Cohen, J., Hebert, P.R., Taylor, J.O., and Hennekens, C.H. (1995). Implications of small reductions in diastolic blood pressure for primary prevention. *Archives of Internal Medicine*, **155**, 701–9.

Cook, R.J. and Sackett, D.L. (1995). The number needed to treat: a clinically useful measure of treatment effect. *British Medical Journal*, **310**, 452–4. [See erratum in *BMJ* (1995), **310**, 1056.]

Coope, J. and Warrender, T.S. (1986). Randomised trial of treatment of hypertension in elderly patients in primary care. *British Medical Journal*, **293**, 1145–8.

Cooper, B. (1991). The epidemiology of dementia. In *Psychiatry in the elderly*, (ed. R. Jacoby and C. Oppenheimer), pp. 574–85. Oxford University Press, Oxford.

Cooperative North Scandinavian Enalapril Survival Study (CONSENSUS) (1987). Effects of enalapril on mortality in severe congestive heart failure. *New England Journal of Medicine*, **316**, 1429–35.

Coppola, W.G., Whincup, P.H., Papacosta, O., Walker, M., and Ebrahim, S. (1995). Scoring system to identify men at high risk of stroke: a strategy for general practice. *British Journal of General Practice*, **45**, 185–9.

Coppola, W.G., Whincup, P.H., Walker, M., and Ebrahim, S. (1997). Identification and management of stroke risk in older people: a national survey of current practice in primary care. *Journal of Human Hypertension*, **11**, 185–91.

Cote, R., Battista, R.N., Wolfson, C., Boucher, J., Adam, J., and Hachinski, V. (1989). The Canadian Neurological Scale: validation and reliability assessment. *Neurology*, **39**, 638–43.

Counsell, C. and Sandercock, P. (1998*a*) . Anticoagulant therapy in patients with in acute presumed ischaemic stroke (Cochrane review). In *Cochrane database of systematic reviews (disc and CD-ROM). Stroke module*, (ed. C.P. Warlow, J. van Gijn, and P.A.G. Sandercock). Update Software/BMJ Publishing, Oxford.

Counsell, C.E. and Sandercock, P.A.G. (1998*b*). Low molecular weight heparins or heparinoids compared to standard unfractionated heparin in acute ischaemic stroke (Cochrane review). In *Cochrane database of systematic reviews (disc and CD-ROM). Stroke module,* (ed. C.P. Warlow, J. van Gijn, and P.A.G. Sandercock). Update Software/ BMJ Publishing, Oxford.

Counsell, C.E., Warlow, C.P., Sandercock, P. *et al.* (1995) The Cochrane Collaboration Stroke Review Group: meeting the need for systematic reviews in stroke care. *Stroke* **26**: 498-502

Croog, S.H., Levine, S., Testa, M.A., Brown, B. *et al.* (1986). The effects of antihypertensive treatment on quality of life. *New England Journal of Medicine*, **314**, 1657–64.

Crouse, J.R., Byngton, R.P., Hoen, H.M., and Furberg, C.T. (1997). Reductase inhibitor monotherapy and stroke prevention. *Archives of Internal Medicine*, **157**, 1305–10.

Cruickshank, J.M., Thorpe, J.M., and Zacharias, F.J. (1987). Benefits and potential harm of lowering high blood pressure. *Lancet*, **i**, 581–584.

Cummins, R.O. (1983). Recent changes in salt use and stroke mortality in England and Wales. Any help for the salt hypertension debate? *Journal of Epidemiology and Community Health*, **37**, 25–8.

Cutler, J.A., Follmann, D., and Allender, P.S. (1997). Randomised trials of sodium reduction: an overview. *American Journal of Clinical Nutrition*, **65**, (Suppl.), 643S– 651S.

D'Agostino, R.B., Wolf, P.A., Belanger, A.J., and Kannel, W.B. (1994). Stroke risk profile: adjustment for antihypertensive medication. The Framingham Study. *Stroke*, **25**, 40–3.

Dahlof, B., Lindholm, L.H., Hansson, L., Schersten, B. *et al.* (1991). Morbidity and mortality in the Swedish Trial in Old Patients with Hypertension (STOP-HT). *Lancet*, **338**, 1281–5.

Dam, M., Tonin, P., De Boni, A. *et al.* (1996). Effects of fluoxetine and maprotiline on functional recovery in poststroke hemiplegic patients undergoing rehabilitation therapy. *Stroke*, **27**, 1211–14.

Davenport, R.J., Dennis, M.S., and Warlow, C.P. (1995). Improving the recording of the clinical assessment of stroke patients using a clerking pro forma. *Age and Ageing*, **24**, 43–8.

Davenport, R.J., Dennis, M.S., and Warlow, C.P. (1996*a*). Effect of correcting outcome data for case mix: an example from stroke medicine. *British Medical Journal*, **312**, 1503–5.

Davenport, R.J., Dennis, M.S., Wellwood, I., and Warlow, C.P. (1996*b*). Complications after acute stroke. *Stroke*, **27**, 415–20.

Daverat, P., Castel, J.P., Dartigues, J.F., and Orgogozo, J.M. (1991). Death and functional outcome after spontaneous intracerebral haemorrhage. A prospective study of 166 cases using multivariate analysis. *Stroke*, **22**, 1–6.

Davey Smith, G. and Ebrahim, S. (1998). Dietary change, cholesterol reduction and the public health: what does meta analysis add? *British Medical Journal*, **316**, 1220.

Davey Smith, G. and Phillips, A. (1992). Confounding in epidemiological studies: why 'independent' effects may not be all they seem. *British Medical Journal*, **305**, 757–9.

Davey Smith, G. and Phillips, A.N. (1996). Inflation in epidemiology: 'the proof and measurement of association between two things' revisited. *British Medical Journal*, **312**, 1659–61.

Davey Smith, G., Phillips, A.N., and Neaton, J.D. (1992). Smoking as 'independent' risk factor for suicide: illustration of an artifact from observational epidemiology? *Lancet*, **340**, 709–12.

Davey Smith, G., Song, F.S., and Sheldon, T. (1993). Cholesterol lowering and mortality: the importance of considering initial level of risk. *British Medical Journal*, **306**, 1367–73.

Davey Smith, G., Frankel, S., and Yarnell, J. (1997). Sex and death: are they related? Findings from the Caerphilly Cohort Study. *British Medical Journal*, **315**, 1641–4.

David, R., Enderby, P., and Bainton, D. (1982). Treatment of acquired aphasia: speech therapists and volunteers compared. *Journal of Neurology, Neurosurgery and Psychiatry*, **45**, 957–61.

Davies, M.J. and Woolf, N. (1993). Atherosclerosis: what is it and why does it occur? *British Heart Journal*, 69, (Suppl.), s3–s11.

Davis, P.H., Dambrosia, J.M., Schoenberg, B.S. *et al.* (1987). Risk factors for ischemic stroke: a prospective study in Rochester, Minnesota. *Annals of Neurology*, **22**, 319–27.

Davis, S.M., Albers, G.W., Diener, H.C., Lees, K.R., and Norris, J. (1997). Termination of Acute Stroke Studies Involving Selfotel Treatment. ASSIST Steering Committee. *Lancet*, **349**, 32.

Dawber, T.R. (1980) *The Framingham Study*. Harvard University Press, London.

Dean, C.M. and Shepherd, R.B. (1997). Task-related training improves performance of seated reaching tasks after stroke. A randomized controlled trial. *Stroke*, **28**, 722–8.

De-Deyn, P.P., Reuck, J.D., Deberdt, W., Vlietink, R., and Orgogozo, J.M. (1997). Treatment of acute ischaemic stroke with piracetam. Members of the Piracetam in Acute Stroke Study (PASS) group. *Stroke*, **28**, 2347–52.

De Faire, U., Friberg, L., and Lundman, T. (1975). Concordance for mortality with special reference to ischaemic heart disease and cerebrovascular disease. *Preventive Medicine*, **4**, 509–17.

De Haan, R., Horn, J., Limburg, M., Van Der Meulen, J., and Bossuyt, P. (1993). A comparison of five stroke scales with measures of disability, handicap, and quality of life. *Stroke*, **24**, 1178–81.

De Haan, R., Limburg, M., Bossuyt, P., Van Der Meulen, J., and Aaronson, N. (1995*a*). The clinical meaning of Rankin 'handicap' grades after stroke. *Stroke*, **26**, 2027–30.

De Haan, R.J., Limburg, M., van der Meulen, J.H., Jacobs, H.M., and Aaronson, N.K. (1995*b*). Quality of life after stroke. Impact of stroke type and lesion location. *Stroke*, **26**, 402–8.

DeJong, G. and Branch, L.G. (1982). Predicting the stroke patient's ability to live independently. *Stroke*, **13**, 648–55.

Del Zoppo, G.J., Wagner, S., and Tagaya, M. (1997). Trends and future developments in the pharmacological treatment of acute ischaemic stroke. *Drugs*, **54**, 9–38.

Denham, M.J., Farran, H., and James, G. (1973). The value of 125-I-fibrinogen in the diagnosis of deep vein thrombosis in hemiplegia. *Age and Ageing*, **2**, 207–10.

Dennis, M.S., Bamford, J.M., Molyneux, A.J., and Warlow, C.P. (1987). Rapid resolution of signs of primary intracerebral haemorrhage in computed tomograms of the brain. *British Medical Journal*, **295**, 379–81.

Dennis, M.S., Bamford, J.M., Sandercock, P.A., and Warlow, C.P. (1989*a*). A comparison of risk factors and prognosis for transient ischemic attacks and minor ischemic strokes. The Oxfordshire Community Stroke Project. *Stroke*, **20**, 1494–9.

Dennis, M.S., Bamford, J.M., Sandercock, P.A., and Warlow, C.P. (1989*b*). Incidence of transient ischemic attacks in Oxfordshire, England. *Stroke*, **20**, 333–9.

Dennis, M., Bamford, J., Sandercock, P., and Warlow, C. (1990). Prognosis of transient ischemic attacks in the Oxfordshire Community Stroke Project. *Stroke*, **21**, 848–53.

Dennis, M.S., Burn, J.P., Sandercock, P.A., Bamford, J.M., Wade, D.T., and Warlow, C.P. (1993). Long-term survival after first-ever stroke: the Oxfordshire Community Stroke Project. *Stroke*, **24**, 796–800.

Dennis, M., O'Rourke, S., Slattery, J., Staniforth, T., and Warlow, C. (1997). Evaluation of a stroke family care worker: results of a randomised controlled trial. *British Medical Journal*, **314**, 1071–6.

Denton, D., Weisinger, R., Mundy, N.I. *et al.* (1995). The effect of increased salt intake on blood pressure of chimpanzees. *Nature Medicine*, **1**, 1009–16.

Desmond, D.W., Moroney, J.T., Sano, M., and Stern, Y. (1996). Recovery of cognitive function after stroke. *Stroke*, **27**, 1798–803.

Diabetes Control and Complications Trial (1995). Effect of intensive diabetes management on macrovascular events and risk factors in the Diabetes Control and Complications Trial. *American Journal of Cardiology*, **75**, 894–903.

Diener, H.C., Cunha, L., Forbes, C., Sivenius, J., Smets, P., and Lowenthal, A. (1996). European Stroke Prevention Study 2-Dipyridamole and acetylsalicylic acid in the secondary prevention of stroke. *Journal of the Neurological Sciences*, **143**, 1–13.

Di Piero, V., Chollet, F.M., MacCarthy, P., Lenzi, G.L., and Frackowiak, R.S. (1992). Motor recovery after acute ischaemic stroke: a metabolic study. *Journal of Neurology, Neurosurgery and Psychiatry*, **55**, 990–6.

DiPietro, L., Ostfeld, A.M., and Rosner, G.L. (1994). Adiposity and stroke among older adults of low socioeconomic status: the Chicago Stroke Study. *American Journal of Public Health*, **84**, 14–19.

Dippel, D.W. and Koudstaal, P.J. (1997). We need stronger predictors of major vascular events in patients with a recent transient ischemic attack or nondisabling stroke. Dutch TIA Trial Study Group. *Stroke*, **28**, 774–6.

Diringer, M.N. (1993). Intracerebral hemorrhage: pathophysiology and management. *Critical Care Medicine*, **21**, 1591–603.

D'Olhaberriague, L., Litvan, I., Mitsias, P., and Mansbach, H.H. (1996). A reappraisal of reliability and validity studies in stroke. *Stroke*, **27**, 2331–6.

Donaldson, S.W., Wagner, C.W., and Gresham, G.E. (1973). A unified ADL evaluation form. *Archives of Physical Medicine and Rehabilitation*, **54**, 175–80.

Donnan, G.A., Davis, S.M., Chambers, B.R. *et al.* (1996). Streptokinase for acute ischemic stroke with relationship to time of administration: Australian Streptokinase (ASK) Trial Study Group. *Journal of the American Medical Association*, **276**, 961–6.

Dorman, P.J. and Sandercock, P.A. (1996). Considerations in the design of clinical trials of neuroprotective therapy in acute stroke. *Stroke*, **27**, 1507–15.

Dorman, P., Slattery, J., Farrell, B., Dennis, M., and Sandercock, P. (1998). Qualitative comparison of the reliability of health status assessments with the EuroQol and SF-36 questionnaires after stroke. United Kingdom Collaborators in the International Stroke Trial. *Stroke*, **29**, 63–8.

Droller, H. (1960). Survival after apoplexy. *Gerontology Clinics*, **2**, 120–8.

Drummond, A.E.R. and Walker, M.F. (1994). Nottingham leisure questionnaire for stroke patients. *British Journal of Occupational Therapy*, **57**, 414–18.

Drummond, A.E.R. and Walker, M.F. (1995). A randomised controlled trial of leisure rehabilitation after stroke. *Clinical Rehabilitation*, **9**, 283–90.

Dudley, H.A.F. (1987). Extracranial–intracranial bypass, one; clinical trials, nil. *British Medical Journal*, **294**, 1501–2.

Duncan, P.W., Goldstein, L.B., Matchar, D., Divine, G.W., and Feussner, J. (1992). Measurement of motor recovery after stroke. Outcome assessment and sample size requirements. *Stroke*, **23**, 1084–9.

Duncan, P.W., Goldstein, L.B., Horner, R.D. *et al.* (1994). Similar motor recovery of upper and lower extremities after stroke. *Stroke*, **25**, 1181–8.

Dunn, R.B. and Lewis, P.A. (1993). Compliance with standardised assessment scales for elderly people among consultant geriatricians in Wessex. *British Medical Journal*, **307**, 606.

Dutch TIA Trial Study Group (1991). A comparison of two doses of aspirin (30mg vs. 283mg a day) in patients after a transient ischemic attack or minor ischemic stroke. *New England Journal of Medicine*, **325**, 1261–6.

Dutch TIA Trial Study Group (1993). Predictors of major vascular events in patients with a transient ischemic attack or nondisabling stroke. *Stroke*, **24**, 527–31.

Dyer, A.R., Elliott, P., Marmot, M., Kesteloot, H., Stamler, R., and Stamler, J. (1996). Commentary: strength and importance of the relation of dietary salt to blood pressure. Intersalt Steering and Editorial Committee. *British Medical Journal*, **312**, 1661–4. [See erratum in *BMJ* (1996), **313**, 222.]

Dyken, M.L., Barnett, H.J., Easton, J.D. *et al.* (1992). Low-dose aspirin and stroke. 'It ain't necessarily so'. *Stroke*, **23**, 1395–9.

Dyker, A.G. and Lees, K.R. (1998). Duration of neuroprotective therapy for ischaemic stroke. *Stroke*, **29**, 535–42.

Ebrahim, S. (1985) Physical disability, health, depressed mood, and use of services after stroke. M.D. thesis, University of Nottingham.

Ebrahim, S. (1995). Clinical and public health perspectives and applications of health-related quality of life measurement. *Social Science and Medicine*, **41**, 1383–94.

Ebrahim, S. (1996). Stroke. In *Epidemiology in old age*, (ed. S. Ebrahim and A. Kalache). BMJ Books/WHO, London.

Ebrahim, S. (1997). Stroke mortality: secular and geographic trends. *Journal of Epidemiology and Community Health*, **51**, 132–3.

Ebrahim, S. (1998). Stroke: pathology and epidemiology. In *Brocklehurst's textbook of geriatric medicine and gerontology*, (5th edn), (ed. R.C. Tallis, J.C. Brocklehurst, and H.M. Fillit). Churchill-Livingstone, Edinburgh.

Ebrahim, S. and Davey Smith, G. (1996). Health promotion in older people for cardiovascular disease prevention: a systematic review and meta-analysis, pp. 1–136. Health Education Authority, London.

Ebrahim, S. and Davey Smith, G. (1998). Lowering blood pressure: a systematic review of non-pharmacological interventions. *Journal of Public Health Medicine*, **20**, 441–448.

Ebrahim, S. and Nouri, F. (1987). Caring for stroke patients at home. *International Rehabilitation Medicine*, **8**, 171–3.

Ebrahim, S., Nouri, F., and Barer, D. (1985). Measuring disability after a stroke. *Journal of Epidemiology and Community Health*, **39**, 86–9.

Ebrahim, S., Barer, D., and Nouri, F. (1986). Use of the Nottingham Health Profile with patients after a stroke. *Journal of Epidemiology and Community Health*, **40**, 166–9.

Ebrahim, S., Barer, D., and Nouri, F. (1987*a*). Affective illness after stroke. *British Journal of Psychiatry*, **151**, 52–6.

Ebrahim, S., Barer, D., and Nouri, F. (1987*b*). An audit of follow-up services for stroke patients after discharge from hospital. *International Disability Studies*, **9**, 103–5.

Ebrahim, S., Dallosso, H., Morgan, K., Bassey, J., Fentem, P., and Arie, T. (1988). Causes of ill health among a random sample of old and very old people: possibilities for prevention. *Journal of the Royal College of Physicians of London*, **22**, 105–7.

Ebrahim, S., Brittis, S., and Wu, A. (1991). The valuation of states of ill-health: the impact of age and disability. *Age and Ageing*, **20**, 37–40.

Ebrahim, S., Thompson, P.W., Baskaran, V., and Evans, K. (1997). Randomised placebo controlled trial of brisk walking in the prevention of postmenopausal osteoporosis. *Age and Ageing*, **26**, 253–60.

Ebrahim, S. and Redfern, J. (1999). Stroke Care-a matter of chance. National survey of stroke services. Stroke Association, London.

EC–IC Bypass Study Group (1985). Failure of extracranial arterial bypass to reduce the risk of ischaemic stroke. *New England Journal of Medicine*, **313**, 1191–200.

Edmans, J.A. and Lincoln, N.B. (1989). Treatment of visual perceptual deficits after stroke: four single case studies. *International Disability Studies*, **11**, 25–33.

Effective Health Care Bulletin (1998). Cholesterol and coronary heart disease: screening and treatment. *Effective Health Care Bulletin*, **4**, 1–16.

Egger, M., Davey Smith, G., Schneider, M., and Minder, C. (1997). Bias in metaanalysis detected by a simple graphical test. *British Medical Journal*, **315**, 629–34.

Egger, M., Schneider, M., Davey Smith, G. (1998). Spurious precision? Meta-analysis of observational studies. *British Medical Journal*, **316**, 140-4.

Eisenberg, H., Morrison, J.T., Sullivan, P., and Foote, F.M. (1964). Cerebrovascular accidents. Incidence and survival rates in a defined population, Middlesex County, Connecticut. *Journal of the American Medical Association*, **189**, 107–12.

Eliasziw, M., Streifler, J.Y., Fox, A.J., Hachinski, V.C., Ferguson, G.G., and Barnett, H.J. (1994). Significance of plaque ulceration in symptomatic patients with high-grade carotid stenosis. North American Symptomatic Carotid Endarterectomy Trial. *Stroke*, **25**, 304–8.

Elliott, P. (1997). Lower sodium for all? *Lancet*, **350**, 825–6.

Elliott, P., Stamler, J., Nichols, R. *et al.* (1996). Intersalt revisited: further analyses of 24 hour sodium excretion and blood pressure within and across populations. Intersalt Cooperative Research Group. *British Medical Journal*, **312**, 1249–53.

European Atrial Fibrillation Trial Study Group (1993). Secondary prevention in non-rheumatic atrial fibrillation after transient ischaemic attack or minor stroke. *Lancet*, **342**, 1255–62.

European Carotid Surgery Trialists Collaborative Group (1991). MRC European Carotid Surgery Trial: interim results for symptomatic patients with severe (70–99%) or with mild (0–29%) carotid stenosis. *Lancet*, **337**, 1235–43.

European Carotid Surgery Trialists (1995). Risk of stroke in the distribution of an asymptomatic carotid artery. *Lancet*, **345**, 209–12.

European Carotid Surgery Trialists Study Group (1996). Endarterectomy for moderate symptomatic carotid stenosis: interim results from the MRC European Carotid Surgery Trial. *Lancet*, **347**, 1591–3.

European Carotid Surgery Trialists (1998). Randomised trial of endarterectomy for recently symptomatic carotid stenosis: final results of the MRC European Carotid Surgery Trial (ECST). *Lancet*, **351**, 1379–87.

EuroQol Group (1990). EuroQol: a new facility for the measurement of health-related quality of life. *Health Policy*, **16**, 199–208.

Evans, J.G. (1987). Blood pressure and stroke in an elderly English population. *Journal of Epidemiology and Community Health*, **41**, 275–82.

Evans, J.G. (1991). Aging and rationing. *British Medical Journal*, **303**, 869–70.

Evans, J.G., Prudham, D., and Wandless, I. (1980). Risk factors for stroke in the elderly. In *The ageing brain. Neurological and mental disturbances*, (ed. G. Barbagallo and A.N. Exton-Smith), pp. 113–26. New York and London, Plenum Press.

Evans, R.L., Matlock, A.L., Bishop, D.S., Stranahan, S., and Pederson, C. (1988). Family intervention after stroke: does counseling or education help? *Stroke*, **19**, 1243–9.

Falkeborn, M., Persson, I., Terent, A., Adami, H.O., Lithell, H., and Bergstrom, R. (1993). Hormone replacement therapy and the risk of stroke. Follow-up of a population-based cohort in Sweden. *Archives of Internal Medicine*, **153**, 1201–9.

Farrell, B., Godwin, J., Richards, S., and Warlow, C. (1991). The United Kingdom transient ischaemic attack (UK-TIA) aspirin trial: final results. *Journal of Neurology, Neurosurgery and Psychiatry*, **54**, 1044–54.

Feigin, V.L., Wiebers, D.O., Nikitin, Y.P., O'Fallon, W.M., and Whisnant, J.P. (1995*a*). Stroke epidemiology in Novosibirsk, Russia: a population-based study. *Mayo Clinic Proceedings*, **70**, 847–52.

Feigin, V.L., Wiebers, D.O., Whisnant, J.P., and O'Fallon, W.M. (1995*b*). Stroke incidence and 30-day case-fatality rates in Novosibirsk, Russia, 1982 through 1992. *Stroke*, **26**, 924–9.

Feinberg, W.M., Seeger, J.F., Carmody, R.F., Anderson, D.C., Hart, R.G., and Pearce, L.A. (1990). Epidemiologic features of asymptomatic cerebral infarction in patients with nonvalvular atrial fibrillation. *Archives of Internal Medicine*, **150**, 2340–4.

Feys, H.M., de Weerdt, W.J., Selz, B.E., and Coxsteck, G.A. (1998). Effect of therapeutic intervention for the hemiplegic upper limb in the acute phase after stroke, a single blind randomised controlled multicentre trial. *Stroke*, **29**, 785–92.

Field, D., Cordle, C.J., and Bowman, G.S. (1983). Coping with stroke at home. *International Rehabilitation Medicine*, **5**, 96–100.

Fisher, C.M. (1982). Disorientation for place. *Archives of Neurology*, **39**, 33–6.

Fletcher, A.E. (1992). In *Measures of the quality of life and the uses to which such measures may be put*. (ed. A. Hopkins), p. 35. Royal College of Physicians, London.

Fogelholm, R., Murros, K., Rissanen, A., and Ilmavirta, M. (1996). Factors delaying hospital admission after acute stroke. *Stroke*, **27**, 398–400.

Folsom, A.R., Prineas, R.J., Kaye, S.A., and Munger, R.G. (1990). Incidence of hypertension and stroke in relation to body fat distribution and other risk factors in older women. *Stroke*, **21**, 701–6.

Folstein, M.F., Folstein, S.E., and McHugh, P.R. (1975). Mini-mental state. A practical method for grading the cognitive state of patients for the clinician. *Journal of Psychiatric Research*, **12**, 189–98.

Folstein, M.F., Maiberger, R., and McHugh, P.R. (1977). Mood disorder as a specific complication of stroke. *Journal of Neurology, Neurosurgery and Psychiatry*, **40**, 1018–20.

Forster, A. and Young, J. (1995). Incidence and consequences of falls due to stroke. A systematic enquiry. *British Medical Journal*, **311**, 83–6.

Forster, A. and Young, J. (1996). Specialist nurse support for patients with stroke in the community: a randomised controlled trial. *British Medical Journal*, **312**, 1642–6.

Franke, C.L., Palm, R., Dalby, M. *et al.* (1996). Flunarizine in stroke treatment (FIST): a double blind placebo controlled trial in Scandinavia and the Netherlands. *Acta Neurologica Scandinavica*, **93**, 56–60.

Frankel, S., Elwood, P., Sweetnam, P., Yarnell, J., and Davey Smith, G. (1996). Birthweight, body-mass index in middle age, and incident coronary heart disease. *Lancet*, **348**, 1478–80.

Frederico, F., Lucivero, V., Lamberti, P., Fiore, A., and Conte, C. (1991). A double blind randomised pilot trial of naloxone in the treatment of acute ischaemic stroke. *Italian Journal of Neurological Sciences*, **12**, 557–63.

Freeling, P., Rao, B.M., Paykel, E.S., Sireling, L.I., and Burton, R.H. (1985). Unrecognised depression in general practice. *British Medical Journal*, **290**, 1880–3.

Friedland, J.F. and McColl, M. (1992). Social support intervention after stroke: results of a randomized trial. *Archives of Physical Medicine and Rehabilitation*, **73**, 573–81.

Friedman, H.S. (1996). Tissue plasminogen activator for acute ischemic stroke. *New England Journal of Medicine*, **334**, 1405.

Friedman, R.C., Bigger, J.T., and Koranfield, D.S. (1971). The intern and sleep loss. *New England Journal of Medicine*, **285**, 201–3.

Frost, C.D., Law, M.R., and Wald, N.J. (1991). By how much does dietary salt reduction lower blood pressure? II–Analysis of observational data within populations. *British Medical Journal*, **302**, 815–18.

Fullerton, K.J., Mackenzie, G., and Stout, R.W. (1988). Prognostic indices in stroke. *Quarterly Journal of Medicine*, **66**, 147–62.

Gage, B.F., Cardinalli, A.B., Albers, G.W., and Owens, D.K. (1995). Cost-effectiveness of warfarin and aspirin for prophylaxis of stroke in patients with nonvalvular atrial fibrillation. *Journal of the American Medical Association*, **274**, 1839–45.

Gage, B.F., Cardinalli, A.B., and Owens, D.K. (1996). The effect of stroke and stroke prophylaxis with aspirin or warfarin on quality of life. *Archives of Internal Medicine*, **156**, 1829–36.

Gagne, P.J., Matchett, J., MacFarland, D. *et al.* (1996). Can the NASCET technique for measuring carotid stenosis be reliably applied outside the trial? *Journal of Vascular Surgery*, **24**, 449–55.

Gagnon, D.R., Zhang, T.J., Brand, F.N., and Kannel, W.B. (1994). Hematocrit and the risk of cardiovascular disease–the Framingham study: a 34-year follow-up. *American Heart Journal*, **127**, 674–82.

Gale, C.R. and Martyn, C.N. (1997). The conundrum of time trends in stroke. *Journal of the Royal Society of Medicine*, **90**, 138–43.

Gale, C.R., Martyn, C.N., Winter, P.D., and Cooper, C. (1995). Vitamin C and risk of death from stroke and coronary heart disease in a cohort of elderly people. *British Medical Journal*, **310**, 1563–6.

Garg, R.K., Nag, D., and Agrawal, A. (1995). A double blind placebo controlled trial of *Ginkgo biloba* extract in acute cerebral ischaemia. *Journal of the Association of Physicians of India*, **43**, 760–3.

Garraway, W.M. and Akhtar, A.J. (1978). Theory and practice of stroke rehabilitation. In

Recent advances in geriatric medicine, (ed. B. Isaacs), pp. 7–20. Churchill Livingstone, London.

Garraway, W.M., Akhtar, A.J., Gore, S.M., Prescott, R.J., and Smith, R.G. (1976). Observer variation in the clinical assessment of stroke. *Age and Ageing,* **5,** 233–40.

Garraway, W.M., Whisnant, J.P., Furlan, A.J., Phillips, L.H. 2d, Kurland, L.T., and O'Fallon, W.M. (1979). The declining incidence of stroke. *New England Journal of Medicine,* **300,** 449–52.

Garraway, W.M., Akhtar, A.J., Hockey, L., and Prescott, R.J. (1980a). Management of acute stroke in the elderly: follow-up of a controlled trial. *British Medical Journal,* **281,** 827–9.

Garraway, W.M., Akhtar, A.J., Prescott, R.J., and Hockey, L. (1980b). Management of acute stroke in the elderly: preliminary results of a controlled trial. *British Medical Journal,* **280,** 1040–3.

Garraway, W.M., Akhtar, A.J., Smith, D.L., and Smith, M.E. (1981). The triage of stroke rehabilitation. *Journal of Epidemiology and Community Health,* **35,** 39–44.

Garraway, W.M., Elverback, L.R., Connolly, D.C., and Whisnant, J.P. (1983). The changing pattern of survival following stroke. *Stroke,* **14,** 699–703.

Gelber, D.A., Good, D.C., Laven, L.J., and Verhulst, S.J. (1993). Causes of urinary incontinence after acute hemispheric stroke. *Stroke,* **24,** 378–82.

Gelmers, H.J., Gorter, K., de Weerdt, C.J., and Wiezer, H.J. (1988a). A controlled trial of nimodipine in acute stroke. *New England Journal of Medicine,* **318,** 203–7.

Gelmers, H.J., Gorter, K., de Weerdt, C.J., and Wiezer, H.J. (1988b). Assessment of interobserver variability in a Dutch multicenter study on acute ischemic stroke. *Stroke,* **19,** 709–11.

Gennser, G., Rymark, P., and Isberg, P.E. (1988). Low birth weight and risk of high blood pressure in adulthood. *British Medical Journal,* **296,** 1498–500.

Genton, E., Barnett, H., and Fields, W. (1977). Cerebral ischaemia: the role of thrombosis and antithrombotic treatment. *Stroke,* **8,** 150–75.

Gill, J.S., Zezulka, A.V., Shipley, M.J., Gill, S.K., and Beevers, D.G. (1986). Stroke and alcohol consumption. *New England Journal of Medicine,* **315,** 1041–6.

Gill, J.S., Shipley, M.J., Tsementzis, S.A. *et al.* (1989). Cigarette smoking. A risk factor for hemorrhagic and nonhemorrhagic stroke. *Archives of Internal Medicine,* **149,** 2053–7.

Gill, J.S., Shipley, M.J., Tsementzis, S.A., *et al.* (1991). Alcohol consumption–a risk factor for hemorrhagic and non-hemorrhagic stroke. *American Journal of Medicine,* **90,** 489–97.

Gillman, M.W., Cupples, L.A., Gagnon, D., *et al.* (1995). Protective effect of fruits and vegetables on development of stroke in men. *Journal of the American Medical Association,* **273,** 1113–17.

Gillum, R.F., Mussolino, M.E., and Ingram, D.D. (1996a). Physical activity and stroke incidence in women and men. The NHANES I Epidemiologic Follow-up Study. *American Journal of Epidemiology,* **143,** 860–9.

Gillum, R.F., Mussolino, M.E., and Madans, J.H. (1996b). The relationship between fish consumption and stroke incidence. The NHANES I Epidemiologic Follow-up Study (National Health and Nutrition Examination Survey). *Archives of Internal Medicine,* **156,** 537–42.

Gladman, J.R., Harwood, D.M., and Barer, D.H. (1992). Predicting the outcome of acute stroke: prospective evaluation of five multivariate models and comparison with simple methods. *Journal of Neurology, Neurosurgery and Psychiatry,* **55,** 347–51.

Gladman, J.R., Lincoln, N.B., and Barer, D.H. (1993). A randomised controlled trial of domiciliary and hospital-based rehabilitation for stroke patients after discharge from hospital. *Journal of Neurology, Neurosurgery and Psychiatry*, **56**, 960–6.

Glanz, M., Klawansky, S., Stason, W., Berkey, C., and Chalmers, T.C. (1996). Functional electrostimulation in poststroke rehabilitation: a meta-analysis of the randomized controlled trials. *Archives of Physical Medicine and Rehabilitation*, **77**, 549–53.

Glanz, M., Klawansky, S., and Chalmers, T. (1997). Biofeedback therapy in stroke rehabilitation: a review. *Journal of the Royal Society of Medicine*, **90**, 33–9.

Glass, R., Allan, A., Uheinhuth, E., Kimball, C., and Borinstein, D. (1978). Psychiatric screening in a medical clinic. *Archives of General Psychiatry*, **35**, 1189–95.

Glass, T.A. and Maddox, G.L. (1992). The quality and quantity of social support: stroke recovery as psycho-social transition. *Social Science and Medicine*, **34**, 1249–61.

Glass, T.A., Matchar, D.B., Belyea, M., and Feussner, J.R. (1993). Impact of social support on outcome in first stroke. *Stroke*, **24**, 64–70.

Goble, R.E.A. (1976). The relevence of the ADL index. *British Journal of Occupational Therapy*, **39**, 12.

Godlee, F. (1996). The food industry fights for salt. *British Medical Journal*, **312**, 1239–40.

Goggenmoos-Holzmann, I. (1993). How reliable are chance corrected measures of agreement? *Statistics in Medicine*, 12, 2191–205.

Gold, G., Giannakopoulos, P., Montes-Paixao Junior, C. *et al.* (1997). Sensitivity and specificity of newly proposed clinical criteria for possible vascular dementia. *Neurology*, **49**, 690–4.

Goldberg, D. and Hillier, V. (1979). A scaled version of the general health questionnaire. *Psychological Medicine*, **9**, 139–45.

Goldstein, L.B. and Samsa, G.P. (1997). Reliability of the National Institutes of Health Stroke Scale. Extension to non-neurologists in the context of a clinical trial. *Stroke*, **28**, 307–10.

Goldstein, L.B., Bertels, C., and Davis, J.N. (1989). Interrater reliability of the NIH stroke scale. *Archives of Neurology*, **46**, 660–2.

Gompertz, P., Pound, P., and Ebrahim, S. (1993). The reliability of stroke outcome measures. *Clinical Rehabilitation*, **7**, 290–6.

Gompertz, P., Dennis, M., Hopkins, A., and Ebrahim, S. (1994a). Development and reliability of the Royal College of Physicians stroke audit form. UK Stroke Audit Group. *Age and Ageing*, **23**, 378–83.

Gompertz, P., Pound, P., and Ebrahim, S. (1994b). Predicting stroke outcome: Guy's prognostic score in practice. *Journal of Neurology, Neurosurgery and Psychiatry*, **57**, 932–35.

Gompertz, P., Pound, P., Briffa, J., and Ebrahim, S. (1995). How useful are non-random comparisons of outcomes and quality of care in purchasing hospital stroke services? *Age and Ageing*, **24**, 137–41.

Gong, L., Zhang, W., Zhu, Y., *et al.* (1996). Shanghai trial of nifedipine in the elderly (STONE). *Journal of Hypertension*, **14**, 1237–45.

Goodwill, C.J. and Chamberlain, M.A. (1988). *Rehabilitation of the physically disabled adult.* Croom Helm, London.

Gordon, C., Hewer, R.L., and Wade, D.T. (1987). Dysphagia in acute stroke. *British Medical Journal*, **295**, 411–14.

Gordon, D.L., Bendixen, B.H., Adams, H.P. Jr, Clarke, W., Kappelle, L.J., and Woolson, R.F. (1993). Interphysician agreement in the diagnosis of subtypes of acute ischemic stroke: implications for clinical trials. The TOAST Investigators. *Neurology*, **43**, 1021–7.

Gorelick, P.B. (1989). The status of alcohol as a risk factor for stroke. *Stroke*, **20**, 1607–10.

Graffagnino, C., Gasecki, A.P., Doig, G.S., and Hachinski, V.C. (1994). The importance of family history in cerebrovascular disease. *Stroke*, **25**, 1599–604.

Grau, A.J., Buggle, F., Heindl, S. *et al.* (1995). Recent infection as a risk factor for cerebrovascular ischemia. *Stroke*, **26**, 373–9.

Gray, C.S., French, J.M., Bates, D., Cartlidge, N.E., Venables, G.S., and James, O.F. (1989). Recovery of visual fields in acute stroke: homonymous hemianopia associated with adverse prognosis. *Age and Ageing*, **18**, 419–21.

Gray, C.S., French, J.M., Bates, D., Cartlidge, N.E., James, O.F., and Venables, G. (1990). Motor recovery following acute stroke. *Age and Ageing*, **19**, 179–84.

Greener, J., Enderby, P., and Whurr, R. (1998) . Speech and language therapy for aphasia following stroke (Cochrane review). In *Cochrane database of systematic reviews (disc and CD-ROM). Stroke module*, (ed. C.P. Warlow, J. van Gijn, and P.A.G. Sandercock). Update Software/BMJ Publishing, Oxford.

Gresham, G.E., Fitzpatrick, T.E., Wolf, P.A. *et al.* (1975). Residual disability in survivors of stroke: the Framingham Study. *New England Journal of Medicine*, **293**, 954–6.

Gresham, G.E., Phillips, T.F., Wolf, P.A. *et al.* (1979). Epidemiological profile of long term stroke disability. The Framingham study. *Archives of Physical Medicine and Rehabilitation*, **60**, 487–90.

Gresham, G.E., Phillips, T.F., and Labi, M.L.C. (1980). ADL status in stroke: relative merits of three standard indexes. *Archives of Physical Medicine and Rehabilitation*, **61**, 355–8.

Greveson, G.C. and James, O.F.W. (1991). Improving long term outcome after stroke: the views of patients and carers. *Health Trends*, **23**, 161–2.

Greveson, G.C., Gray, C.S., French, J.M., and James, O.F. (1991). Long-term outcome for patients and carers following hospital admission for stroke. *Age and Ageing*, **20**, 337–44.

Gross, C.R., Shinar, D., Mohr, J.P. *et al.* (1986). Interobserver agreement in the diagnosis of stroke type. *Archives of Neurology*, **43**, 893–8.

Grotta, J. (1997). Lubeluzole treatment of acute ischaemic stroke. The US and Canadian Lubeluzole Ischaemic Stroke Study group. *Stroke*, **28**, 2338–46.

Grotta, J., Clark, W., Coull, B. *et al.* (1995). Safety and tolerability of the glutamate antagonist CGS 19755 (Selfotel) in patients with acute ischaemic stroke. Results of a phase IIa randomised trial. *Stroke*, **26**, 602–5.

Grover, S., Gray-Donald, K., Joseph, L., and Abrahamowicz, M. (1994). Life expectancy following dietary modifications or smoking cessation. Estimating the benefits of a prudent life style. *Archives of Internal Medicine*, **154**, 1697–704.

Gurling, H.M.D. (1984). Genetic epidemiology in medicine: recent twin research. *British Medical Journal*, **288**, 3–5.

Gustafsson, C., Asplund, K., Britton, M., Norrving, B., Olsson, B., and Marke, L.A. (1992). Cost effectiveness of primary stroke prevention in atrial fibrillation: Swedish national perspective. *British Medical Journal*, **305**, 1457–60.

Guyatt, G., Sackett, D., and Taylor, D.W. (1986). Determining optimal therapy: randomised trials in individual patients. *New England Journal of Medicine*, **314**, 889–92.

Haberman, S., Capildeo, R., and Rose, F.C. (1978). The changing mortality of cerebrovascular disease. *Quarterly Journal of Medicine*, **47**, 71–88.

Haberman, S., Capildeo, R., and Rose, F.C. (1981). The seasonal variation in mortality from cerebrovascular disease. *Journal of Neurological Science*, **52**, 25–36.

Haberman, S., Capildeo, R., and Rose, F.C. (1982). Diverging trends in cerebrovascular disease and ischaemic heart disease mortality. *Stroke*, **13**, 582–9.

Hachinski, V.S., Cliff, L.D., Zilkha, E. *et al.* (1975). Cerebral blood flow in dementia. *Archives of Neurology*, **32**, 632–7.

Hacke, W., Kaste, M., Fieschi, C. *et al.* (1995). Intravenous thrombolysis with recombinant tissue plasminogen activator for acute hemispheric stroke. The European Cooperative Acute Stroke Study (ECASS). *Journal of the American Medical Association*, **274**, 1017–25.

Hacke, W., Kaste, M., Fieschi, C. *et al.* (1998). Randomised double blind placebo controlled trial of thrombolytic therapy with intravenous alteplase in acute ischaemic stroke (ECASS-II). *Lancet* **352**:1245-51

Haerer, A.F., Gotshall, R.A., Conneally, P.M. *et al.* (1977). Cooperative study of hospital frequency and character of transient ischaemic attacks. *Journal of the American Medical Association*, **238**, 142–6.

Haheim, L.L., Holme, I., Hjermann, I., and Leren, P. (1996). Smoking habits and risk of fatal stroke: 18 years follow up of the Oslo Study. *Journal of Epidemiology and Community Health*, **50**, 621–4.

Haley, E.C., Alves, W., Kassell, N.F. *et al.* (1996). A randomised trial of tirilazad mesylate in patients with acute stroke (RANTTAS). *Stroke*, **27**, 1453–8.

Hampton, J. (1981). Presentation and analysis of the results of clinical trials in cardiovascular disease. *British Medical Journal*, **282**, 1371–3.

Hankey, G.J. and Warlow, C.P. (1990). Symptomatic carotid ischaemic events: safest and most cost effective way of selecting patients for angiography, before carotid endarterectomy. *British Medical Journal*, **300**, 1485–91.

Hankey, G.J., Warlow, C.P., and Molyneux, A.J. (1990*a*). Complications of cerebral angiography for patients with mild carotid territory ischaemia being considered for carotid endarterectomy. *Journal of Neurology, Neurosurgery and Psychiatry*, **53**, 542–8.

Hankey, G.J., Warlow, C.P., and Sellar, R.J. (1990*b*). Cerebral angiographic risk in mild cerebrovascular disease. *Stroke*, **21**, 209–22.

Hankey, G.J., Slattery, J.M., and Warlow, C.P. (1991). The prognosis of hospital-referred transient ischaemic attacks. *Journal of Neurology, Neurosurgery and Psychiatry*, **54**, 793–802.

Hankey, G.J., Slattery, J.M., and Warlow, C.P. (1992). Transient ischaemic attacks: which patients are at high (and low) risk of serious vascular events? *Journal of Neurology, Neurosurgery and Psychiatry*, **55**, 640–52.

Hankey, G.J., Dennis, M.S., Slattery, J.M., and Warlow, C.P. (1993*a*). Why is the outcome of transient ischaemic attacks different in different groups of patients? *British Medical Journal*, **306**, 1107–11.

Hankey, G.J., Slattery, J.M., and Warlow, C.P. (1993*b*). Can the long term outcome of individual patients with transient ischaemic attacks be predicted accurately? *Journal of Neurology, Neurosurgery and Psychiatry*, **56**, 752–9.

Hanley, S., Bevan, J., Cockbill, S., and Heptinstall, S. (1981). Differential inhibition of low dose aspirin of human venous prostacyclin synthesis and platelet thromboxane synthesis. *Lancet*, **i**, 969–71.

Hanlon, R.E. (1996). Motor learning following unilateral stroke. *Archives of Physical Medicine and Rehabilitation*, **77**, 811–15.

Hannaford, P.C., Croft, P.R., and Kay, C.R. (1994). Oral contraception and stroke. Evidence from the Royal College of General Practitioners' Oral Contraception Study. *Stroke*, **25**, 935–42.

Hanneman, R. (1996). Intersalt: hypertension risk with age revisited. *British Medical Journal*, **312**, 1283–4.

Hansagi, H., Romelsjo, A., Gerhardsson de Verdier, M., Andreasson, S., and Leifman, A. (1995). Alcohol consumption and stroke mortality. 20-year follow-up of 15,077 men and women. *Stroke*, **26**, 1768–73.

Hansson, L. (1998). Effects of intensive blood pressure lowering and low dose aspirin in patients with hypertension. Principal results of the Hypertension Optimal Treatment (HOT) randomised trial. *Lancet*, **351**, 1755–62.

Hantson, L., De Weerdt, W., De Keyser, J. *et al.* (1994). The European Stroke Scale. *Stroke*, **25**, 2215–19.

Harmsen, P. and Wilhelmsen, L. (1984). Stroke registration in Goteberg, Sweden,1971–5. Clinical profile and prognosis. *Acta Medica Scandinavica*, **215**, 239–48.

Harmsen, P., Rosengren, A., Tsipogianni, A., and Wilhelmsen, L. (1990). Risk factors for stroke in middle-aged men in Goteborg, Sweden. *Stroke*, **21**, 223–9.

Harmsen, P., Tsipogianni, A., and Wilhelmsen, L. (1992). Stroke incidence rates were unchanged, while fatality rates declined, during 1971–1987 in Goteborg, Sweden. *Stroke*, **23**, 1410–15.

Harper, G.D., Haigh, R.A., Potter, J.F., and Castleden, C.M. (1992). Factors delaying hospital admission after stroke in Leicestershire. *Stroke*, **23**, 835–8.

Harrison, M.J.G. (1980). Clinical distinction of cerebral haemorrhage and infarction. *Postgraduate Medical Journal*, **56**, 629–32.

Hart, R.G. and Harrison, M.J. (1996). Aspirin wars: the optimal dose of aspirin to prevent stroke. *Stroke*, **27**, 585–7.

Hart, R.G., Boop, B.S., and Anderson, D.C. (1995). Oral anticoagulants and intracranial hemorrhage. Facts and hypotheses. *Stroke*, **26**, 1471–7.

Harvey, R.L., Roth, E.J., Yarnold, P.R., Durham, J.R., and Green, D. (1996). Deep vein thrombosis in stroke. The use of plasma D-dimer level as a screening test in the rehabilitation setting. *Stroke*, **27**, 1516–20.

Harwood, R.H. and Ebrahim, S. (1995). *Manual of the London Handicap Scale*. University of Nottingham, Nottingham.

Harwood, R.H., Gompertz, P., and Ebrahim, S. (1994a). Handicap one year after a stroke: validity of a new scale. *Journal of Neurology, Neurosurgery and Psychiatry*, **57**, 825–9.

Harwood, R.H., Jitapunkul, S., Dickinson, E., and Ebrahim, S. (1994b). Measuring handicap: motives, methods and a model. *Quality in Health Care*, **3**, 53–7.

Harwood, R.H., Rogers, A., Dickinson, E., and Ebrahim, S. (1994c). Measuring handicap: the London Handicap Scale, a new outcome measure for chronic disease. *Quality in Health Care*, **3**, 11–16.

Harwood, R.H., Gompertz, P., Pound, P., and Ebrahim, S. (1997). Determinants of handicap 1 and 3 years after a stroke. *Disability and Rehabilitation*, **19**, 205–11.

Harwood, R.H., Prince, M., Mann, A., and Ebrahim, S. (1998). Associations between diagnoses, impairments, disability and handicap in a population of elderly people. *International Journal of Epidemiology*, **27**, 261–8.

Hatano, S., Shigematsu, I. and Strasser, T. (1976). *Hypertension and stroke control in the community*. World Health Organization, Geneva.

Havlik, R.J., Garrison, R.J., Feinleb, M. *et al.* (1979). Blood pressure aggregation in families. *American Journal of Epidemiology*, **110**, 304–12.

Hawton, K. (1981). The long term outcome of psychiatric morbidity detected in general medical patients. *Journal of Psychosomatic Research*, **25**, 237–43.

Haynes, R.B., Taylor, D.W., Sackett, D.L., Thorpe, K., Ferguson, G.G., and Barnett, H.J. (1994). Prevention of functional impairment by endarterectomy for symptomatic high-grade carotid stenosis. North American Symptomatic Carotid Endarterectomy Trial Collaborators. *Journal of the American Medical Association*, **271**, 1256–9.

Heasman, M.A. and Lipworth, L. (1966). Accuracy of certification of cause of death. In *Studies on medical and population subjects*, No. 20, pp. 23–24. HMSO, London.

Heinemann, L.A.J., Lewis, M.A., Thorogood, M., Spitzer, W.O. *et al.* (1996). Case control study of oral contraceptives and risk of thrombo embolic stroke: results from international study. *British Medical Journal*, **315**, 1502–4.

Heiss, W.D. and Graf, R. (1994). The ischemic penumbra. *Current Opinion in Neurology*, **7**, 11–19.

Helgason, C.M. (1988). Blood glucose and stroke. *Stroke*, **19**, 1049–53.

Henley, S., Pettit, S., Todd-Pokropek, A., and Tupper, A. (1985). Who goes home? Predictive factors in stroke recovery. *Journal of Neurology, Neurosurgery and Psychiatry*, **48**, 1–6.

Hennekens, C.H. and Buring, J.E. (1987). *Epidemiology in Medicine*. Little Brown, Boston.

Herderschee, D., Hijdra, A., Algra, A., Koudstaal, P.J., Kappelle, L.J., and van Gijn, J. (1992). Silent stroke in patients with transient ischemic attack or minor ischemic stroke. The Dutch TIA Trial Study Group. *Stroke*, **23**, 1220–4.

Herman, B., Schulte, B.P.M., Van Luijk, J.H., and Leyten, A.C.M. (1980). Epidemiology of stroke in Tilberg, The Netherlands. The population-based stroke incidence register. 1. Introduction and preliminary results. *Stroke*, **11**, 162–5.

Herman, B., Leyten, A.C.M., Van Luijk, J.H. *et al.* (1982a). Epidemiology of stroke in Tilberg, The Netherlands. The population based stroke incidence register: 2. Incidence, initial clinical picture and medical care, and three week case fatality. *Stroke*, **13**, 629–34.

Herman, B., Leyten, A.C.M., Van Luijk, J.H. *et al.* (1982b). An evaluation of risk factors for stroke in a Dutch Community. *Stroke*, **13**, 334–9.

Hertanu, J.S., Demopoulos, J.T., Yang, W.L. *et al.* (1984). Stroke rehabilitation: correlation and prognostic value of computerised tomography and sequential functional assessments. *Archives of Physical Medicine and Rehabilitation*, **65**, 505–8.

Hewer, R.L. (1973). Stroke rehabilitation: some current problems. *Proceedings of the Royal Society of Medicine*, **66**, 882–4.

Hewer, R.L. (1987). Dysphagia after stroke. *British Medical Journal*, **295**, 1137.

Heyman, A., Wilkinson, E.E., Hurvitz, B.J. *et al.* (1984). Risk of ischaemic heart disease in patients with TIA. *Neurology*, **34**, 626–30.

Hier, D.B., Foulkes, M.A., Swiontoniowski, M. *et al.* (1991). Stroke recurrence within 2 years after ischemic infarction. *Stroke*, **22**, 155–61.

Hill, A.B. (1965). The environment and disease: association or causation. *Proceedings of the Royal Society of Medicine*, **58**, 295–300.

Hill, A.B., Marshall, J., and Shaw, D. (1962). Cerebrovascular disease: trial of long term anticoagulant therapy. *British Medical Journal*, **2**, 1003–5.

Hilton, P. and Stanton, S. (1981). Algorithmic method for assessing urinary incontinence in elderly women. *British Medical Journal*, **282**, 940–2.

Hirsch, J.A., Langlotz, C.P., Lee, J., Tanio, C.P., Grossman, R.I., and Schulman, K.A. (1996). Clinical assessment of MR of the brain in nonsurgical inpatients. *American Journal of Neuroradiology*, **17**, 1245–53.

Hobson, R.W., Weiss, D.G., Fields, W.S. *et al.* (1993). Efficacy of carotid endarterectomy for asymptomatic carotid stenosis. The Veterans Affairs Cooperative Study Group. *New*

England Journal of Medicine, **328**, 221–7.

Hodkinson, H.M. (1972). Evaluation of a mental test score for assessment of mental impairment in the elderly. *Age and Ageing*, **1**, 233–8.

Holmqvist, L.W., Von Koch, L., Kostulas, V., and Holm, M. (1998). A randomised controlled trial of rehabilitation at home after stroke in South West Stockholm. *Stroke*, **29**, 591–7.

Homer, D., Whisnant, J.P., and Schoenberg, B.S. (1987). Trends in the incidence rates of stroke in Rochester, Minnesota, since 1935. *Annals of Neurology*, **22**, 245–51.

Homocysteine Lowering Trialists Collaboration (1998). Lowering blood homocysteine with folic acid based supplements. Meta-analysis of randomised trials. *British Medical Journal*, **316**, 894–8.

Hopkins, A. (1975). The need for speech therapy for dysphasia following stroke. *Health Trends*, **7**, 58–60.

House, A. (1987*a*). Depression after stroke. *British Medical Journal*, **294**, 76–8.

House, A. (1987*b*). Mood disorders after stroke: a review of the evidence. *International Journal of Geriatric Psychiatry*, **2**, 211–21.

House, A. and Ebrahim, S. (1991). Psychological aspects of physical disease. In *Psychiatry in the Elderly*, (ed. R. Jacoby and C. Oppenheimer), pp. 437–60. Oxford University Press, Oxford.

House, A., Dennis, M., Hawton, K., and Warlow, C. (1989*a*). Methods of identifying mood disorders in stroke patients: experience in the Oxfordshire Community Stroke Project. *Age and Ageing*, **18**, 371–9.

House, A., Dennis, M., Molyneux, A., Warlow, C., and Hawton, K. (1989*b*). Emotionalism after stroke. *British Medical Journal*, **298**, 991–4.

House, A., Dennis, M., Mogridge, L., Hawton, K., and Warlow, C. (1990*a*). Life events and difficulties preceding stroke. *Journal of Neurology, Neurosurgery and Psychiatry*, **53**, 1024–8.

House, A., Dennis, M., Warlow, C., Hawton, K., and Molyneux, A. (1990*b*). Mood disorders after stroke and their relation to lesion location. A CT scan study. *Brain*, **113**, 1113–29.

House, A., Dennis, M., Warlow, C., Hawton, K., and Molyneux, A. (1990*c*). The relationship between intellectual impairment and mood disorder in the first year after stroke. *Psychological Medicine*, **20**, 805–14.

House, A., Dennis, M., Mogridge, L., Warlow, C., Hawton, K., and Jones, L. (1991). Mood disorders in the year after first stroke. *British Journal of Psychiatry*, **158**, 83–92.

Howard, D. (1984). Speech therapy for aphasic stroke patients. *Lancet*, **i**, 1413–14.

Howard, G., Russell, G.B., Anderson, R. *et al.* (1995). Role of social class in excess black stroke mortality. *Stroke*, **26**, 1759–63.

Hulley, S., Grady, D., Bush, T. *et al.* (1998). Randomised trial of estrogen plus progestin for secondary prevention of coronary heart disease in postmenopausal women. *Journal of the American Medical Association*, **280**, 605–13.

Hunt, S.M., McEwan, J., and McKenna, S.P. (1986). *Measuring health status*. Croom Helm, London.

Hurwitz, L.J. and Adams, G.F. (1972). Rehabilitation of hemiplegia: indices of assessment and prognosis. *British Medical Journal*, **1**, 94–8.

Hypertension Stroke Co-operative Study Group (1974). Effects of antihypertensive treatment on stroke recurrence. *Journal of the American Medical Association*, **229**, 409–18.

Indredavik, B., Bakke, F., Solberg, R., Rokseth, R., Haaheim, L.L., and Holme, I. (1991). Benefit of a stroke unit: a randomized controlled trial. *Stroke*, **22**, 1026–31.

Indredavik, B., Bakke, F., Slovdahl, S.A., Rokseth, R., and Haheim, L.L. (1998). Stroke Unit treatment improves long term quality of life. A randomised controlled trial. *Stroke*, **29**, 895–9.

INJECT Group (1995). Randomised, double-blind comparison of reteplase double-bolus administration with streptokinase in acute myocardial infarction (INJECT): trial to investigate equivalence. International Joint Efficacy Comparison of Thrombolytics. *Lancet*, **346**, 329–36.

International Stroke Trial Collaborative Group (1997). The International Stroke Trial (IST): a randomised trial of aspirin, subcutaneous heparin, both, or neither among 19435 patients with acute ischaemic stroke. *Lancet*, **349**, 1569–81.

Intersalt Cooperative Research Group (1988). Intersalt: an international study of electrolyte excretion and blood pressure. Results for 24 hour urinary sodium and potassium excretion. *British Medical Journal*, **297**, 319–28.

Iribarren, C., Reed, D.M., Burchfiel, C.M., and Dwyer, J.H. (1995). Serum total cholesterol and mortality. Confounding factors and risk modification in Japanese-American men. *Journal of the American Medical Association*, **273**, 1926–32.

Isaacs, B. and Marks, R. (1973). Determinants of outcome of stroke rehabilitation. *Age and Ageing*, **2**, 139–49.

Isaacs, B., Neville, Y., and Rushford, I. (1976). The stricken: the social consequenses of stroke. *Age and Ageing*, **5**, 188–92.

Isard, P.A. and Forbes, J.F. (1992). Cost of stroke to the National Health Service in Scotland. *Cerebrovascular Diseases*, **2**, 47–50.

ISIS-4 Collaborative Group (1995). ISIS-4: a randomised controlled trial assessing early oral captopril, oral mononitrate, and intravenous magnesium sulphate in 58,050 patients with suspected acute myocardial infarction. *Lancet*, **345**, 669–85.

Iso, H., Jacobs, D.R. Jr, Wentworth, D., Neaton, J.D., and Cohen, J.D. (1989). Serum cholesterol levels and six-year mortality from stroke in 350,977 men screened for the multiple risk factor intervention trial. *New England Journal of Medicine*, **320**, 904–10.

Italian Acute Stroke Study Group (1988). Hemodilution in acute stroke: results of the Italian haemodilution trial. *Lancet*, **i**, 318–21.

Jakovljevic, D., Salomaa, V., Sivenius, J. *et al.* (1996). Seasonal variation in the occurrence of stroke in a Finnish adult population. The FINMONICA Stroke Register. Finnish Monitoring Trends and Determinants in Cardiovascular Disease. *Stroke*, **27**, 1774–9.

James, W.P., Ralph, A., and Sanchez-Castillo, C.P. (1987). The dominance of salt in manufactured food in the sodium intake of affluent societies. *Lancet*, **i**, 426–9.

Jamrozik, K., Broadhurst, R.J., Anderson, C.S., and Stewart-Wynne, E.G. (1994). The role of lifestyle factors in the etiology of stroke. A population-based case-control study in Perth, Western Australia. *Stroke*, **25**, 51–9.

Jansen, P., Gribnau, F., Schulte, B., and Poels, E. (1986*a*). Contribution of inappropriate treatment for hypertension to pathogenesis of stroke in the elderly. *British Medical Journal*, **293**, 914–17.

Jansen, P., Schulte, B., Meyboom, R., and Gribnau, F. (1986*b*). Antihypertensive treatment as a possible cause of strokes in the elderly. *Age and Ageing*, **15**, 129–38.

Jarvik, L.F. and Matsuyama, S.S. (1983). Parental stroke: risk factor for multi-infarct dementia? *Lancet*, **ii**, 1025.

Jay, P. (1976). How the Association sought a standard way to record assessment. *British*

Journal of Occupational Therapy, **39**, 36.

Jha, P., Flather, M., Lonn, E., Farkouh, M., and Yusuf, S. (1995). The antioxidant vitamins and cardiovascular disease. A critical review of epidemiologic and clinical trial data. *Annals of Internal Medicine*, **123**, 860–72.

Johansson, B.B. and Grabowski, M. (1994). Functional recovery after brain infarction: plasticity and neural transplantation. *Brain Pathology*, **4**, 85–95.

Johansson, K., Lindgren, I., Widner, H., Wiklund, I., and Johansson, B.B. (1993). Can sensory stimulation improve the functional outcome in stroke patients? *Neurology*, **43**, 2189–92.

Johnston, J., Beevers, G., Dunn, F., Larkin, H., and Titterington, D. (1981). The importance of good blood pressure control in the prevention of stroke recurrence in hypertensive patients. *Postgraduate Medical Journal*, **57**, 690–3.

Johnston, K.C., Li, J.Y., Lynden, P.D., Hanson, S.K., Feasby, T.E. *et al.* (1998). Medical and neurological complications of ischaemic stroke. *Stroke*, **29**, 447.

Jonas, S. (1988). Anticoagulant therapy in cerebrovascular disease: review and meta-analysis. *Stroke*, **19**, 1043–8. [See erratum in *Stroke* (1989), **20**, 562.]

Jones, D. and Vetter, N.J. (1985). Formal and informal support received by carers of elderly dependents. *British Medical Journal*, **291**, 643–5.

Joosens, J.V., Kestelloot, H., and Amery, A. (1979). Salt intake and mortality from stroke. *New England Journal of Medicine*, **300**, 1396.

Jorgensen, H.S., Plesner, A.M., Hubbe, P., and Larsen, K. (1992). Marked increase of stroke incidence in men between 1972 and 1990 in Frederiksberg, Denmark. *Stroke*, **23**, 1701–4.

Jorgensen, H.S., Nakayama, H., Raaschou, H.O., Gam, J., and Olsen, T.S. (1994). Silent infarction in acute stroke patients. Prevalence, localization, risk factors, and clinical significance: the Copenhagen Stroke Study . *Stroke*, **25**, 97–104.

Jorgensen, H.S., Nakayama, H., Raaschou, H.O., and Olsen, T.S. (1995*a*). Recovery of walking function in stroke patients: the Copenhagen Stroke Study. *Archives of Physical Medicine and Rehabilitation*, **76**, 27–32.

Jorgensen, H.S., Nakayama, H., Raaschou, H.O., Vive-Larsen, J., Stoier, M., and Olsen, T.S. (1995*b*). Outcome and time course of recovery in stroke. Part I: Outcome. The Copenhagen Stroke Study. *Archives of Physical Medicine and Rehabilitation*, **76**, 399–405.

Jorgensen, H.S., Nakayama, H., Raaschou, H.O., Vive-Larsen, J., Stoier, M., and Olsen, T.S. (1995*c*). Outcome and time course of recovery in stroke. Part II: Time course of recovery. The Copenhagen Stroke Study. *Archives of Physical Medicine and Rehabilitation*, **76**, 406–12.

Jorgensen, H.S., Nakayama, H., Reith, J., Raaschou, H.O., and Olsen, T.S. (1996). Factors delaying hospital admission in acute stroke: the Copenhagen Stroke Study. *Neurology*, **47**, 383–7.

Jorgensen, H.S., Nakayama, H., Reith, J., Raaschou, H.O., and Olsen, T.S. (1997). Stroke recurrence: predictors, severity, and prognosis. The Copenhagen Stroke Study. *Neurology*, **48**, 891–5.

Jousilahti, P., Rastenyte, D., Tuomilehto, J., Sarti, C., and Vartiainen, E. (1997). Parental history of cardiovascular disease and risk of stroke. A prospective follow-up of 14371 middle-aged men and women in Finland. *Stroke*, **28**, 1361–6.

Juby, L.C., Lincoln, N.B., and Berman, P. (1996). The effect of a stroke rehabilitation unit on functional and psychological outcomes: a randomised controlled trial.

Cerebrovascular Diseases, **6**, 106–10.

Juvela, S., Hillbom, M., and Palomaki, H. (1995). Risk factors for spontaneous intracerebral hemorrhage. *Stroke*, **26**, 1558–64.

Kagan, A., Yano, K., Rhoads, G. *et al.* (1979). Is the reported high mortality from cerebrovascular disease in Japan really an artefact? *Journal of Chronic Diseases*, **32**, 153–6.

Kalra, L. (1994a). The influence of stroke unit rehabilitation on functional recovery from stroke. *Stroke*, **25**, 821–5.

Kalra, L. (1994b). Does age affect benefits of stroke unit rehabilitation? *Stroke*, **25**, 346–51.

Kalra, L. and Eade, J. (1995). Role of stroke rehabilitation units in managing severe disability after stroke. *Stroke*, **26**, 2031–4.

Kalra, L., Dale, P., and Crome, P. (1993a). Improving stroke rehabilitation. A controlled study. *Stroke*, **24**, 1462–7.

Kalra, L., Smith, D.H., and Crome, P. (1993b). Stroke in patients aged over 75 years: outcome and predictors. *Postgraduate Medical Journal*, **69**, 33–6.

Kalra, L., Yu, G., Wilson, K., and Roots, P. (1995). Medical complications during stroke rehabilitation. *Stroke*, **26**, 990–4.

Kalra, L., Perez, I., Gupta, S., and Wittink, M. (1997). The influence of visual neglect on stroke rehabilitation. *Stroke*, **28**, 1386–91.

Kannel, W.B., Wolf, P.A., and Verter, J. (1983). Manifestations of coronary disease predisposing to stroke. The Framingham study. *Journal of the American Medical Association*, **250**, 2942–6.

Kannel, W.B., Wolf, P.A., Castelli, W.P., and D'Agostino, R.B. (1987). Fibrinogen and risk of cardiovascular disease. The Framingham Study. *Journal of the American Medical Association*, **258**, 1183–6.

Kaplan, R.M., Bush, J.W., and Berry, C.C. (1976). Health status: types of validity and the index of well-being. *Health Services Research*, **11**, 478–507.

Kappelle, L.J., van Latum, J.C., Van Swieten, J.C., Algra, A., Koudstaal, P.J., and van Gijn, J. (1995). Recurrent stroke after transient ischaemic attack or minor ischaemic stroke: does the distinction between small and large vessel disease remain true to type? Dutch TIA Trial Study Group. *Journal of Neurology, Neurosurgery and Psychiatry*, **59**, 127–31.

Kaste, M., Palomaki, H., and Sarna, S. (1995). Where and how should elderly stroke patients be treated? A randomized trial. *Stroke*, **26**, 249–53.

Kawachi, I., Colditz, G.A., Stampfer, M.J. *et al.* (1993). Smoking cessation and decreased risk of stroke in women. *Journal of the American Medical Association*, **269**, 232–6.

Kawamata, T., Speliotes, E.K., and Finklestein, S.P. (1997). The role of polypeptide growth factors in recovery from stroke. *Advances in Neurology*, **73**, 377–82.

Keatinge, W.R. (1986). Seasonal mortality among elderly people with unrestricted home heating. *British Medical Journal*, **293**, 732–3.

Keatinge, W.R., Coleshaw, S.R.K., Cotter, F., Mattock, M., Murphy, M., and Chelliah, R. (1984). Increases in platelet and red cell counts, blood viscosity, and arterial pressure during mild surface cooling: factors in mortality from coronary and cerebral thrombosis in winter. *British Medical Journal*, **289**, 1405–8.

Keith, R.A. and Cowell, K.S. (1987). Time use of stroke patients in three rehabilitation hospitals. *Social Science and Medicine*, **24**, 529–33.

Keli, S., Bloemberg, B., and Kromhout, D. (1992). Predictive value of repeated systolic blood pressure measurements for stroke risk. The Zutphen Study. *Stroke*, **23**, 347–51.

Keli, S.O., Feskens, E.J., and Kromhout, D. (1994). Fish consumption and risk of stroke. The Zutphen Study. *Stroke*, **25**, 328–32.

Keli, S.O., Hertog, M.G., Feskens, E.J., and Kromhout, D. (1996). Dietary flavonoids, antioxidant vitamins, and incidence of stroke: the Zutphen study. *Archives of Internal Medicine*, **156**, 637–42.

Kelly-Hayes, M., Wolf, P.A., Kase, C.S., Brand, F.N., McGuirk, J.M., and D'Agostino, R.B. (1995). Temporal patterns of stroke onset. The Framingham Study. *Stroke*, **26**, 1343–7.

Kelman, H.R. and Willner, A. (1962). Problems of measurement and evaluation in rehabilitation. *Archives of Physical Medicine and Rehabilitation*, **4**, 172–81.

Kent, K.C., Kuntz, K.M., Patel, M.R. *et al.* (1995). Perioperative imaging strategies for carotid endarterectomy. An analysis of morbidity and cost-effectiveness in symptomatic patients. *Journal of the American Medical Association*, **274**, 888–93.

Kenton, A.R., Martin, P.J., Abbott, R.J., and Moody, A.R. (1997). Comparison of transcranial color-coded sonography and magnetic resonance angiography in acute stroke. *Stroke*, **28**, 1601–6.

Kertesz, A., Black, S.E., Nicholson, L., and Carr, T. (1987). The sensitivity and specificity of MRI in stroke. *Neurology*, **37**, 1580–5.

Khaw, K.T. (1996). Epidemiology of stroke. *Journal of Neurology, Neurosurgery and Psychiatry*, **61**, 333–8.

Khaw, K.T. and Barrett-Connor, E. (1986). Family history of stroke as an independent predictor of ischaemic heart disease in men and stroke in women. *American Journal of Epidemiology*, **123**, 59–66.

Khaw, K.T. and Barrett-Connor, E. (1987). Dietary potassium and stroke-associated mortality. A 12-year prospective population study. *New England Journal of Medicine*, **316**, 235–40.

Khaw, K.T. and Woodhouse, P. (1995). Interrelation of vitamin C, infection, haemostatic factors, and cardiovascular disease. *British Medical Journal*, **310**, 1559–63.

Kidd, D., Lawson, J., Nesbitt, R., and MacMahon, J. (1995). The natural history and clinical consequences of aspiration in acute stroke. *Quarterly Journal of Medicine*, **88**, 409–13.

Kiely, D.K., Wolf, P.A., Cupples, L.A., Beiser, A.S., and Myers, R.H. (1993). Familial aggregation of stroke. The Framingham Study. *Stroke*, **24**, 1366–71.

Kiely, D.K., Wolf, P.A., Cupples, L.A., Beiser, A.S., and Kannel, W.B. (1994). Physical activity and stroke risk: the Framingham Study. *American Journal of Epidemiology*, **140**, 608–20. [See erratum in *Am. J. Epidemiol.* (1995), **141**, 178.]

King, R.B. (1996). Quality of life after stroke. *Stroke*, **27**, 1467–72.

Kinsella, G. and Ford, B. (1985). Hemi-inattention and the recovery patterns of stroke patients. *International Rehabilitation Medicine*, **7**, 102–6.

Kirkwood, B.R. (1988). *Essentials of medical statistics*. Blackwell Scientific, Oxford.

Kittner, S.J., Stern, B.J., Feeser, B.R. *et al.* (1996). Pregnancy and the risk of stroke. *New England Journal of Medicine*, **335**, 768–74.

Kiyohara, Y., Kato, I., Iwamoto, H., Nakayama, K., and Fujishima, M. (1995). The impact of alcohol and hypertension on stroke incidence in a general Japanese population. The Hisayama Study. *Stroke*, **26**, 368–72.

Klag, M.J., Whelton, P.K., and Seidler, A.J. (1989). Decline in US stroke mortality. Demographic trends and antihypertensive treatment. *Stroke*, **20**, 14–21.

Klatsky, A.L., Freidman, G.D., Siegelaub, A.B., and Gerard, M.J. (1977). Alcohol consumption and blood pressure. Kaiser–Permanente Multiphasic Health Examination

Data. *New England Journal of Medicine*, **296**, 1194–200.

Knauth, M., von Kummer, R., Jansen, O., Hahnel, S., Dorfler, A., and Sartor, K. (1997). Potential of CT angiography in acute ischemic stroke. *American Journal of Neuroradiology*, **18**, 1001–10.

Knights, E. and Folstein, M.F. (1977). Unsuspected emotional and cognitive disturbance in medical patients. *Annals of Internal Medicine*, **87**, 723–4.

Knox, E.G. (1981). Meteorological associations of cerebrovascular disease mortality in England and Wales. *Journal of Epidemiology and Community Health*, **35**, 220–3.

Kobayashi, S., Okada, K., and Yamashita, K. (1991). Incidence of silent lacunar lesions in normal adults and its relation to cerebral blood flow. *Stroke*, **22**, 1379–83.

Koistinaho, J. and Hokfelt, T. (1997). Altered gene expression in brain ischemia. *Neuroreport*, **8**, i–viii.

Kopitnik, T.A. and Samson, D.S. (1993). Management of subarachnoid haemorrhage. *Journal of Neurology, Neurosurgery and Psychiatry*, **56**, 947–59.

Koroshetz, W.J. and Gonzalez, G. (1997). Diffusion-weighted MRI: an ECG for 'brain attack'? *Annals of Neurology*, **41**, 565–6.

Korv, J., Roose, M., and Kaasik, A.E. (1996). Changed incidence and case-fatality rates of first-ever stroke between 1970 and 1993 in Tartu, Estonia. *Stroke*, **27**, 199–203.

Koskenvuo, M., Kaprio, J., Telakivi, T., Partinen, M., Heikkila, K., and Sarna, S. (1987). Snoring as a risk factor for ischaemic heart disease and stroke in men. *British Medical Journal*, **294**, 16–19.

Kotila, M., Waltimo, O., Niemi, M.L., Laaksonen, R., and Lempinen, M. (1984). The profile of recovery from stroke and factors influencing outcome. *Stroke*, **15**, 1039–44.

Kotila, M., Niemi, M.L., and Laaksonen, R. (1986*a*). Four-year prognosis of stroke patients wih visuospatial inattention. *Scandinavian Journal of Rehabilitation Medicine*, **18**, 177–9.

Kotila, M., Waltimo, O., Niemi, M.L., and Laaksonen, R. (1986*b*). Dementia after stroke. *European Neurology*, **25**, 134–40.

Kuh, D. and Ben-Shlomo, Y. (1997). *A life course approach to chronic disease epidemiology*. Oxford University Press, Oxford.

Kuller, L.H., Ockene, J.K., Meilahn, E., Wentworth, D.N., Svendsen, K.H., and Neaton, J.D. (1991). Cigarette smoking and mortality. MRFIT Research Group. *Preventive Medicine*, **20**, 638–54.

Kuntz, K.M. and Kent, K.C. (1996). Is carotid endarterectomy cost-effective? An analysis of symptomatic and asymptomatic patients. *Circulation*, **94**, II194–8.

Kwakkel, G., Wagenaar, R.C., Kollen, B.J., and Lankhorst, G.J. (1996). Predicting disability in stroke–a critical review of the literature. *Age and Ageing*, **25**, 479–89.

Kwakkel, G., Wagenaar, R.C., Koelman, T.W., Lankhorst, G.J., and Koetsier, J.C. (1997). Effects of intensity of rehabilitation after stroke. A research synthesis. *Stroke*, **28**, 1550–6.

Landefeld, C.S. and Beyth, R.J. (1993). Anticoagulant-related bleeding: clinical epidemiology, prediction and prevention. *American Journal of Medicine*, **95**, 315–28.

Landis, J.R. and Koch, G.G. (1977). The measurement of observer agreement for categorical data. *Biometrics*, **33**, 159–74.

Langhorne, P., Williams, B.O., Gilchrist, W., and Howie, K. (1993). Do stroke units save lives? *Lancet*, **342**, 395–8.

Langhorne, P., Wagenaar, R., and Partridge, C. (1996). Physiotherapy after stroke: more is better? *Physiotherapy Research International*, **1**, 75–88.

Lapidus, L. and Bengtsson, C. (1986). Socioeconomic factors and physical activity in relation to cardiovascular disease and death. A 12 year follow up of participants in a population study of women in Gothenburg, Sweden. *British Heart Journal*, **55**, 295–301.

Larsson, B., Svardsudd, K., Welin, L. *et al.* (1984). Abdominal adipose tissue distribution, obesity, and risk of cardiovascular disease and death: 13 year follow up of participants in the study of men born in 1913. *British Medical Journal*, **288**, 1401–4.

LaRue, L.J., Alter, M., Traven, N.D., Sterman, A.B., Sobel, E., and Kleiner, J. (1988). Acute stroke therapy trials: problems in patient accrual. *Stroke*, **19**, 950–4.

Lau, J., Antman, E.M., Jimenez-Silva, J., Kupelnick, B., Mosteller, F., and Chalmers, T.C. (1993). Cumulative meta-analysis of therapeutic trials for myocardial infarction. *New England Journal of Medicine*, **327**, 248–54.

Lauritzen, J.B., Petersen, M.M., and Lund, B. (1993). Effect of external hip protectors on hip fractures. *Lancet*, **341**, 11–13.

Law, M. (1996). Evidence on salt is consistent. *British Medical Journal*, **312**, 1284–5.

Law, M.R., Frost, C.D., and Wald, N.J. (1991*a*). By how much does dietary salt reduction lower blood pressure? I–Analysis of observational data among populations. *British Medical Journal*, **302**, 811–15.

Law, M.R., Frost, C.D., and Wald, N.J. (1991*b*). By how much does dietary salt reduction lower blood pressure? III–Analysis of data from trials of salt reduction. *British Medical Journal*, **302**, 819–24. [See erratum in *BMJ* (1991), **302**, 939.]

Lee, M.C., Heaney, L.M., Jacobson, R.L., and Klassen, A.C. (1975). Cerebrospinal fluid in cerebral haemorrhage and infarction. *Stroke*, **6**, 638–41.

Lee, T.K., Huang, Z.S., Ng, S.K. *et al.* (1995). Impact of alcohol consumption and cigarette smoking on stroke among the elderly in Taiwan. *Stroke*, **26**, 790–4.

Lee, T.T., Solomon, N.A., Heidenreich, P.A., Oehlert, J., and Garber, A.M. (1997). Cost-effectiveness of screening for carotid stenosis in asymptomatic persons. *Annals of Internal Medicine*, **126**, 337–46.

Lees, K.R. (1998). Does neuroprotection improve stroke outcome? *Lancet*, **351**, 1447–8.

Legh-Smith, J.A., Denis, R., Enderby, P.M., Wade, D.T., and Hewer, R.L. (1987). Selection of aphasic stroke patients for intensive speech therapy. *Journal of Neurology, Neurosurgery and Psychiatry*, **50**, 1488–92.

Lendrum, W. and Lincoln, N.B. (1985). Spontaneous recovery of language in patients with aphasia between 4 and 34 weeks after stroke. *Journal of Neurology, Neurosurgery and Psychiatry*, **48**, 743–8.

Leon, D.A., Koupilova, I., Lithell, H.O. *et al.* (1996). Failure to realise growth potential *in utero* and adult obesity in relation to blood pressure in 50 year old Swedish men. *British Medical Journal*, **312**, 401–6.

Leon, D.A., Chenet, L., Shkolnikov, V.M. *et al.* (1997). Huge variation in Russian mortality rates 1984–94: artefact, alcohol, or what? *Lancet*, **350**, 383–8.

Lewis, C.E., Grandits, G.A., Flack, J., and McDonald, R. (1996). Efficacy and tolerance of antihypertensive treatment in men and women with stage one diastolic hypertension. *Archives of Internal Medicine*, **156**, 377–85.

Libman, R.B., Wirkowski, E., Alvir, J., and Rao, T.H. (1995). Conditions that mimic stroke in the emergency department: implications for acute stroke trials. *Archives of Neurology*, **52**, 1119–22.

Lin, C.H., Shimizu, Y., Kato, H. *et al.* (1984). Cerebrovascular diseases in a fixed population of Hiroshima and Nagasaki, with special reference to relationship between type and risk factors. *Stroke*, **15**, 653–60.

Lin, H.J., Wolf, P.A., Kelly-Hayes, M. *et al.* (1996). Stroke severity in atrial fibrillation. The Framingham Study. *Stroke*, **27**, 1760–4.

Lincoln, N.B., McGuirk, E., Lendrum, W., Jones, A.C., and Mitchell, J.R.A. (1984). Effectiveness of speech therapy for aphasic stroke patients. *Lancet*, **i**, 1197–200.

Lincoln, N.B., Willis, D., Philips, S.A., Juby, L.C., and Berman, P. (1996). Comparison of rehabilitation practice on hospital wards for stroke patients. *Stroke*, **27**, 18–23.

Lindenstrom, E., Boysen, G., and Nyboe, J. (1993). Lifestyle factors and risk of cerebrovascular disease in women. The Copenhagen City Heart Study. *Stroke*, **24**, 1468–72.

Lindenstrom, E., Boysen, G., and Nyboe, J. (1994). Influence of total cholesterol, high density lipoprotein cholesterol, and triglycerides on risk of cerebrovascular disease: the Copenhagen City Heart Study. *British Medical Journal*, **309**, 11–15. [See erratum in *BMJ* (1994), **309**,1619.]

Lindgren, A., Norrving, B., Rudling, O., and Johansson, B.B. (1994a). Comparison of clinical and neuroradiological findings in first ever stroke: a population based study. *Stroke*, **25**, 1371–7.

Lindgren, A., Roijer, A., Rudling, O. *et al.* (1994b). Cerebral lesions on magnetic resonance imaging, heart disease, and vascular risk factors in subjects without stroke. A population-based study. *Stroke*, **25**, 929–34.

Lindley, R.I., Warlow, C.P., Wardlaw, J.M., Dennis, M.S., Slattery, J., and Sandercock, P.A. (1993). Interobserver reliability of a clinical classification of acute cerebral infarction. *Stroke*, **24**, 1801–4.

Lindley, R.I., Amayo, E.O., Marshall, J., Sandercock, P.A., Dennis, M., and Warlow, C.P. (1995). Acute stroke treatment in UK hospitals: the Stroke Association survey of consultant opinion. *Journal of the Royal College of Physicians of London*, **29**, 479–84.

Lipsey, J.R., Robinson, R.G., Pearlson, G.D., Rao, K., and Price, T.R. (1984). Nortriptyline treatment of post-stroke depression: a double blind study. *Lancet*, **i**, 297–300.

Lipsey, J.R., Robinson, R.G., Pearlson, G.D., Rao, K., and Price, T.R. (1985). The dexamethasone suppression test and mood following stroke. *American Journal of Psychiatry*, **142**, 318–23.

Liu, M., Counsell, C.E., and Wardlaw, J.M. (1998). Fibrinogen depleting agents in acute ischaemic stroke (Cochrane review). In *Cochrane database of systematic reviews (disc and CD-ROM). Stroke module,* (ed. C.P. Warlow, J. van Gijn, and P.A.G. Sandercock). Update Software/BMJ Publishing, Oxford.

Lodder, J., Bamford, J.M., Sandercock, P.A., Jones, L.N., and Warlow, C.P. (1990). Are hypertension or cardiac embolism likely causes of lacunar infarction? *Stroke*, **21**, 375–81.

Logan, P.A., Ahern, J., Gladman, J.R., and Lincoln, N.B. (1997). A randomized controlled trial of enhanced Social Service occupational therapy for stroke patients. *Clinical Rehabilitation*, **11**, 107–13.

Lorenze, E.J., Simon, H., and Linden, J. (1959). Urological problems in the rehabilitation of hemiplegic patients. *Journal of the American Medical Association*, **169**, 1042–6.

Lowe, G.D., Jaap, A.J., and Forbes, C.D. (1983). Relation of atrial fibrillation and high haematocrit to mortality in acute stroke. *Lancet*, **i**, 784–6.

Lutsep, H.C., Albers, G.W., DeCrespigny, A., Kamat, G.N. *et al.* (1997). Clinical utility of diffusion weighted MRI in the assessment of ischaemic stroke. *Annals of Neurology*, **41**, 574–80.

Lyden, P.D. and Lau, G.T. (1991). A critical appraisal of stroke evaluation and rating scales. *Stroke*, **22**, 1345–52.

McAvoy, B.R. (1986). Death after bereavement. *British Medical Journal*, **293**, 835–6.

McCarron, D.A. (1998). Diet and blood pressure: the paradigm shift. *Science*, **281**, 933–4.

McCarthy, S.T. and Turner, J. (1986). Low-dose subcutaneous heparin in the prevention of deep-vein thrombosis and pulmonary emboli following acute stroke. *Age and Ageing*, **15**, 84–8.

McCarthy, S.T., Turner, J.J., Robertson, D., Hawkey, C.J., and Macey, D.J. (1977). Low dose heparin after acute stroke. *Lancet*, **ii**, 800–1.

MacClure, M. and Willett, W.C. (1987). Misinterpretation and misuse of the kappa statisitic. *American Journal of Epidemiology*, **126**, 161–9.

McGovern, P.G., Burke, G.L., Sprafka, J.M., Xue, S., Folsom, A.R., and Blackburn, H. (1992). Trends in mortality, morbidity, and risk factor levels for stroke from 1960 through 1990. The Minnesota Heart Survey. *Journal of the American Medical Association*, **268**, 753–9.

McGovern, P.G., Pankow, J.S., Burke, G.L. *et al.* (1993). Trends in survival of hospitalized stroke patients between 1970 and 1985. The Minnesota Heart Survey. *Stroke*, **24**, 1640–8.

MacGuire, G., Julier, D., Hawton, K., and Bancroft, J. (1974). Psychiatric morbidity and referral in two general medical wards. *British Medical Journal*, **1**, 268–70.

Mackey, F., Ada, L., Heard, R., and Adams, R. (1996). Stroke rehabilitation: are highly structured units more conducive to physical activity than less structured units? *Archives of Physical Medicine and Rehabilitation*, **77**, 1066–70.

MacMahon, S., Peto, R., Cutler, J. *et al.* (1990). Blood pressure, stroke, and coronary heart disease. Part 1, Prolonged differences in blood pressure: prospective observational studies corrected for the regression dilution bias. *Lancet*, **335**, 765–74.

Madden, K.P., Karanjia, P.N., Adams, H.P. Jr, and Clarke, W.R. (1995). Accuracy of initial stroke subtype diagnosis in the TOAST study. Trial of ORG 10172 in Acute Stroke Treatment. *Neurology*, **45**, 1975–9.

Maheswaran, R., Strachan, D.P., Elliott, P., and Shipley, M.J. (1997). Trends in stroke mortality in Greater London and south east England: evidence for a cohort effect? *Journal of Epidemiology and Community Health*, **51**, 121–6.

Mahon, J., Laupacis, A., Donner, A., and Wood, T. (1996). Randomised study of n of l trials versus standard practice. *British Medical Journal*, **312**, 1069–74. [See erratum in *BMJ* (1996), **312**, 1392.]

Mahoney, F.I. and Barthel, D.W. (1965). Functional evaluation: the Barthel Index. *Maryland State Medical Journal*, **14**, 61–5.

Malinow, M.R., Duell, P.B., Hess, D.L. *et al.* (1998). Reduction in plasma homocysteine levels by breakfast cereal fortified with folic acid in patients with coronary heart disease. *New England Journal of Medicine*, **338**, 1009–15.

Malmgren, R., Warlow, C., Bamford, J., and Sandercock, P. (1987). Geographical and secular trends in stroke incidence. *Lancet*, **ii**, 1196–200.

Manning, W.J. (1997). Role of transesophageal echocardiography in the management of thromboembolic stroke. *American Journal of Cardiology*, **80**, 19D–28D.

Manson, J.E., Colditz, G.A., Stampfer, M.J. *et al.* (1991). A prospective study of maturity-onset diabetes mellitus and risk of coronary heart disease and stroke in women. *Archives of Internal Medicine*, **151**, 1141–7.

Markus, H.S., Thomson, N.D., and Brown, M.M. (1995). Asymptomatic cerebral embolic signals in symptomatic and asymptomatic carotid artery disease. *Brain*, **118**, 1005–11.

Markus, H.S., Clifton, A., Buckenham, T., Taylor, R., and Brown, M.M. (1996). Improvement in cerebral hemodynamics after carotid angioplasty. *Stroke*, **27**, 612–16.

Marmot, M.G. and McDowall, M.E. (1986). Mortality decline and widening social inequalities. *Lancet*, **ii**, 274–6. [See erratum in *Lancet* (1987), **i**, 394.]

Marmot, M.G. and Poulter, N.R. (1992). Primary prevention of stroke. *Lancet*, **339**, 344–7.

Marmot, M.G., Syme, S.L., Kagan, A., Kato, H., Cohen, J.B., and Belsky, J. (1975). Epidemiologic studies of coronary heart disease and stroke in Japanese men living in Japan, Hawaii, and California: prevalence of coronary and hypertensive heart disease and associated risk factors. *American Journal of Epidemiology*, **102**, 514–25.

Marmot, M.G., Adelstein, A.M., and Bulusu, L. (1984). Lessons from the study of immigrant mortality. *Lancet*, **i**, 1455–8.

Marquardsen, J. (1969). *The natural history of acute cerebrovascular disease*. Munksgaard, Copenhagen.

Marshall, J. and Shaw, D.A. (1959). The natural history of cerebrovascular disease. *British Medical Journal*, **1**, 1614–17.

Martin, J., Meltzer, H., and Elliot, D. (1988). *The prevalence of disability among adults*. HMSO, London.

Martyn, C.N., Barker, D.J., and Osmond, C. (1996). Mothers' pelvic size, fetal growth, and death from stroke and coronary heart disease in men in the UK. *Lancet*, **348**, 1264–8.

Matsumoto, N., Whisnant, J.P., Kurland, L.T., and Okazati, H. (1973). Natural history of stroke in Rochester, Minnesota, 1955 through 1969: an extension of a previous study, 1945 through 1954. *Stroke*, **4**, 20–9.

Mattilla, K., Haavisto, M., Rajala, S., and Heikinheimo, R. (1988). Blood pressure and survival in the very old. *British Medical Journal*, **296**, 887–9.

Maxwell, R. (1984). Quality assessment in health care. *British Medical Journal*, **288**, 1470–2.

Maynard, A. (1992). The economics of hypertension control: some basic issues. *Journal of Human Hypertension*, **6**, 417–20.

Meade, T.W. (1977). Problems for the research worker in rehabilitation studies. *Rheumatology and Rehabilitation*, **16**, 254–6.

Meade, T.W., Gardner, M.J., and Cannon, P. (1968). Observer variability in the recording of peripheral pulses. *British Heart Journal*, **30**, 661–5.

Medical Research Council Working Party (1985). MRC trial of treatment of mild hypertension: principal results. *British Medical Journal*, **291**, 97–104.

Medical Research Council Working Party (1988). Stroke and coronary heart disease in mild hypertension: risk factors and the value of treatment. *British Medical Journal*, **296**, 1565–70.

Medical Research Council Working Party (1992). Medical Research Council trial of treatment of hypertension in older adults: principal results. MRC Working Party. *British Medical Journal*, **304**, 405–12.

Medrano, M.J., Lopez-Abente, G., Barrado, M.J., Pollan, M., and Almazan, J. (1997). Effect of age, birth cohort, and period of death on cerebrovascular mortality in Spain, 1952 through 1991. *Stroke*, **28**, 40–4.

Meikle, M., Wechsler, E., Tupper, A. *et al.* (1979). Comparative trial of volunteer and professional treatments of dysphasia after stroke. *British Medical Journal*, **2**, 87–9.

Meissner, I., Whisnant, J.P., and Garraway, W.M. (1988). Hypertension management and stroke recurrence in a community (Rochester, Minnesota, 1950–1979). *Stroke*, **19**, 459–63.

Merikangas, K.R., Fenton, B.T., Cheng, S.H., Stolar, M.J., and Risch, N. (1997). Association between migraine and stroke in a large-scale epidemiological study of the United States. *Archives of Neurology*, **54**, 362–8.

Merrett, J.D. and Adams, G.F. (1966). Comparison of mortality rates in elderly hypertensive and normotensive patients. *British Medical Journal*, **2**, 802–5.

Miall, W.E. and Oldham, P.D. (1963). The hereditary factor in arterial blood pressure. *British Medical Journal*, **1**, 75–80.

Miall, W.E., Henage, P., Kholsa, T., Lovell, H.G., and Moore, F. (1967). Factors influencing the degree of resemblance in arterial pressure of close relatives. *Clinical Science*, **33**, 271–83.

Michaels, J.A. (1988). Surgical audit and carotid endarterectomy. *Lancet*, **ii**, 110–11.

Midgley, J.P., Matthew, A.G., Greenwood, C.M., and Logan, A.G. (1996). Effects of reduced dietary sodium on blood pressure. A meta analysis of randomised controlled trials. *Journal of the American Medical Association*, **275**, 1590–7.

Mittl, R.L., Broderick, M., Carpenter, J.P., Goldberg, H.I. *et al.* (1994). Blinded reader comparison of magnetic resonance angiography and duplex ultrasongraphy for carotid artery bifurcation stenosis. *Stroke*, **25**, 4–10.

Mitusch, R., Doherty, C., Wucherpfennig, H. *et al.* (1997). Vascular events during follow-up in patients with aortic arch atherosclerosis. *Stroke*, **28**, 36–9.

Mohiuddin, A.A., Bath, F.J., and Bath, P.M.W. (1998). Theophylline, aminophylline, caffeine and analogues, in acute ischaemic stroke (Cochrane review). In *Cochrane database of systematic reviews (disc and CD-ROM). Stroke module*, (ed. C.P. Warlow, J. van Gijn, and P.A.G. Sandercock). Update Software/BMJ Publishing, Oxford.

Molloy, J. and Markus, H.S. (1996). Multigated Doppler ultrasound in the detection of emboli in a flow model and embolic signals in patients. *Stroke*, **27**, 1548–52.

Moreland, J.D., Thompson, M.A., and Fuoco, A.R. (1998). Electromyographic feedback to improve lower extremity function after stroke: a meta-analysis. *Archives of Physical Medicine and Rehabilitation*, **79**, 134–40.

Morgan, K., Dallosso, H., and Ebrahim, S. (1985). A brief self report scale for assessing personal engagement in the elderly: reliability and validity. In *Ageing: recent advances and creative responses*, (ed. A. Butler), pp. 298–304. Croom Helm, London.

Morris, M.C., Manson, J.E., Rosner, B., Buring, J.E., Willett, W.C., and Hennekens, C.H. (1995). Fish consumption and cardiovascular disease in the physicians' health study: a prospective study. *American Journal of Epidemiology*, **142**, 166–75.

Morris, P.L., Raphael, B., and Robinson, R.G. (1992). Clinical depression is associated with impaired recovery from stroke. *Medical Journal of Australia*, **157**, 239–42.

Morris, P.L., Robinson, R.G., Andrzejewski, P., Samuels, J., and Price, T.R. (1993). Association of depression with 10-year poststroke mortality. *American Journal of Psychiatry*, **150**, 124–9.

Muir, K.W. and Lees, K.R. (1995). A randomized, double-blind, placebo-controlled pilot trial of intravenous magnesium sulfate in acute stroke. *Stroke*, **26**, 1183–8.

Mulley, G.P. (1982). Avoidable complications of stroke. *Journal of the Royal College of Physicians of London*, **16**, 94–7.

Mulley, G.P., Wilcock, R.G., and Mitchell (1978). Dexamethasone in acute stroke. *British Medical Journal*, **ii**, 994–6.

Mulrow, C.D., Cornell, J.A., Herrera, C.R. *et al.* (1995). Hypertension in the elderly:

implications and generalisability of randomized trials. *Journal of the American Medical Association*, **272**, 1932–8.

Multicentre Acute Stroke Trial Europe (MAST-E) Study Group (1996). Thrombolytic therapy with streptokinase in acute ischaemic stroke. *New England Journal of Medicine*, **335**, 145–50.

Multicentre Acute Stroke Trial-Italy (1995). Randomised controlled trial of streptokinase, aspirin and combination of both in treatment of acute ischaemic stroke. *Lancet*, **346**, 1509–16.

Murphy, E. (1982). Social origins of depression in old age. *British Journal of Psychiatry*, **141**, 135–42.

Nabarro, J. (1984). Unrecognised psychiatric illness in medical patients. *British Medical Journal*, **289**, 635–6.

Nakayama, H., Jorgensen, H.S., Raaschou, H.O., and Olsen, T.S. (1994). Compensation in recovery of upper extremity function after stroke: the Copenhagen Stroke Study. *Archives of Physical Medicine and Rehabilitation*, **75**, 852–7.

Nakayama, H., Jorgensen, H.S., Pedersen, P.M., Raaschou, H.O., and Olsen, T.S. (1997). Prevalence and risk factors of incontinence after stroke. The Copenhagen Stroke Study. *Stroke*, **28**, 58–62.

Naylor, A.R., London, N.J., and Bell, P.R. (1997). Carotid endarterectomy versus carotid angioplasty. *Lancet*, **349**, 203–4.

Neaton, J.D., Blackburn, H., Jacobs, D. *et al.* (1992). Serum cholesterol level and mortality findings for men screened in the Multiple Risk Factor Intervention Trial. Multiple Risk Factor Intervention Trial Research Group. *Archives of Internal Medicine*, **152**, 1490–500.

Newall, J.T., Wood, V.A., Hewer, R.L., and Tinson, D.J. (1997). Development of a neurological rehabilitation environment: an observational study. *Clinical Rehabilitation*, **11**, 146–55.

Newman, G. and Mitchell, J.R.A. (1984). Homocystinuria presenting as multiple arterial occlusions. *Quarterly Journal of Medicine*, **53**, 251–8.

NHS Research and Development Programme (1997) *NHS Research and Development Programme*, 1 August 1997. NHS Executive Northern and Yorkshire Region.

Nicholls, E.S. and Johansen, H.L. (1983). Implications of the changing trends in cerebrovascular and ischemic heart disease mortality. *Stroke*, **14**, 153–5.

Niemi, M.L., Laaksonen, R., Kotila, M., and Waltimo, O. (1988). Quality of life 4 years after stroke. *Stroke*, **19**, 1101–7.

NINDS rt-PA Stroke Study Group (1995). Tissue plasminogen activator for acute ischemic stroke. The National Institute of Neurological Disorders and Stroke rt-PA Stroke Study Group. *New England Journal of Medicine*, **333**, 1581–7.

NINDS t-PA Stroke Study Group (1997). A systems approach to immediate evaluation and management of hyperacute stroke. Experience at eight centers and implications for community practice and patient care. The National Institute of Neurological Disorders and Stroke (NINDS) rt-PA Stroke Study Group. *Stroke*, **28**, 1530–40.

Nitti, V.W., Adler, H., and Combs, A.J. (1996). The role of urodynamics in the evaluation of voiding dysfunction in men after cerebrovascular accident. *Journal of Urology*, **155**, 263–6.

Norris, J.W. and Hachinski, V.C. (1982). Misdiagnosis of stroke. *Lancet*, **i**, 328–31.

Norris, J.W., Zhu, C.Z., Bornstein, N.M., and Chambers, B.R. (1991). Vascular risks of asymptomatic carotid stenosis. *Stroke*, **22**, 1485–90.

North American Symptomatic Carotid Endarterectomy Trial Collaborators (1991). Beneficial effect of carotid endarterectomy in symptomatic patients with high-grade carotid stenosis. *New England Journal of Medicine*, **325**, 445–53.

Norton, B., Homer-Ward, M., Donnelly, M.T., Long, R.G., and Holmes, G.K. (1996). A randomised prospective comparison of percutaneous endoscopic gastrostomy and nasogastric tube feeding after acute dysphagic stroke. *British Medical Journal*, **312**, 13–16.

Nouri, F.M. and Lincoln, N.B. (1987). An extended activities of daily living scale for stroke patients. *Clinical Rehabilitation*, **1**, 301–5.

Numminen, H., Kotila, M., Waltimo, O., Aho, K., and Kaste, M. (1996). Declining incidence and mortality rates of stroke in Finland from 1972 to 1991. Results of three population-based stroke registers. *Stroke*, **27**, 1487–91.

O'Boyle, C.A., McGee, H., Hickey, A., O'Malley, K., and Joyce, C.R.B. (1992). Individual quality of life in patients undergoing hip replacement. *Lancet*, **339**, 1088–91.

O'Brien, J.R. (1980). Platelets and vessel wall. How much aspirin? *Lancet*, **i**, 372–3.

O'Brien, P.A., Ryder, D.Q., and Twomey, C. (1987). The role of computed tomography brain scan in the diagnosis of acute stroke in the elderly. *Age and Ageing*, **16**, 319–22.

Ogren, M., Hedblad, B., Isacsson, S.O., Janzon, L., Jungquist, G., and Lindell, S.E. (1995). Ten year cerebrovascular morbidity and mortality in 68 year old men with asymptomatic carotid stenosis. *British Medical Journal*, **310**, 1294–8.

O'Neill, P.A., Davies, I., Fullerton, K.J., and Bennett, D. (1991). Stress hormone and blood glucose response following acute stroke in the elderly. *Stroke*, **22**, 842–7.

Orencia, A.J., Daviglus, M.L., Dyer, A.R., Shekelle, R.B., and Stamler, J. (1996). Fish consumption and stroke in men. 30-year findings of the Chicago Western Electric Study. *Stroke*, **27**, 204–9.

O'Rourke, S., MacHale, S., Signorini, G., and Dennis, M. (1998). Detecting psychiatric morbidity after stroke: comparison of the GHQ and HAD scales. *Stroke*, **29**, 980–5.

Ostfeld, A.M. (1980). A review of stroke epidemiology. *Epidemiologic Reviews*, **2**, 136–52.

Overstall, P.W. (1995). Falls after strokes. *British Medical Journal*, **311**, 74–5.

Oxbury, J.M., Greenhall, R.C.D., and Grainger, K.M.R. (1975). Predicting the outcome of stroke: acute stage after cerebral infarction. *British Medical Journal*, **iii**, 125–7.

Oxfordshire Community Stroke Project (1985). Incidence of stroke in Oxfordshire: first year's experience of a community stroke register. *British Medical Journal*, **287**, 713–17.

Paffenbarger, R.S., Laughlin, M.E., Gima, A.S., and Black, R.A. (1970). Work activity of longshoremen as related to death from coronary heart disease and stroke. *New England Journal of Medicine*, **282**, 1109–14.

Paganini-Hill, A., Ross, R.K., and Henderson, B.E. (1988). Postmenopausal oestrogen treatment and stroke: a prospective study. *British Medical Journal*, **297**, 519–22.

Palomaki, H. (1991). Snoring and the risk of ischemic brain infarction. *Stroke*, **22**, 1021–5.

Palomaki, H. and Kaste, M. (1993). Regular light-to-moderate intake of alcohol and the risk of ischemic stroke. Is there a beneficial effect? *Stroke*, **24**, 1828–32.

Palomaki, H., Partinen, M., Juvela, S., and Kaste, M. (1989). Snoring as a risk factor for sleep-related brain infarction. *Stroke*, **20**, 1311–15.

Pan, W.H., Li, L.A., and Tsai, M.J. (1995). Temperature extremes and mortality from coronary heart disease and cerebral infarction in elderly Chinese. *Lancet*, **345**, 353–5.

Parikh, R.M., Robinson, R.G., Lipsey, J.R. *et al.* (1990). The impact of poststroke depression on recovery in activities of daily living over a 2-year follow-up. *Archives of Neurology*, **47**, 785–9.

Parker, C.J., Gladman, J.R., and Drummond, A.E. (1997). The role of leisure in stroke rehabilitation. *Disability and Rehabilitation*, **19**, 1–5.

Partridge, C.J., Johnston, M., and Edwards, S. (1987). Recovery from physical disability after stroke: normal patterns as a basis for evaluation. *Lancet*, **i**, 373–5.

Patrono, C. and Roth, G.J. (1996). Aspirin in ischemic cerebrovascular disease. How strong is the case for a different dosing regimen? *Stroke*, **27**, 756–60.

Patten, J. (1977). *Neurological differential diagnosis*. Harold Starke, Springer Verlag, London.

Pearson, T.C. and Wetherley-Mein, G. (1978). Vascular occlusive epsiodes and venous haematocrit in primary proliferative polycythaemia. *Lancet*, **ii**, 1219–22.

Pedersen, P.M., Jorgensen, H.S., Nakayama, H., Raaschou, H.O., and Olsen, T.S. (1995). Aphasia in acute stroke: incidence, determinants, and recovery. *Annals of Neurology*, **38**, 659–66.

Pedersen, P.M., Jorgensen, H.S., Nakayama, H., Raaschou, H.O., and Olsen, T.S. (1997). Hemineglect in acute stroke: incidence and prognostic implications. The Copenhagen Stroke Study. *American Journal of Physical Medicine and Rehabilitation*, **76**, 122–7.

Perry, I.J., Refsum, H., Morris, R.W., Ebrahim, S., Ueland, P.M., and Shaper, A.G. (1995). Prospective study of serum total homocysteine concentration and risk of stroke in middle-aged British men. *Lancet*, **346**, 1395–8.

Persson, U., Silverberg, R., Lindgren, B. *et al.* (1990). Direct costs of stroke for a Swedish population. *International Journal of Technology Assessment in Health Care*, **6**, 125–37.

Peto, R. (1982). Long term and short term beta-blockade after myocardial infarction. *Lancet*, **i**, 1159–61.

Peto, R., Pike, M.C., Armitage, P. *et al.* (1976). Design and analysis of randomised clinical trials requiring prolonged observation of each patient. Part I. *British Journal of Cancer*, **34**, 585–612.

Peto, R., Pike, M.C., Armitage, P. *et al.* (1977). Design and analysis of randomised clinical trials requiring prolonged observation of each patient. Part II. *British Journal of Cancer*, **35**, 1–39.

Philipp, T., Anlauf, M., Distler, A., Holzgreve, H., Michaelis, J., and Wellek, S. (1997). Randomised, double blind, multicentre comparison of hydrochlorothiazide, atenolol, nitrendipine, and enalapril in antihypertensive treatment: results of the HANE study. *British Medical Journal*, **315**, 154–9.

Phillips, A.N. and Davey Smith, G. (1991). How independent are 'independent' effects? Relative risk estimation when correlated exposures are measured imprecisely. *Journal of Clinical Epidemiology*, **44**, 1223–31.

Phillips, A.N. and Davey Smith, G. (1992). Bias in relative odds estimation owing to imprecise measurement of correlated exposures. *Statistics in Medicine*, **11**, 953–61.

Pocock, S.J. (1983). *Clinical Trials. A practical approach*. John Wiley and Sons, Chichester.

Pocock, S.J. (1992). When to stop a clinical trial. *British Medical Journal*, **305**, 235–40.

Pohjasvaara, T., Erkinjuntti, T., Vataja, R., and Kaste, M. (1997). Dementia three months after stroke. Baseline frequency and effect of different definitions of dementia in the Helsinki Stroke Aging Memory Study (SAM) cohort. *Stroke*, **28**, 785–92.

Pound, P., Bury, M., and Ebrahim, S. (1993). From apoplexy to stroke. *Age and Ageing*, **26**, 331–7.

Pound, P., Bury, M., Gompertz, P., and Ebrahim, S. (1994). Views of survivors of stroke on benefits of physiotherapy. *Quality in Health Care*, **3**, 69–74.

Pound, P., Bury, M., Gompertz, P., and Ebrahim, S. (1995). Stroke patients' views on their admission to hospital . *British Medical Journal*, **311**, 18–22.

Pound, P., Sabin, C., and Ebrahim, S. (1999). Observing the process of care: a stroke unit, elderly care unit and general medical ward compared. *Age and Ageing*, in press.

Poungvarin, N., Viriyavejakul, A., and Komontri, C. (1991). Siriraj stroke score and validation study to distinguish supratentorial intracerebral haemorrhage from infarction. *British Medical Journal*, **302**, 1565–7.

Power, M.J., Fullerton, K.J., and Stout, R.W. (1988). Blood glucose and prognosis of acute stroke. *Age and Ageing*, **17**, 164–70.

Prencipe, M., Culasso, F., Rasura, M., Anzini, A., Beccia, M. *et al.* (1998). Long term prognosis after a minor stroke: 10 year mortality and major stroke recurrence rates in a hospital based cohort. *Stroke*, **29**, 126–32.

Prescott, R.J., Garraway, W.M., and Akhtar, A.J. (1982). Predicting functional outcome following acute stroke using a standard clinical examination. *Stroke*, **13**, 641–7.

Prince, M.J., Harwood, R.H., Blizard, R.A., Thomas, A., and Mann, A.H. (1997). Impairment, disabilty and handicap as risk factors for depression in old age. The Gospel Oak Project. *Psychological Medicine*, **27**, 311–21.

Prospective Studies Collaboration (1995). Cholesterol, diastolic blood pressure, and stroke: 13,000 strokes in 450,000 people in 45 prospective cohorts. *Lancet*, **346**, 1647–53.

Pulsinelli, W. (1992). Pathophysiology of acute ischaemic stroke. *Lancet*, **339**, 533–6.

Qizilbash, N., Jones, L., Warlow, C., and Mann, J. (1991). Fibrinogen and lipid concentrations as risk factors for transient ischaemic attacks and minor ischaemic strokes. *British Medical Journal*, **303**, 605–9.

Qizilbash, N., Lewington, S.L., and Lopez-Arrieta, J.M. (1998). Corticosteroids following acute presumed ischaemic stroke (Cochrane review). In *Cochrane database of systematic reviews (disc and CD-ROM)*. *Stroke module*, (ed. C.P. Warlow, J. van Gijn, and P.A.G. Sandercock). Update Software/BMJ Publishing, Oxford.

Raftery, J. (1995). Stroke services purchasing-present and future. In *Best buy for stroke. Procedings of a seminar for purchasers*, (ed. S. Law and J. Mant). London School of Hygiene and Tropical Medicine, London.

Rankin, J. (1957). Cerebral vascular accidents in patients over the age of 60. 2. Prognosis. *Scottish Medical Journal*, **2**, 200–15.

Reding, M.J. and Potes, E. (1988). Rehabilitation outcome following initial unilateral hemispheric stroke. Life table analysis approach. *Stroke*, **19**, 1354–8.

Reding, M.J., Orto, L.A., Winter, S.W., Fortuna, I.M., Di Ponte, P., and McDowell, F.H. (1986). Antidepressant therapy after stroke. A double-blind trial. *Archives of Neurology*, **43**, 763–5.

Reith, J., Jorgensen, H.S., Pedersen, P.M. *et al.* (1996). Body temperature in acute stroke: relation to stroke severity, infarct size, mortality, and outcome. *Lancet*, **347**, 422–5.

Rentzhog, L., Stanton, S.L., Cardozo, L., Nelson, E., Fall, M., and Abrams, P. (1998). Efficacy and safety of tolterodine in patients with detrusor instability: a dose ranging study. *British Journal of Urology*, **81**, 42–8.

Reuben, D.B., Borok, G.M., Wolde-Tsadik, G., *et al.* (1995). Randomised trial of comprehensive geriatric assessment in the care of hospitalised patients. *New England Journal of Medicine*, **332**, 1345–50.

Ricci, S., Celani, M.G., La Rosa, F., Righetti, E., Duca, E., and Caputo, N. (1993). Silent brain infarctions in patients with first-ever stroke. A community-based study in Umbria, Italy. *Stroke*, **24**, 647–51.

Rich-Edwards, J.W., Stampfer, M.J., Manson, J.E. *et al.* (1997). Birth weight and risk of cardiovascular disease in a cohort of women followed up since 1976. *British Medical Journal*, **315**, 396–400.

Ridker, P.M., Hennekens, C.H., Stampfer, M.J., Manson, J.E., and Vaughan, D.E. (1994). Prospective study of endogenous tissue plasminogen activator and risk of stroke. *Lancet*, **343**, 940–3.

Ridker, P.M., Cushman, M., Stampfer, M.J., Tracy, R.P., and Hennekens, C.H. (1997). Inflammation, aspirin, and the risk of cardiovascular disease in apparently healthy men. *New England Journal of Medicine*, **336**, 973–9. [See erratum in *NEJM* (1997), **337**, 356.]

Ringelstein, E.B., Droste, D.W., Babikian, V.L. *et al.* (1998). Consensus on microembolus detection by TCD. International Consensus Group on Microembolus Detection. *Stroke*, **29**, 725–9.

Ritchie, K. (1988). The screening of cognitive impairment in the elderly. *Journal of Clinical Epidemiology*, **41**, 635–43.

Robbins, A.S., Manson, J.E., Lee, I.M., Satterfield, S., and Hennekens, C.H. (1994). Cigarette smoking and stroke in a cohort of U.S. male physicians. *Annals of Internal Medicine*, **120**, 458–62.

Roberts, L. and Counsell, C. (1998). Assessment of clinical outcomes in acute stroke trials. *Stroke*, **29**, 986–91.

Robertson, I.H., Ridgeway, V., Greenfield, E., and Parr, A. (1997). Motor recovery after stroke depends on intact sustained attention: a 2-year follow-up study. *Neuropsychology*, **11**, 290–5.

Robinson, R.G. and Price, T.R. (1982). Post stroke depressive disorders: a follow up study of 103 patients. *Stroke*, **13**, 635–41.

Robinson, R.G., Kubos, K.L., Starr, L.B., Rao, K., and Price, T.R. (1984). Mood disorders in stroke patients. Importance of location of lesion. *Brain*, **107**, 81–93.

Roden-Jullig, A., Britton, M., Gustafsson, C., and Fugl-Meyer, A. (1994). Validation of four scales for the acute stage of stroke. *Journal of Internal Medicine*, **236**, 125–36.

Rodgers, A., MacMahon, S., Gamble, G., Slattery, J., Sandercock, P., and Warlow, C. (1996). Blood pressure and risk of stroke in patients with cerebrovascular disease. The United Kingdom Transient Ischaemic Attack Collaborative Group. *British Medical Journal*, **313**, 147.

Rodgers, H., Soutter, J., Kaiser, W., Pearson, P. *et al.* (1997). Early supported hospital discharge following stroke: pilot study results. *Clinical Rehabilitation*, **11**, 280–7.

Rogvi-Hansen, B. and Boysen, G. (1998). Glycerol treatment in acute ischaemic stroke (Cochrane review). In *Cochrane database of systematic reviews (disc and CD-ROM). Stroke module*, (ed. C.P. Warlow, J. van Gijn, and P.A.G. Sandercock). Update Software/ BMJ Publishing, Oxford.

Roman, C.G., Tatemichi, T.K., Erkinjuntti, T. *et al.* (1993). Vascular dementia: diagnostic criteria for research studies. *Neurology*, **43**, 250–60.

Ronning, O.M. and Guldrog, V. (1998). Outcome of subacute stroke rehabilitation: a randomised controlled trial. *Stroke*, **29**, 779–84.

Rose, G. (1981). Strategy of prevention: lessons from cardiovascular disease. *British Medical Journal*, **280**, 1847–51.

Rose, G. (1992). *The strategy of preventive medicine*. OUP, Oxford.

Rothrock, J.F., Lyden, P.D., Hesselink, J.R., Brown, J.J., and Healy, M.E. (1987). Brain magnetic resonance imaging in the evaluation of lacunar stroke. *Stroke*, **18**, 781–6.

Rothwell, P.M., Gibson, R.J., Slattery, J., Sellar, R.J., and Warlow, C.P. (1994*a*).

Equivalence of measurements of carotid stenosis. A comparison of three methods on 1001 angiograms. European Carotid Surgery Trialists' Collaborative Group. *Stroke*, **25**, 2435–9.

Rothwell, P.M., Gibson, R.J., Slattery, J., and Warlow, C.P. (1994*b*). Prognostic value and reproducibility of measurements of carotid stenosis. A comparison of three methods on 1001 angiograms. European Carotid Surgery Trialists' Collaborative Group. *Stroke*, **25**, 2440–4.

Royal College of Physicians of London (1974). Report of Geriatrics Committee Working Group on Strokes. Royal College of Physicians, London.

Rubenstein, L., Calkins, D.R., Young, R.T. *et al.* (1989). Improving patient function: a randomised trial of functional disability screening. *Annals of Internal Medicine*, **111**, 836–42.

Rudd, A.G., Wolfe, C.D.A., Tilling, K., and Beech, R. (1997). Randomised controlled trial to evaluate early discharge scheme for patients with stroke. *British Medical Journal*, **315**, 1039–44.

Ruff, R.L. and Dougherty, J.H. (1981). Evaluation of acute cerebral ischaemia for anticoagulant therapy: computed tomography or lumbar puncture. *Neurology*, **31**, 736–40.

Ruggieri, P.M., Masaryk, T.J., and Ross, J.S. (1992). Magnetic resonance angiography. Cerebrovascular applications. *Stroke*, **23**, 774–80.

Rupright, J., Singh, A., Stonnington, H. *et al.* (1997). Correlation of functional independence measure (FIM) and SPECT Iofetamine (I-123) as a predictor of functional return in stroke. *Brain Injury*, **11**, 49–57.

Russell, R.W. (1975). How does blood-pressure cause stroke? *Lancet*, **ii**, 1283–5.

Rutan, G.H., Kuller, L.H., Neaton, J.D., Wentworth, D.N., McDonald, R.H., and Smith, W.M. (1988). Mortality associated with diastolic hypertension and isolated systolic hypertension among men screened for the Multiple Risk Factor Intervention Trial. *Circulation*, **77**, 504–14.

Sacco, R., Wolf, P., Kannel, W., and McNamara, P. (1982). Survival and recurrence following stroke. The Framingham Study. *Stroke*, **13**, 290–5.

Sacco, R.L., Ellenberg, J.H., Mohr, J.P. *et al.* (1989). Infarcts of undetermined cause. The NINCDS Stroke Data Bank. *Annals of Neurology*, **25**, 35–41.

Sackett, D.L. (1979). Bias in analytic research. *Journal of Chronic Diseases*, **32**, 51–63.

Sackett, D.L., Haynes, R.B., and Tugwell, P. (1985). *Clinical epidemiology; a basic science for clinical medicine*, (1st edn). Little Brown, Boston.

Sacquegna, T., de Carolis, P., Andreoli, A. *et al.* (1984). Long term prognosis after occlusion of the middle cerebral artery. *British Medical Journal*, **288**, 1490–1.

Safar, P. (1980). Amelioration of post-ischaemic brain damage with barbiturates. *Stroke*, **11**, 565–8.

Sagar, G., Riley, P., and Vohrah, A. (1996). Is admission chest radiography of any clinical value in acute stroke patients? *Clinical Radiology*, **51**, 499–502.

Sage, J. and Uitert, R. (1983). Risk of recurrent stroke in patients with atrial fibrillation and non-valvular heart disease. *Stroke*, **14**, 537–40.

Sainsbury, S. (1973). *Measuring disability*. Bell, London.

Sakakibara, R., Hattori, T., Yasuda, K., and Yamanishi, T. (1996). Micturitional disturbance after acute hemispheric stroke: analysis of the lesion site by CT and MRI. *Journal of the Neurological Sciences*, **137**, 47–56.

Sakamoto-Momiyama, M. (1978). Changes in the seasonality of human mortality: a medico-geographical study. *Social Science and Medicine*, **12**, 29–42.

Salonen, J.T., Puska, P., Tuomilheto, J., and Homan, K. (1982). Relation of blood pressure, serum lipids, and smoking to the risk of cerebral stroke. *Stroke*, **13**, 327–33.

SALT Collaborative Group (1991). Swedish Aspirin Low-Dose Trial (SALT) of 75mg aspirin as secondary prophylaxis after cerebrovascular ischaemic events. The SALT Collaborative Group. *Lancet*, **338**, 1345–9.

Samuelsson, M., Soderfeldt, B., and Olsson, G.B. (1996). Functional outcome in patients with lacunar infarction. *Stroke*, **27**, 842–6.

Sandercock, P.A. and Warlow, C.P. (1985). The prevention of stroke in the elderly. In *Prevention of disease in the elderly*, (ed. J.A.M. Gray), pp. 130–55. Churchill Livingstone, London.

Sandercock, P.A., Molyneux, A., and Warlow, C. (1985a). Value of computed tomography in patients with stroke: Oxfordshire Community Stroke Project. *British Medical Journal*, **290**, 193–7.

Sandercock, P.A., Allen, C.M., Corston, R.N., Harrison, M.J., and Warlow, C.P. (1985b). Clinical diagnosis of intracranial haemorrhage using Guy's Hospital score. *British Medical Journal*, **291**, 1675–7.

Sandercock, P.A., Warlow, C., Bamford, J., Peto, R., and Starkey, I. (1986). Is a controlled trial of long-term oral anticoagulants in patients with stroke and non-rheumatic atrial fibrillation worthwhile? *Lancet*, **i**, 788–92.

Sandercock, P.A., Warlow, C.P., Jones, L.N., and Starkey, I.R. (1989). Predisposing factors for cerebral infarction: the Oxfordshire community stroke project. *British Medical Journal*, **298**, 75–80.

Sandercock, P.A., Bamford, J., Dennis, M. *et al.* (1992). Atrial fibrillation and stroke: prevalence in different types of stroke and influence on early and long term prognosis (Oxfordshire community stroke project). *British Medical Journal*, **305**, 1460–5.

Sandercock, P.A., van den Belt, A.G., Lindley, R.I., and Slattery, J. (1993). Antithrombotic therapy in acute ischaemic stroke: an overview of the completed randomised trials. *Journal of Neurology, Neurosurgery and Psychiatry*, **56**, 17–25.

Sarti, C., Tuomilehto, J., Sivenius, J. *et al.* (1993). Stroke mortality and case-fatality rates in three geographic areas of Finland from 1983 to 1986. *Stroke*, **24**, 1140–7.

Sato, Y., Maruoka, H., and Oizumi, K. (1997). Amelioration of hemiplegia-associated osteopenia more than 4 years after stroke by 1 alpha-hydroxyvitamin D3 and calcium supplementation. *Stroke*, **28**, 736–9.

Saunders, J.B. (1987). Alcohol: an important cause of hypertension. *British Medical Journal*, **294**, 1045–6.

Scandinavian Stroke Study Group (1987). Multicenter trial of hemodilution in acute ischemic stroke. I. Results in the total patient population. Scandinavian Stroke Study Group. *Stroke*, **18**, 691–9.

Scandinavian Stroke Study Group (1988). Multicenter trial of hemodilution in acute ischemic stroke. Results of subgroup analyses. Scandinavian Stroke Study Group. *Stroke*, **19**, 464–71.

Schneider, L.B., Libman, R.B., and Kanner, R. (1996). Utility of repeat brain imaging in stroke. *American Journal of Neuroradiology*, **17**, 1259–63.

Schwartz, D. and Lellouch, J. (1967). Explanatory and pragmatic attitudes in therapeutic trials. *Journal of Chronic Diseases*, **20**, 637–48.

Scmidt, E.V., Smirnov, V.E., and Ryabova, V.S. (1988). Results of the seven-year prospective study of stroke patients. *Stroke*, **19**, 942–9.

Seale, C. and Davies, P. (1987). Outcome measurement in stroke rehabilitation research. *International Disability Studies*, **9**, 155–60.

Segal, M.E. and Schall, R.R. (1995). Assessing handicap of stroke survivors. A validation study of the Craig Handicap Assessment and Reporting Technique. *American Journal of Physical Medicine and Rehabilitation*, **74**, 276–86.

Sekita, Y. (1985). Cost-benefit evaluation of comprehensive medical care for cerebral strokes. *Medical Informatics*, **10**, 59–71.

Selley, W.G. (1985). Swallowing difficulties in stroke patients: a new treatment. *Age and Ageing*, **14**, 361–5.

Sever, P., Beevers, G., Bulpitt, C. *et al.* (1993). Management guidelines in essential hypertension: report of the second working party of the British Hypertension Society. *British Medical Journal*, **306**, 983–7.

Shah, S., Vanclay, F., and Cooper, B. (1990). Efficiency, effectiveness, and duration of stroke rehabilitation. *Stroke*, **21**, 241–6.

Shah, S., Vanclay, F., and Cooper, B. (1991). Stroke rehabilitation: Australian patient profile and functional outcome. *Journal of Clinical Epidemiology*, **44**, 21–8.

Shahar, E., McGovern, P.G., Sprafka, J.M. *et al.* (1995). Improved survival of stroke patients during the 1980s. The Minnesota Stroke Survey. *Stroke*, **26**, 1–6.

Shaper, A.G., Phillips, A.N., Pocock, S.J., Walker, M., and Macfarlane, P.W. (1991). Risk factors for stroke in middle aged British men. *British Medical Journal*, **302**, 1111–15.

Sharpe, M., Hawton, K., House, A. *et al.* (1990). Mood disorders in long-term survivors of stroke: associations with brain lesion location and volume. *Psychological Medicine*, **20**, 815–28.

Sharpe, M., Hawton, K., Seagroatt, V. *et al.* (1994). Depressive disorders in long-term survivors of stroke. Associations with demographic and social factors, functional status, and brain lesion volume. *British Journal of Psychiatry*, **164**, 380–6.

Sheikh, K., Smith, D.S., Meade, T.W. *et al.* (1979). Repeatability and validity of a modified ADL index in studies of chronic disability. *International Journal of Rehabilitation Medicine*, **1**, 51–8.

Sheikh, K., Brennan, P.J., Meade, T.W., Smith, D.S., and Goldenberg, E. (1983). Predictors of mortality and disability in stroke. *Journal of Epidemiology and Community Health*, **37**, 70–4.

SHEP Co-operative Research Group (1991). Prevention of stroke by antihypertensive drug treatment in older persons with isolated systolic hypertension. Final results of the Systolic Hypertension in the Elderly Program (SHEP). *Journal of the American Medical Association*, **265**, 3255–64.

Sherman, D.G., Hart, R.G., and Easton, J.D. (1986). The secondary prevention of stroke in patients with atrial fibrillation. *Archives of Neurology*, **43**, 68–70.

Shinar, D., Gross, C.R., Mohr, J.P. *et al.* (1985). Interobserver variability in the assessment of neurologic history and examination in the stroke data bank. *Archives of Neurology*, **42**, 557–65.

Shinar, D., Gross, C.R., Hier, D.B. *et al.* (1987). Interobserver reliability in the interpretation of computed tomographic scans of stroke patients. *Archives of Neurology*, **44**, 149–55.

Shinkawa, A., Ueda, K., Kiyohara, Y. *et al.* (1995). Silent cerebral infarction in a community-based autopsy series in Japan. The Hisayama Study. *Stroke*, **26**, 380–5.

Shintani, S., Kikuchi, S., Hamaguchi, H., and Shiigai, T. (1993). High serum lipoprotein(a) levels are an independent risk factor for cerebral infarction. *Stroke*, **24**, 965–9.

Shinton, R. (1992) Lifestyle and the risk of stroke. M.D. thesis, University of Cambridge.

Shinton, R. and Beevers, G. (1989). Meta-analysis of relation between cigarette smoking and stroke. *British Medical Journal*, **298**, 789–94.

Shinton, R. and Sagar, G. (1993). Lifelong exercise and stroke. *British Medical Journal*, **307**, 231–4. [See erratum in *BMJ* (1993), **307**, 706.]

Shinton, R., Shipley, M., and Rose, G. (1991). Overweight and stroke in the Whitehall study. *Journal of Epidemiology and Community Health*, **45**, 138–42.

Shrier, D.A., Tanaka, H., Numaguchi, Y., Konno, S., Patel, U., and Shibata, D. (1997). CT angiography in the evaluation of acute stroke. *American Journal of Neuroradiology*, **18**, 1011–20.

Shuaib, A. and Hachinski, V.C. (1991). Mechanisms and management of stroke in the elderly. *Canadian Medical Association Journal*, **145**, 433–43.

Shuaib, A., Lee, D., Pelz, D., Fox, A., and Hachinski, V.C. (1992). The impact of magnetic resonance imaging on the management of acute ischemic stroke. *Neurology*, **42**, 816–18.

Siesjo, B.K. (1992). Pathophysiology and treatment of focal cerebral ischemia. Part I: Pathophysiology. *Journal of Neurosurgery*, **77**, 169–84.

Sigurdsson, G., Sigfusson, N., Thorsteinsson, T., Olafsson, O., Davidsson, D., and Samuelsson, S. (1983). Screening for health risks. How useful is a questionnaire response showing a family history of myocardial infarction, hypertension, or stroke? *Acta Medica Scandinavica*, **213**, 45–50.

Sila, C.A. and Furlan, A.J. (1988). Drug treatment of stroke. Current status and future prospects. *Drugs*, **35**, 468–76.

Simpson, F.O. (1979). Salt and hypertension: a sceptical review of the evidence. *Clinical Science*, **57**, 463s–480s.

Sinyor, D., Jacques, P., Kaloupek, D.G., Becker, R., Goldenberg, M., and Coopersmith, H. (1986). Poststroke depression and lesion location. An attempted replication. *Brain*, **109**, 537–46.

Sivenius, J., Pyorala, K., Heinonen, O.P., Salonen, J.T., and Reikkinen, P. (1985). The significance of intensity of rehabilitation of stroke: a controlled trial. *Stroke*, **16**, 928–31.

Skilbeck, C.E., Wade, D.T., Hewer, R.L., and Wood, V.A. (1983). Recovery after stroke. *Journal of Neurology, Neurosurgery and Psychiatry*, **46**, 5–8.

Sloan, M.A. (1987). Thrombolysis and stroke. Past and future. *Archives of Neurology*, **44**, 748–68.

Smith, D.S., Goldenberg, E., Ashburn, A. *et al.* (1981). Remedial therapy after stroke: a randomised controlled trial. *British Medical Journal*, **282**, 517–20.

Smith, G.T. (1990). The economics of hypertension and stroke. *American Heart Journal*, **119**, (Pt 2), 725–7.

Smith, P., Arnesen, H., and Holme, I. (1990). The effect of warfarin on mortality and reinfarction after myocardial infarction. *New England Journal of Medicine*, **323**, 147–52.

Smith, W.C.S., Lee, A.J., Crombie, I.K., and Tunstall-Pedoe, H. (1990). Control of blood pressure in Scotland: the rule of halves. *British Medical Journal*, **300**, 981–3.

Smithard, D.G., O'Neill, P.A., Parks, C., and Morris, J. (1996). Complications and outcome after acute stroke. Does dysphagia matter? *Stroke*, **27**, 1200–4.

Sneeuw, K.C.A., Aaronson, N.K., de Haan, R.J., and Limberg, M. (1997). Assessing quality of life after stroke. The value and limitations of proxy ratings. *Stroke*, **28**, 1541–9.

Solomon, N.A., Glick, H.A., Russo, C.J., Lee, J., and Schulman, K.A. (1994). Patient preferences for stroke outcomes. *Stroke*, **25**, 1721–5.

Sotaniemi, K.A., Pyhtinen, J., and Myllyla, V.V. (1990). Correlation of clinical and computed tomographic findings in stroke patients. *Stroke*, **21**, 1562–6.

Sox, H.J., Margulies, I., and Sox, C. (1981). Psychologically mediated effects of diagnostic tests. *Annals of Internal Medicine*, **95**, 680–5.

Spiteri, M.A., Cook, D.G., and Clarke, S.W. (1988). Reliability of eliciting physical signs in the examination of the chest. *Lancet*, **i**, 873–5.

Squire, I.B., Lees, K.R., Pryse, P.W. *et al.* (1996). The effects of lifarizine in acute cerebral infarction: a pilot safety study. *Cerebrovascular Diseases*, **6**, 156–60.

Srinivasan, J., Mayberg, M.R., Weiss, D.G., and Eskridge, J. (1995). Duplex accuracy compared with angiography in the Veterans Affairs Cooperative Studies Trial for Symptomatic Carotid Stenosis. *Neurosurgery*, **36**, 648–53.

Staessen, J.A., Fagard, R., Thijs, L. *et al.* (1997). Randomised double-blind comparison of placebo and active treatment for older patients with isolated systolic hypertension. The Systolic Hypertension in Europe (Syst-Eur) Trial Investigators. *Lancet*, **350**, 757–64.

Stamler, J., Elliott, P., Dyer, A. *et al.* (1993). Sodium and blood pressure in the Intersalt Study and other studies-in reply to the Salt Institute. *British Medical Journal*, **312**, 1285–7.

Stamler, R., Stamler, J., Gosch, F.C., Civinelli, J. *et al.* (1989). Primary prevention of hypertension by nutritional hygienic means: final report of a randomised controlled trial. *Journal of the American Medical Association*, **262**, 1801–7.

Stampfer, M.J., Willet, W.C., Colditz, G.A. *et al.* (1988a). A prospective study of oral contraceptive agents and risk of cardiovascular disease. *New England Journal of Medicine*, **319**, 1313–17.

Stampfer, M.J., Colditz, G.A., Willett, W.C., Speizer, F.E., and Hennekens, C.H. (1988b). A prospective study of moderate alcohol consumption and the risk of coronary disease and stroke in women. *New England Journal of Medicine*, **319**, 267–73.

Stampfer, M.J., Colditz, G.A., Willett, W.C. *et al.* (1991). Postmenopausal estrogen therapy and cardiovascular disease. Ten-year follow-up from the nurses' health study. *New England Journal of Medicine*, **325**, 756–62.

Stanner, S.A., Bulmer, K., Andres, C. *et al.* (1997). Does malnutrition *in utero* determine diabetes and coronary heart disease in adulthood? Results from the Leningrad siege study, a cross sectional study. *British Medical Journal*, **315**, 1342–8.

Starkey, I. and Warlow, C. (1986). The secondary prevention of stroke in patients with atrial fibrillation. *Archives of Neurology*, **43**, 66–8.

Starkstein, S.E., Fedoroff, J.P., Price, T.R., Leiguarda, R., and Robinson, R.G. (1993). Apathy following cerebrovascular lesions. *Stroke*, **24**, 1625–30.

Stegmayr, B. and Asplund, K. (1996). Exploring the declining case fatality in acute stroke. Population-based observations in the northern Sweden MONICA Project. *Journal of Internal Medicine*, **240**, 143–9.

Stein, R.E.K., Gortmaker, S.L., Perrin, E.C. *et al.* (1987). Severity of illness: concepts and measurements. *Lancet*, **ii**, 1506–9.

Steiner, T.J. and Rose, F.C. (1986). Towards a model stroke trial. The single-centre naftidrofuryl study. *Neuroepidemiology*, **5**, 121–47.

Stemmermann, G.N., Hayashi, T., Resch, J.A., Chung, C.S., Reed, D.M., and Rhoads, G.G. (1984). Risk factors related to ischemic and hemorrhagic cerebrovascular disease at autopsy: the Honolulu Heart Study. *Stroke*, **15**, 23–8.

Stephan, K.M. and Frackowiak, R.S. (1997). Recovery from subcortical stroke–PET activation patterns in patients compared with healthy subjects. *Advances in Neurology*, **73**, 311–20.

Stevens, R. and Ambler, N.R. (1982). The incidence and survival of stroke patients in a defined community. *Age and Ageing*, **11**, 266–74.

Stevens, R.S., Ambler, N.R., and Warren, M.D. (1984). A randomized controlled trial of a stroke rehabilitation ward. *Age and Ageing*, **13**, 65–75.

Stineman, M.G., Maislin, G., Fiedler, R.C., and Granger, C.V. (1997). A prediction model for functional recovery in stroke. *Stroke*, **28**, 550–6.

STIPAS Study Group (1994). Safety study of tirilazad mesylate in patients with acute ischemic stroke (STIPAS). *Stroke*, **25**, 418–23.

Stout, R.W. and Crawford, V. (1991). Seasonal variations in fibrinogen concentrations among elderly people. *Lancet*, **338**, 9–13.

Strachan, D.P. (1991). Ventilatory function as a predictor of fatal stroke. *British Medical Journal*, **302**, 84–7.

Strand, T., Asplund, K., Eriksson, S. *et al.* (1984). A randomised controlled trial of haemodilution therapy in acute stroke. *Stroke*, **15**, 980–9.

Streifler, J.Y., Eliasziw, M., Benavente, O.R. *et al.* (1995). The risk of stroke in patients with first-ever retinal vs hemispheric transient ischemic attacks and high-grade carotid stenosis. North American Symptomatic Carotid Endarterectomy Trial. *Archives of Neurology*, **52**, 246–9.

Stroke Prevention in Atrial Fibrillation Investigators (1990*a*). Preliminary report of the Stroke Prevention in Atrial Fibrillation Study. *New England Journal of Medicine*, **322**, 863–8.

Stroke Prevention in Atrial Fibrillation Investigators (1990*b*). Design of a multicenter randomized trial for the Stroke Prevention in Atrial Fibrillation Study. *Stroke*, **21**, 538–45.

Stroke Prevention in Atrial Fibrillation Investigators (1991). Stroke Prevention in Atrial Fibrillation Study. Final results. *Circulation*, **84**, 527–39.

Stroke Prevention in Atrial Fibrillation Investigators (1993*a*). Predictors of thromboembolism in atrial fibrillation: I. Clinical features of patients at risk. *Annals of Internal Medicine*, **116**, 1–5.

Stroke Prevention in Atrial Fibrillation Investigators (1993*b*). Predictors of thromboembolism in atrial fibrillation: II. Echocardiographic features of patients at risk. *Annals of Internal Medicine*, **116**, 6–12.

Stroke Prevention in Atrial Fibrillation Investigators (1994). Warfarin versus aspirin for prevention of thromboembolism in atrial fibrillation: Stroke Prevention in Atrial Fibrillation II Study. *Lancet*, **343**, 687–91.

Stroke Prevention in Atrial Fibrillation Investigators (1996). Bleeding during antithrombotic therapy in patients with atrial fibrillation. *Archives of Internal Medicine*, **156**, 409–16.

Stroke Prevention in Reversible Ischaemia (SPIRIT) Study Group (1997). A randomised trial of anticoagulants versus aspirin after cerebral ischaemia of presumed arterial origin. *Annals of Neurology*, **42**, 857–65.

Stroke Unit Trialists Collaboration (1997). Collaborative systematic review of the randomised trials of organised inpatient (stroke unit) care after stroke. *British Medical Journal*, **314**, 1151–9.

Stuck, A.W., Sui, A.L., Wieland, G.D., Adams, J., and Rubenstein, L.Z. (1993). Comprehensive geriatric assessment: a meta-analysis of controlled trials. *Lancet*, **342**, 1032–6.

Sudlow, C.L. and Warlow, C.P. (1996). Comparing stroke incidence worldwide: what makes studies comparable? *Stroke*, **27**, 550–8.

Sudlow, C.L. and Warlow, C.P. (1997). Comparable studies of the incidence of stroke and its pathological types: results from an international collaboration. International Stroke Incidence Collaboration. *Stroke*, **28**, 491–9.

Sunderland, A., Wade, D.T., and Hewer, R.L. (1987). The natural history of visual neglect after stroke. Indications from two methods of assessment. *International Disability Studies*, **9**, 55–9.

Sunderland, A., Tinson, D.J., Bradley, E.L., Fletcher, D., Hewer, R.L., and Wade, D.T. (1992). Enhanced physical therapy improves recovery of arm function after stroke. A randomised controlled trial. *Journal of Neurology, Neurosurgery and Psychiatry*, **55**, 530–5.

Svanborg, A. (1988). The health of the elderly population: results from longitudinal studies with age-cohort comparisons. In *Research and the ageing population*, (ed. D. Evered and J. Whelan), pp. 3–16. John Wiley, Chichester.

Swales, J.D. (1989). Salt saga continued. *British Medical Journal*, **297**, 307–8.

Swets, J.A., Pickett, R.M., Whitehead, S.F. *et al.* (1979). Assessment of diagnostic technologies. *Science*, **205**, 753–9.

Syrjanen, J., Valtonen, V.V., Iivanainen, M., Kaste, M., and Huttunen, J.K. (1988). Preceding infection as an important risk factor for ischaemic brain infarction in young and middle aged patients. *British Medical Journal*, **296**, 1156–60.

Szczepura, A.K., Fletcher, J., and Fitz-Patrick, J.D. (1991). Cost-effectiveness of MRI in the neurosciences. *British Medical Journal*, **303**, 1435–9.

Tanaka, H., Ueda, Y., Date, C. *et al.* (1981). Incidence of stroke in Shibata, Japan: 1976–1978. *Stroke*, **12**, 460–6.

Tanaka, H., Ueda, Y., Hayashi, M. *et al.* (1982). Risk factors for cerebral haemorrhage and cerebral infarction in a Japanese rural community. *Stroke*, **13**, 62–73.

Tatemichi, T.K., Desmond, D.W., Paik, M. *et al.* (1993). Clinical determinants of dementia related to stroke. *Annals of Neurology*, **33**, 568–75.

Taub, N.A., Wolfe, C.D., Richardson, E., and Burney, P.G. (1994). Predicting the disability of first-time stroke sufferers at 1 year. 12-month follow-up of a population-based cohort in southeast England. *Stroke*, **25**, 352–7.

Taubes, G. (1998). The (political) science of salt. *Science*, **281**, 898–907.

Taylor, S.J., Whincup, P.H., Cook, D.G., Papacosta, O., and Walker, M. (1997). Size at birth and blood pressure: cross sectional study in 8–11 year old children. *British Medical Journal*, **314**, 475–80.

Tennant, A., Geddes, J.M., Fear, J., Hillman, M., and Chamberlain, M.A. (1997). Outcome following stroke. *Disability and Rehabilitation*, **19**, 278–84.

Terent, A. (1988). Increasing incidence of stroke among Swedish women. *Stroke*, **19**, 598–603.

Terent, A. (1989). Survival after stroke and transient ischemic attacks during the 1970s and 1980s. *Stroke*, **20**, 1320–6.

Thomas, D.J. (1984). Treatment of acute stroke. *British Medical Journal*, **288**, 2–3.

Thompson, S.G. and Pocock, S.J. (1991). Can meta-analyses be trusted? *Lancet*, **338**, 1127–30.

Thompson, S.G., Greenberg, G., and Meade, T.W. (1989). Risk factors for stroke and myocardial infarction in women in the United Kingdom as assessed in general practice: a case-control study. *British Heart Journal*, **61**, 403–09.

Thornbury, J.R. (1994). Clinical efficacy of diagnostic imaging. *American Journal of Roentgenology*, **162**, 1–8.

Thorogood, M., Mann, J., Murphy, M., and Vessey, M. (1992). Fatal stroke and use of oral contraceptives: findings from a case-control study. *American Journal of Epidemiology*, **136**, 35–45.

Thorvaldsen, P., Asplund, K., Kuulasmaa, K., Rajakangas, A.M., and Schroll, M. (1995). Stroke incidence, case fatality, and mortality in the WHO MONICA project. World Health Organization Monitoring Trends and Determinants in Cardiovascular Disease. *Stroke*, **26**, 361–7. [See erratum in *Stroke* (1995), **26**, 1504.]

Thorvaldsen, P., Kuulasmaa, K., Rajakangas, A.M., Rastenyte, D., Sarti, C., and Wilhelmsen, L. (1997). Stroke trends in the WHO MONICA project. *Stroke*, **28**, 500–6.

Tinetti, M.E., Speechley, M., and Ginter, S.F. (1988). Risk factors for falls among elderly persons living in the community. *New England Journal of Medicine*, **319**, 1701–7.

Tinetti, M.E., Baker, D.I., McAvay, G. *et al.* (1994). A multifactorial intervention to reduce the risk of falling among elderly people living in the community. *New England Journal of Medicine*, **331**, 821–7.

Tinson, D.J. and Lincoln, N.B. (1987). Subjective memory impairment after stroke. *International Disability Studies*, **9**, 6–9.

Toghi, H., Mochizuki, H., Yamanouchi, H. *et al.* (1981). A comparison between the computed tomogram and neuropathological findings in cerebrovascular disease. *Journal of Neurology*, **224**, 211–20.

Tomasello, F., Mariani, F., Fieschi, C. *et al.* (1982). Assessment of inter-observer differences in the Italian multicenter study on reversible cerebral ischemia. *Stroke*, **13**, 32–5.

Tomlinson, B.E., Blessed, G., and Roth, M. (1970). Observations on the brains of demented old people. *Journal of Neurological Science*, **11**, 205–42.

Toni, D., Del Duca, R., Fiorelli, M. *et al.* (1994). Pure motor hemiparesis and sensorimotor stroke. Accuracy of very early clinical diagnosis of lacunar strokes. *Stroke*, **25**, 92–6.

Torrance, G.W. (1976). Toward a utility theory foundation for health status index models. *Health Services Research*, **11**, 349–69.

Townsend, J., Piper, M., Frank, A.O., Dyer, S., North, W.R.S., and Meade, T.W. (1988). Reduction in hospital readmission stay of elderly patients by a community based discharge scheme: a randomised controlled trial. *British Medical Journal*, **297**, 544–7.

Treasure, T. and MacRae, K.D. (1998). Minimisation: the platinum standard for trials? *British Medical Journal*, **317**, 362–3.

Treves, T.A., Karepov, V.G., Aronovich, B.D., Gorbulev, A.Y., Bornstein, N.M., and Korczyn, A.D. (1994). Interrater agreement in evaluation of stroke patients with the unified neurological stroke scale. *Stroke*, **25**, 1263–4.

Trials of Hypertension Prevention Collaborative Research Group (1997). Effects of weight loss and sodium reduction intervention on blood pressure and hypertension incidence in overweight people with high-normal blood pressure. The Trials of Hypertension Prevention, phase II. *Archives of Internal Medicine*, **157**, 657–67.

TRUST Study Group (1990). Randomised, double-blind, placebo-controlled trial of nimodipine in acute stroke. *Lancet*, **336**, 1205–9.

Tuomilehto, J., Nissinen, A., and Wold, E. (1985). Effectiveness of treatment with anti-hypertensive drugs and trends in mortality from stroke in the community. *British Medical Journal*, **291**, 857–60.

Tuomilehto, J., Geboers, J., Salonen, J.T. *et al.* (1986). Decline in cardiovascular mortality in North Karelia and other parts of Finland. *British Medical Journal*, **293**, 1068–71.

Tuomilehto, J., Bonita, R., Stewart, A., Nissinen, A., and Salonen, J.T. (1991).

Hypertension, cigarette smoking, and the decline in stroke incidence in eastern Finland. *Stroke*, **22**, 7–11.

Tuomilehto, J., Rastenyte, D., Jousilahti, P., Sarti, C., and Vartiainen, E. (1996*a*). Diabetes mellitus as a risk factor for death from stroke. Prospective study of the middle-aged Finnish population. *Stroke*, **27**, 210–15.

Tuomilehto, J., Rastenyte, D., Sivenius, J. *et al.* (1996*b*). Ten-year trends in stroke incidence and mortality in the FINMONICA Stroke Study. *Stroke*, **27**, 825–32.

Turpie, A.G., Levine, M.N., Hirsh, J. *et al.* (1987). Double-blind randomised trial of Org 10172 low-molecular-weight heparinoid in prevention of deep-vein thrombosis in thrombotic stroke. *Lancet*, **i**, 523–6.

Tutuarima, J.A., van der Meulen, J.H., de Haan, R.J., Van Straten, A., and Limburg, M. (1997). Risk factors for falls of hospitalized stroke patients. *Stroke*, **28**, 297–301.

Tzourio, C., Iglesias, S., Hubert, J.B. *et al.* (1993). Migraine and risk of ischaemic stroke: a case-control study . *British Medical Journal*, **307**, 289–92.

Ueda, K., Omae, T., and Hirota, Y.E. (1981). Decreasing trend in incidence and mortality from stroke in Hisayama Residents, Japan. *Stroke*, **12**, 154–60.

UKPDS (1998). Tight blood pressure control and risk of macrovascular and microvascular complications in type 2 diabetes. UK Prospective Diabetes Study Group. *British Medical Journal* **317**: 703-13.

UK-TIA Study Group (1983). Variation in use of angiography and carotid endarterectomy by neurologists in the UK-TIA trial. *British Medical Journal* **286**: 574-17.

UK-TIA Study Group (1988). United Kingdom transient ischaemic attack (UK-TIA) aspirin trial: interim results. *British Medical Journal*, **296**, 316–20.

Vallance, P. and Martin, J. (1997). Drug therapy for coronary heart disease: the Sheffield table. *Lancet*, **350**, 1854.

Vandenbroucke, J.P. (1988). Passive smoking and lung cancer: a publication bias? *British Medical Journal*, **296**, 391–2.

Van Gijn, J. (1992). Subarachnoid haemorrhage. *Lancet*, **339**, 653–5.

Van Gijn, J. and Warlow, C.P. (1992). Down with stroke scales! *Cerebrovascular diseases* 2:244-6

Van Merwijk, G., Lodder, J., Bamford, J., and Kester, A.D. (1990). How often is non-valvular atrial fibrillation the cause of brain infarction? *Journal of Neurology*, **237**, 205–7.

Vanninen, R.L., Manninen, H.I., Partanen, P.K., Tulla, H., and Vainio, P.A. (1996). How should we estimate carotid stenosis using magnetic resonance angiography? *Neuroradiology*, **38**, 299–305.

Van Ruiswyk, J., Noble, H., and Sigmann, P. (1990). The natural history of carotid bruits in elderly persons. *Annals of Internal Medicine*, **112**, 340–3. [See erratum in Ann. Int. Med. (1990), **112**, 967.]

Van Swieten, J.C., Koudstaal, P.J., and Visser, M.C. (1988). Inter-observer agreement for the assessment of handicap in stroke patients. *Stroke*, **19**, 604–7.

Vartiainen, E., Sarti, C., Tuomilehto, J., and Kuulasmaa, K. (1995). Do changes in cardiovascular risk factors explain changes in mortality from stroke in Finland? *British Medical Journal*, **310**, 901–4.

Verhey, F.R.J., Lodder, J., Rozendaal, N., and Jolles, J. (1996). Comparison of seven sets of criteria used for the diagnosis of vascular dementia. *Neuroepidemiology*, **15**, 166–72.

Verhoef, P., Hennekens, C.H., Malinow, M.R., Kok, F.J., Willett, W.C., and Stampfer, M.J.

(1994). A prospective study of plasma homocyst(e)ine and risk of ischemic stroke. *Stroke*, **25**, 1924–30.

Vessey, M.P., Villard-Mackintosh, L., McPherson, K., and Yeates, D. (1989). Mortality among oral contraceptive users: 20 year follow up of women in a cohort study. *British Medical Journal*, **299**, 1487–91.

Viitanen, M., Eriksson, S., Asplund, K., Wester, P.O., and Winblad, B. (1987*a*). Determinants of long-term mortality after stroke. *Acta Medica Scandinavica*, **221**, 349–56.

Viitanen, M., Winblad, B., and Asplund, K. (1987*b*). Autopsy-verified causes of death after stroke. *Acta Medica Scandinavica*, **222**, 401–8.

von Arbin, M., Britton, M., de Faire, U., Helmers, C., Miah, K., and Murray, V. (1981). Accuracy of bedside diagnosis of stroke. *Stroke*, **12**, 288–93.

von Arbin, M., Britton, M., and de Faire, U. (1992). Mortality and recurrences during eight years following stroke. *Journal of Internal Medicine*, **231**, 43–8.

Wade, D.T. (1987). Extracranial–intracranial bypass, one; clinical trials, nil. *British Medical Journal*, **295**, 212.

Wade, D.T. and Collin, C. (1988). The Barthel ADL Index: a standard measure of physical disability? *International Disability Studies*, **10**, 64–7.

Wade, D.T. and Hewer, R.L. (1983). Why admit stroke patients to hospital? *Lancet*, **i**, 807–9.

Wade, D.T. and Hewer, R.L. (1985*a*). Hospital admission for acute stroke: who, for how long, and to what effect? *Journal of Epidemiology and Community Health*, **39**, 347–52.

Wade, D.T. and Hewer, R.L. (1985*b*). Outlook after an acute stroke: urinary incontinence and loss of consciousness compared in 532 patients. *Quarterly Journal of Medicine*, **56**, 601–8.

Wade, D.T. and Hewer, R.L. (1987). Functional abilities after stroke: measurement, natural history and prognosis. *Journal of Neurology, Neurosurgery and Psychiatry*, **50**, 177–82.

Wade, D.T., Hewer, R.L., Wood, V.A., Skilbeck, C.E., and Ismail, H.M. (1983*a*). The hemiplegic arm after stroke: measurement and recovery. *Journal of Neurology, Neurosurgery and Psychiatry*, **46**, 521–4.

Wade, D.T., Skilbeck, C.E., and Hewer, R.L. (1983*b*). Predicting Barthel ADL score at 6 months after an acute stroke. *Archives of Physical Medicine and Rehabilitation*, **64**, 24–8.

Wade, D.T., Skilbeck, C.E., Wood, V.A., and Hewer, R.L. (1984). Long-term survival after stroke. *Age and Ageing*, **13**, 76–82.

Wade, D.T., Hewer, R.L., Skilbeck, C.E., Bainton, D., and Burns-Cox, C. (1985*a*). Controlled trial of a home-care service for acute stroke patients. *Lancet*, **i**, 323–6.

Wade, D.T., Hewer, R.L., Skilbeck, C.E., and David, R.M. (1985*b*). *Stroke: a critical approach to diagnosis, treatment and management*. Chapman & Hall, London.

Wade, D.T., Legh-Smith, J., and Hewer, R.L. (1985*c*). Social activities after stroke: measurement and natural history using the Frenchay Activities Index. *International Rehabilitation Medicine*, **7**, 176–81.

Wade, D.T., Legh-Smith, J., and Hewer, R.L. (1986*a*). Effects of living with and looking after survivors of a stroke. *British Medical Journal*, **293**, 418–20.

Wade, D.T., Parker, V., and Hewer, R.L. (1986*b*). Memory disturbance after stroke: frequency and associated losses. *International Rehabilitation Medicine*, **8**, 60–4.

Wade, D.T., Collen, F.M., Robb, G.F., and Warlow, C.P. (1992). Physiotherapy intervention late after stroke and mobility. *British Medical Journal*, **304**, 609–13.

Walker, J.W. (1977). Changing US life style and declining vascular mortality: cause or coincidence? *New England Journal of Medicine*, **297**, 163–65.

Walker, M., Whincup, P.H., Shaper, A.G., Lennon, L.T., and Thompson, A.G. (1998). Validation of patient recall of doctor diagnosed heart attack and stroke. *American Journal of Epidemiology*, **148**, 355–61.

Walker, M.F. and Lincoln, N.B. (1991). Factors influencing dressing performance after stroke. *Journal of Neurology, Neurosurgery and Psychiatry*, **54**, 699–701.

Walker, S.R. and Rosser, R.M. (1988). *Quality of life: assessment and application*. MTP Press, Lancaster.

Wannamethee, G. and Shaper, A.G. (1992). Physical activity and stroke in British middle aged men. *British Medical Journal*, **304**, 597–601.

Wannamethee, S.G. and Shaper, A.G. (1996). Patterns of alcohol intake and risk of stroke in middle-aged British men. *Stroke*, **27**, 1033–9.

Wannamethee, S.G., Shaper, A.G., and Ebrahim, S. (1995a). Respiratory function and risk of stroke. *Stroke*, **26**, 2004–10.

Wannamethee, S.G., Shaper, A.G., Whincup, P.H., and Walker, M. (1995b). Smoking cessation and the risk of stroke in middle-aged men. *Journal of the American Medical Association*, **274**, 155–60.

Wannamethee, S.G., Shaper, A.G., and Ebrahim, S. (1996). History of parental death from stroke or heart trouble and the risk of stroke in middle-aged men. *Stroke*, **27**, 1492–8.

Wannamethee, S.G., Shaper, A.G., and Walker, M. (1998). Changes in physical activity, mortality and incidence of coronary heart disease in older men. *Lancet*, **351**, 1603–8.

Warach, S., Boska, M., and Welch, K.M. (1997). Pitfalls and potential of clinical diffusion-weighted MR imaging in acute stroke. *Stroke*, **28**, 481–2.

Ward, G., Jamrozik, K., and Stewart-Wynne, E. (1988). Incidence and outcome of cerebrovascular disease in Perth, Western Australia. *Stroke*, **19**, 1501–6.

Wardlaw, J.M. and Sellars, R. (1993). A simple practical classification of cerebral infarction on CT and its interobserver reliability. *American Journal of Neuroradiology*, **15**, 1933–9.

Wardlaw, J.M. and Warlow, C.P. (1992). Thrombolysis in acute ischemic stroke: does it work? *Stroke*, **23**, 1826–39.

Wardlaw, J.M., Dennis, M.S., Lindley, R.I., Sellar, R.J., and Warlow, C.P. (1996). The validity of a simple clinical classification of acute ischaemic stroke. *Journal of Neurology*, **243**, 274–9.

Wardlaw, J., Warlow, C.P., and Counsell, C. (1997). Systematic review of evidence on thrombolytic therapy for acute ischaemic stroke. *Lancet*, **350**, 607–14.

Wardlaw, J.M., Yamaguchi, T., and del Zoppo, G. (1998). Thrombolytic therapy versus control in acute ischaemic stroke (Cochrane review). In *Cochrane database of systematic reviews (disc and CD-ROM). Stroke module*, (ed. C.P. Warlow, J. van Gijn, and P.A.G. Sandercock). Update Software/BMJ Publishing, Oxford.

Ware, J.E., Snow, K., Kosinski, M., and Gandek, B. (1993). *SF-36 health survey manual and interpretation guide*. The Health Institute, New England Medical Center, Boston, MA.

Warlow, C.P. (1984). Carotid endarterectomy: does it work?. *Stroke*, **15**, 1068–76.

Warlow, C.P. (1996). Cerebrovascular disease. In *Oxford Textbook of Medicine*, (3rd edn), (ed. D.J. Weatherall, J.G.G. Ledingham, and D.A. Warrell), pp. 3946–64. Oxford University Press, Oxford.

Warlow, C.P. and Peto, R. (1987). Extracranial–intracranial bypass, one; clinical trials, nil. *British Medical Journal*, **295**, 211.

Warlow, C.P., Ogsten, D., and Douglas, A.S. (1972). Venous thrombosis following strokes. *Lancet*, **i**, 1305–6.

Warlow, C.P., Van Gijn, J., and Sandercock, P. (1998). *Cochrane database of systematic reviews: Stroke module.* Update Software/BMJ Publishing, Oxford.

Waterreus, A., Blanchard, M., and Mann, A. (1994). Community psychiatric nurses for the elderly: well tolerated, few side-effects and effective in the treatment of depression. *Journal of Clinical Nursing*, **3**, 299–306.

Weddell, J.M. and Beresford, S.A.A. (1979). *Planning for stroke patients. A four year descriptive study of home and hospital care.* HMSO, London.

Weingarten, S., Bolus, R., Riedinger, M.S. *et al.* (1990). The principle of parsimony: Glasgow Coma Scale score predicts mortality as well as the APACHE II score for stroke patients. *Stroke*, **21**, 1280–2.

Weir, C.J., Murray, G.D., Adams, F.G., Muir, K.W., Grosset, D.G., and Lees, K.R. (1994). Poor accuracy of stroke scoring systems for differential clinical diagnosis of intracranial haemorrhage and infarction. *Lancet*, **344**, 999–1002.

Weir, C.J., Murray, G.D., Dyker, A.G., and Lees, K.R. (1997). Is hyperglycaemia an independent predictor of poor outcome after acute stroke? Results of a long-term follow up study. *British Medical Journal*, **314**, 1303–6.

Weisberg, L.A. and Nice, C.N. (1977). Intracranial tumours simulating the presentation of cerebrovascular syndromes. Early detection with cranial computed tomography (CCT). *American Journal of Medicine*, **63**, 517–24.

Weksler, B. and Lewin, M. (1983). Anticoagulation in cerebral ischaemia. *Stroke*, **14**, 658–63.

Welin, L., Svardsudd, K., Wilhelmsen, L., Larsson, B., and Tibblin, G. (1987). Analysis of risk factors for stroke in a cohort of men born in 1913. *New England Journal of Medicine*, **317**, 521–6.

Wellwood, I., Dennis, M.S., and Warlow, C.P. (1995). A comparison of the Barthel Index and the OPCS disability instrument used to measure outcome after acute stroke. *Age and Ageing*, **24**, 54–7.

Wetherley-Mein, G., Pearson, T.C., Burney, P., and Morris, R.W. (1987). Polycythaemia study. A project of the Royal College of Physicians Research Unit. 1. Objectives, background and design. *Journal of Royal College of Physicians London*, **21**, 7–15.

Wetle, T., Scherr, P., Branch, L.G., Resnick, N.M., Harris, T. *et al.* (1995). Difficulty with holding urine among older persons in a geographically defined community: prevalence and correlates. *Journal of the American Geriatrics Society*, **43**, 349–55.

Wetterling, T., Kanitz, R.D., and Borgis, K.J. (1996). Comparison of different diagnostic criteria for vascular dementia (ADDTC, DSM-IV, ICD-10, NINDS-AIREN). *Stroke*, **27**, 30–6.

Whisnant, J.P. (1984). The decline of stroke. *Stroke*, **15**, 160–8.

Whisnant, J.P., Fitzgibbons, J.P., Kurland, L.T., and Sayre, G.P. (1971). Natural history of stroke in Rochester, Minnesota, 1945 through 1954. *Stroke*, **2**, 11–22.

Whitehouse, G. (1987). Radiological diagnosis of deep vein thrombosis. *British Medical Journal*, **295**, 801–2.

Whiteneck, G.G., Charlifue, S.W., Gerhart, K.A., Overholser, J.D., and Richardson, G.N. (1992). Quantifying handicap: a new measure of long-term rehabilitation outcomes. *Archives of Physical Medicine and Rehabilitation*, **73**, 519–26.

Wiart, L., Come, A.B., Debelleix, X. *et al.* (1997). Unilateral neglect syndrome rehabilitation by trunk rotation and scanning training. *Archives of Physical Medicine and Rehabilitation*, **78**, 424–9.

Wiebers, D.O., Whisnant, J.P., Sandok, B.A., and O'Fallon, W.M. (1990). Prospective comparison of a cohort with asymptomatic carotid bruit and a population-based cohort without carotid bruit. *Stroke*, **21**, 984–8.

Wikstrand, J., Warnold, I., Olsson, G., Tuomilehto, J., Elmfeldt, D., and Berglund, G. (1988). Primary prevention with metoprolol in patients with hypertension. Mortality results from the MAPHY study. *Journal of the American Medical Association*, **259**, 1976–82.

Wilcox, R.G., Mitchell, J.R.A., and Hampton, J.R. (1986). Treatment of high blood pressure: should clinical practice be based on results of clinical trials? *British Medical Journal*, **293**, 433–7.

Wilhelmsen, L., Svardsudd, K., Korsan-Bengtsen, K., Larsson, B., Welin, L., and Tibblin, G. (1984). Fibrinogen as a risk factor for stroke and myocardial infarction. *New England Journal of Medicine*, **311**, 501–5.

Wilhelmsen, L., Berglund, G., Elmfeldt, D. *et al.* (1987). Beta-blockers versus diuretics in hypertensive men: main results from the HAPPHY trial. *Journal of Hypertension*, **5**, 561–72.

Wilkin, D. (1987). Conceptual problems in dependency research. *Social Science and Medicine*, **24**, 867–73.

Wilkinson, G., Falloon, I., and Sen, B. (1985). Chronic mental disorders in general practice. *British Medical Journal*, **291**, 1302–4.

Wilkinson, P.R., Wolfe, C.D., Warburton, F.G. *et al.* (1997). A long-term follow-up of stroke patients. *Stroke*, **28**, 507–12.

Williams, J., Wenden, F., and Jenkins, D.G. (1984). Speech therapy for aphasic stroke patients. *Lancet*, **i**, 1413.

Wilson, B. (1982). Success and failure in memory training following a cerebral vascular accident. *Cortex*, **18**, 581–94.

Wilson, P.W., Garrison, R.J., and Castelli, W.P. (1985). Postmenopausal estrogen use, cigarette smoking, and cardiovascular morbidity in women over 50. The Framingham Study. *New England Journal of Medicine*, **313**, 1038–43.

Winslow, C.M., Solomon, D.H., Chassin, M.R., Kosecoff, J., Merrick, N.J., and Brook, R.H. (1988). The appropriateness of carotid endarterectomy. *New England Journal of Medicine*, **318**, 721–7.

Wityk, R.J., Pessin, M.S., Kaplan, R.F., and Caplan, L.R. (1994). Serial assessment of acute stroke using the NIH Stroke Scale. *Stroke*, **25**, 362–5. [See erratum in *Stroke* (1994), **25**, 1300.]

Wolf, P.A., Kannel, W.B., Sorlie, P., and McNamara, P. (1981). Asymptomatic carotid bruit and risk of stroke. The Framingham study. *Journal of the American Medical Association*, **245**, 1442–5.

Wolf, P.A., Abbott, R.D., and Kannel, W.B. (1987). Atrial fibrillation: a major contributor to stroke in the elderly. The Framingham Study. *Archives of Internal Medicine*, **147**, 1561–4.

Wolf, P.A., D'Agostino, R.B., Kannel, W.B., Bonita, R., and Belanger, A.J. (1988). Cigarette smoking as a risk factor for stroke. The Framingham Study. *Journal of the American Medical Association*, **259**, 1025–9.

Wolf, P.A., Abbott, R.D., and Kannel, W.B. (1991*a*). Atrial fibrillation as an independent risk factor for stroke: the Framingham Study. *Stroke*, **22**, 983–8.

Wolf, P.A., D'Agostino, R.B., Belanger, A.J., and Kannel, W.B. (1991*b*). Probability of stroke: a risk profile from the Framingham Study. *Stroke*, **22**, 312–18.

Wolf, P.A., D'Agostino, R.B., O'Neal, M.A. *et al.* (1992). Secular trends in stroke incidence and mortality. The Framingham Study. *Stroke*, **23**, 1551–5.

Wolfe, C.D. and Burney, P.G. (1992). Is stroke mortality on the decline in England? *American Journal of Epidemiology*, **136**, 558–65.

Wolfe, C.D., Taub, N.A., Woodrow, J., Richardson, E., Warburton, F.G., and Burney, P.G. (1993). Does the incidence, severity, or case fatality of stroke vary in southern England? *Journal of Epidemiology and Community Health*, **47**, 139–43.

Woo, E., Ma, J.T., Robinson, J.D., and Yu, Y.L. (1988). Hyperglycemia is a stress response in acute stroke. *Stroke*, **19**, 1359–64.

Woo, J., Lam, C.W., Kay, R., Wong, A.H., Teoh, R., and Nicholls, M.G. (1990). The influence of hyperglycemia and diabetes mellitus on immediate and 3-month morbidity and mortality after acute stroke. *Archives of Neurology*, **47**, 1174–7.

Woo, J., Lau, E., Lam, C.W. *et al.* (1991). Hypertension, lipoprotein (a), and apolipoprotein A-I as risk factors for stroke in the Chinese. *Stroke*, **22**, 203–8.

Wood, P. and Badley, E. (1978). An epidemiological appraisal of disablement. In *Recent advances in community medicine*, (ed. A.E. Bennett). Churchill-Livingstone, London.

Woodhouse, P.R., Khaw, K.T., Plummer, M., Foley, A., and Meade, T.W. (1994). Seasonal variations of plasma fibrinogen and factor VII activity in the elderly: winter infections and death from cardiovascular disease. *Lancet*, **343**, 435–9.

Woods, K.L. (1995). Mega-trials and management of acute myocardial infarction. *Lancet*, **346**, 611–14.

World Health Organization (1978). *Cerebrovascular disease: a clinical and research classification*. Offset Series No. 43. WHO, Geneva.

World Health Organization (1980). *International classification of impairments, disabilities and handicaps*. WHO, Geneva.

World Health Organization (1993). *ICD-10 Classification of mental and behavioural disorders*. WHO, Geneva.

World Health Organization (1997). *ICIDH-2. Draft for field trials*. WHO, Geneva.

WHO Collaborative Study (1996*a*). Ischaemic stroke and combined oral contraceptives: results of an international, multicentre, case-control study. WHO Collaborative Study of Cardiovascular Disease and Steroid Hormone Contraception. *Lancet*, **348**, 498–505.

WHO Collaborative Study (1996*b*). Haemorrhagic stroke, overall stroke risk, and combined oral contraceptives: results of an international, multicentre, case-control study. WHO Collaborative Study of Cardiovascular Disease and Steroid Hormone Contraception. *Lancet*, **348**, 505–10.

Wroe, S.J., Sandercock, P., Bamford, J., Dennis, M., Slattery, J., and Warlow, C. (1992). Diurnal variation in incidence of stroke: Oxfordshire community stroke project. *British Medical Journal*, **304**, 155–7.

Wylie, C.M. (1962). Late survival following cerebrovascular accidents. *Archives of Physical Medicine and Rehabilitation*, **43**, 297–300.

Wylie, C.M. (1967). Measuring end results of rehabilitation of patients with stroke. *Public Health Reports*, **82**, 893–8.

Yamaguchi, T., Sano, K., Takakura, K. *et al.* (1998). Ebselen in acute ischaemic stroke: a placebo-controlled, double-blind clinical trial. Ebselen study group. *Stroke*, **29**, 12–17.

Yano, K., Reed, D.M., and Maclean, C.J. (1989). Serum cholesterol and hemorrhagic stroke in the Honolulu Heart Program. *Stroke*, **20**, 1460–5.

Yatsu, F.M. (1991). Strokes in Asians and Pacific-Islanders, Hispanics, and Native Americans. *Circulation*, **83**, 1471–2.

Yekutiel, M. and Guttman, E. (1993). A controlled trial of the retraining of the sensory function of the hand in stroke patients. *Journal of Neurology, Neurosurgery and Psychiatry*, **56**, 241–4.

Young, G.R., Sandercock, P.A., Slattery, J., Humphrey, P.R., Smith, E.T., and Brock, L. (1996). Observer variation in the interpretation of intra-arterial angiograms and the risk of inappropriate decisions about carotid endarterectomy. *Journal of Neurology, Neurosurgery and Psychiatry*, **60**, 152–7.

Young, J. (1994). Is stroke better managed in the community? Community care allows patients to reach their full potential. *British Medical Journal*, **309**, 1356–7.

Young, J. and Forster, A. (1992). The Bradford community stroke trial: results at six months. *British Medical Journal*, **304**, 1085–9.

Zhang, Z.F., Yu, S.Z., and Zhou, G.D. (1988). Indoor air pollution of coal fumes as a risk factor of stroke, Shanghai. *American Journal of Public Health*, **78**, 975–7.

Index

Printed in the United Kingdom
by Lightning Source UK Ltd.
104117UKS00001B/84